The Jossey-Bass Health Series brings together the most current information and ideas in health care from the leaders in the field. Titles from the Jossey-Bass Health Series include these essential health care resources:

Collaborating to Improve Community Health: Workbook and Guide to Best Practices in Creating Healthier Communities and Populations, **Kathryn Johnson, Wynne Grossman, Anne Cassidy,** Editors

Designing Health Care for Populations: Applied Epidemiology in Health Care Administration, **Peter J. Fos, David J. Fine**

Health Issues in the Black Community, **Ronald L. Braithwaite, Sandra E. Taylor,** Editors

Immigrant Women's Health, **Elizabeth J. Kramer, Susan L. Ivey, Yu-Wen Ying,** Editors

Informing American Health Care Policy: The Dynamics of Medical Expenditure and Insurance Surveys, 1977–1996, **Alan C. Monheit, Renate Wilson, Ross H. Arnett III,** Editors

Managed Care in the Inner City: The Uncertain Promise for Providers, Plans, and Communities, **Dennis P. Andrulis, Betsy Carrier**

People in Crisis: Understanding and Helping, **Lee Ann Hoff**

Regulating Managed Care: Theory, Practice, and Future Options, **Stuart H. Altman, Uwe E. Reinhardt, David Shactman,** Editors

Risk Management Handbook for Health Care Organizations, **Roberta Carroll,** Editor

Status One: Breakthroughs in High Risk Population Health Management, **Samuel Forman, Matthew Kelliher**

AT RISK IN AMERICA

AT RISK IN AMERICA

The Health and Health Care Needs of Vulnerable Populations in the United States

SECOND EDITION

Lu Ann Aday

Foreword by Ronald M. Andersen

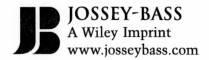

JOSSEY-BASS
A Wiley Imprint
www.josseybass.com

Published by Jossey-Bass
A Wiley Imprint
989 Market Street, San Francisco, CA 94103-1741 www.josseybass.com

Jossey-Bass books and products are available through most bookstores. To contact Jossey-Bass directly call our Customer Care Department within the U.S. at 800-956-7739, outside the U.S. at 317-572-3986, or fax 317-572-4002.

Jossey-Bass also publishes its books in a variety of electronic formats. Some content that appears in print may not be available in electronic books.

Library of Congress Cataloging-in-Publication Data

Aday, Lu Ann.
    At risk in America: the health and health care needs of vulnerable populations in the United States/ Lu Ann Aday. — 2nd ed.
        p. cm. — (The Jossey-Bass health series)
    Includes bibliographical references and indexes.
    ISBN 0-7879-4986-8 (alk. paper)
    1. Poor—Medical care—United States. 2. Poor—Medical care—Government policy—United States. 3. Socially handicapped—Medical care—United States. 4. Socially handicapped—Medical care—Government policy—United States. I. Title. II. Series.
    RA418.5.P6 A3 2001
    362. 1′0425′0973—dc21

                                                                                00-048758

Printed in the United States of America
FIRST EDITION
HB Printing   10 9 8 7

THE JOSSEY-BASS HEALTH SERIES

CONTENTS

FIGURES AND TABLES

Figures

Tables

FOREWORD

The first edition of Lu Ann Aday's *At Risk in America: The Health and Health Care Needs of Vulnerable Populations in the United States* was published in early 1993. Why should you read and own this second edition, published some eight years later? The intervening years have been "good years" for the general welfare of the country according to key economic indicators: increasing per capita income, gross national product, and stock market value, with generally low unemployment and interest rates. You need Aday's new edition to find out if the vulnerable populations of the United States have shared in this increasing largess of the nation—particularly as it applies to health and health care.

You will find that in some ways, for some vulnerable groups, there has been improvement—but in far too many instances there has been stagnation or decline in health indices for vulnerable populations. Even in instances where conditions have not deteriorated, the status of vulnerable populations is often worse than what might be considered acceptable and feasibly obtained according to external norms and guidelines, such as those provided in *Healthy People 2000* (Public Health Service, 1990). Aday points out that social systems promote, in varying degrees, individual rights and the common good. Perhaps, vulnerable populations in the United States would fare better if the system placed relatively more emphasis on the common good.

This new edition of *At Risk in America* provides extensive descriptions and analyses of trends during the 1990s, elaborates and extends Aday's theoretical framework of vulnerability, provides a systematic assessment of research needed to advance our understanding of the vulnerable and the health problems they face, and outlines a policy and plan of action to address these problems.

Aday's concept of vulnerability is a sociological one: "[B]oth the origins and remedies of vulnerability are rooted in the bonds of human communities . . . [T]o be vulnerable to others is to be in a position of being hurt or ignored as well as helped by them . . . [A]s members of human communities we are all potentially vulnerable." Populations are vulnerable that have low social status and limited social or human capital. Key vulnerable populations Aday explores in detail include: high-risk mothers and infants, the chronically ill and disabled, those with HIV/AIDS, the mentally ill and disabled, alcohol and substance abusers, the suicide and homicide prone, abusing families, the homeless, and immigrants and refugees. For all these groups she provides a careful assessment of the extent of their vulnerability, the adequacy of the programs that serve them, and the accessibility, quality, and costs of the care they receive.

This second edition of Aday's comprehensive analysis of vulnerable populations deserves to be on your bookshelf. It is a must for policymakers, health care practitioners, teachers, researchers, and students concerned about the people she describes. It will help us all to think about the nature of the problems of vulnerable populations; it provides a comprehensive source of relevant, up-to-date data and references and carefully considered suggestions for improving the condition of vulnerable populations.

January 2001   Ronald M. Andersen
                                        Wasserman Professor and Chair
                                        Department of Health Services, School of Public Health
                                        Professor, Department of Sociology
                                        University of California at Los Angeles

PREFACE

Policy developments early in the twentieth century led to the expansion of the U.S. health care system and to improved access for many of the traditionally medically and socioeconomically disadvantaged segments of the U.S. population. However, progress has not been without its price. A corresponding acceleration in the rate of expenditures for medical care has accompanied these changes. Public and private providers and third-party payers responded by encouraging initiatives to cut back on the resources spent on health care and to develop innovative organizational models for the cost-effective practice of medicine.

These changes have had a profound impact on slowing or reversing many of the favorable trends of improved access for groups for whom the doors of the health care system were historically more likely to be closed, such as the poor, minorities, the uninsured, and those without a usual medical provider. Further, the increasing visibility of sociomedical morbidities, such as HIV/AIDS, drug and alcohol addiction, family violence, and homelessness, among others, have highlighted categories of individuals with needs, who are particularly vulnerable to restrictive social, economic, and health policies. The solutions to addressing the needs of these diverse groups have been fragmented and categorical—resulting in many particularly at-risk individuals slipping through the cracks of the existing health and social service systems.

The research in this area is often categorical and fragmented, not systematically related to other bodies of information, and fails to identify issues that cut across different professional or service delivery domains. No source has pulled together, in a systematic fashion, the array of information and identified the cross-cutting policy and research issues for the seemingly growing numbers of the vulnerable.

At Risk in America provides this needed integration and synthesis. It presents (1) a framework for identifying and studying vulnerable populations, (2) data on the needs of these populations and on the trends and correlates in the growth of these populations over time, (3) issues regarding the access, cost, and quality of their care, (4) policies and programs that have been developed to address their needs, and (5) research and policy initiatives that could be undertaken to ameliorate vulnerability.

This second edition of the book updates the data and sources presented in Chapters Two through Nine and Resources A and B of the first edition, as well as any corollary conclusions regarding the status of the primary groups that are the focus of the book: high-risk mothers and infants, chronically ill and disabled, persons living with HIV/AIDS, mentally ill and disabled, alcohol or substance abusers, suicide or homicide prone, abusing families, homeless persons, and immigrants and refugees. Other groups may well be identified to be of concern. The framework introduced here, however, is intended to provide a guide for identifying relevant needs and likely programs to address them for these and other groups, focusing particularly on the social determinants of health and illness.

The remaining chapters focus on refining and updating the conceptual framework (Chapter One), research needs (Chapter Ten), and policy implications (Chapter Eleven) introduced in the first edition, based on the latest theoretical, empirical, and policy developments in this area.

Since the publication of the first edition, there has been an increasing interest in the social determinants of health and the design and implementation of new methodologies for tracing aggregate or societal influences on individuals' health and well-being. The accelerating transformation of the health care system to a managed care–driven environment, and the corresponding challenges to redefine the role of public health, have led to a re-examination of the medical and nonmedical remedies for improving the health of populations. The second edition of *At Risk in America* reviews these recent and emerging trends and their implications for addressing the needs of the most vulnerable.

Audience

Public health, health care, social science, social work, and policy analysis professionals, academicians, and researchers will be interested in this book. *At Risk in America* can serve as a reference for legislative staff, policymakers, health professionals, program administrators and students, as well as provide a framework for guiding subsequent research and program development in this area.

This book can acquaint students with the literature in the field and provide a framework to use in identifying vulnerable groups and their specific and common problems. The book can be used as a text for public health, health administration, medical sociology, behavioral science, and social work students, as well as students in the health care professions in courses dealing with the operation and evaluation of the health care system.

At Risk in America can provide health and public health professionals with the background information they will need in developing or evaluating programs to address the needs of vulnerable groups in their own states or communities. The book can serve as a reference source for policymakers and their staffs who need a quick and timely review of the issues for selected target groups. And, finally, this book can also provide a vision of who the most vulnerable are likely to be in the future, what programs or policies can anticipate and address their needs, and what systemic solutions should be considered to address the deepening access, cost, and quality crises in the U.S. health care system.

Overview of the Contents

Each chapter in this book poses a question to explore with respect to the health and health care of vulnerable populations. Vulnerable populations are defined as being at risk of poor physical, psychological, or social health, based on the World Health Organization's definition of health as a "state of complete *physical, mental,* and *social* well-being" (World Health Organization, 1948, p. 1). Selected groups are highlighted throughout the book to illustrate and examine the applicability of the framework for studying vulnerability developed here. The nine vulnerable population groups, based on the primacy of the different types of needs, that will be the primary focus of the book, are as follows: physical needs—high-risk mothers and infants, chronically ill and disabled, persons living with HIV/AIDS; psychological needs—mentally ill and disabled, alcohol or substance abusers, the suicide or homicide prone; social needs—abusing families, homeless persons, immigrants and refugees. The rationale for choosing these groups is discussed in Chapter One.

At Risk in America is organized to facilitate an overview of the cross-cutting issues across the array of groups examined, as well as to provide specific details on a particular group of interest. The first chapter describes the conceptual framework to guide the presentation of material to address the questions regarding the health and health care of vulnerable populations posed in each of the chapters that follow. The final chapter (Chapter Eleven) discusses the principles and parameters of a more community-oriented health policy to ameliorate vulnerability to poor physical, psychological, and social health.

Each of the other chapters (Two through Ten) is divided into three main sections: (1) an introduction to the main question that will be addressed in the chapter and the approach used to assemble and organize the evidence to answer it, (2) a synopsis of the cross-cutting issues identified across all of the vulnerable populations examined, and (3) a population-specific overview of the evidence for each group. In each of these chapters, summary tables are provided to highlight key findings.

Readers may elect to focus on the summary or overview sections of each chapter, or to examine the evidence for a specific question or group within or across chapters.

Chapter One asks who are the vulnerable. The framework for defining and studying vulnerable populations that serves as the basis for the perspective on vulnerability developed in subsequent chapters is presented.

Chapter Two asks how many are vulnerable. National estimates on the number and growth of vulnerable populations are summarized, and the extent to which there is an overlap in these groups is highlighted.

Chapter Three poses the question of who is most vulnerable. Data on demographic subgroups of each of the nine major vulnerable population groups are presented, focusing particularly on breakdowns by age, sex, race, income, and education.

Chapter Four asks why different groups are particularly vulnerable. This discussion provides an overview of the major political, cultural, social, and economic changes in the United States that have given rise to growth in the number and categories of vulnerable populations. The impact of the availability of resources resulting from differences in social status (prestige and power), social capital (social support), and human capital (jobs, schools, and housing) are examined in explaining the differential vulnerability of different subgroups of the population.

Chapter Five asks what programs there are to address the needs of vulnerable populations. Major programs and services are highlighted in the context of a continuum of preventive, treatment, and long-term care services.

Chapter Six asks who pays for care. The discussion focuses on the public and private third-party sources of financing that have been available to pay for the services provided.

Chapter Seven explores how good access to care is. Evidence of organizational and financial barriers to obtaining needed services is reviewed.

Chapter Eight asks how much care costs. A summary of what is known about the total and out-of-pocket costs of care and the cost benefit and cost-effectiveness of alternative program and care arrangements is provided. This chapter illuminates the personal and societal costs of providing care to vulnerable populations, and it considers the efficiency of alternative programs and policies to address the needs of these populations.

Chapter Nine reviews what is known about the quality of care. In this chapter, data are presented on structure, process, and outcome dimensions of the quality of care currently being provided to vulnerable populations, through the medical care, as well as other, service delivery sectors.

Chapter Ten raises the question of what still needs to be known about the health and health care of vulnerable populations. Descriptive, analytic, and evaluative research priorities are identified, and proposals for the type of information needed to make informed decisions, and how to obtain the required information, are presented.

Chapter Eleven asks what programs and policies are needed. This final chapter presents a community-oriented health policy paradigm, based on the perspective on vulnerability developed in previous chapters, as a basis for recommendations regarding how best to address the health and health care needs of vulnerable populations.

An extensive set of references as well as a resource describing the major national data sources on vulnerable populations and a second resource containing detailed source notes on the data tables in this book are provided.

The unique contribution *At Risk in America* makes is to synthesize existing information on the array of vulnerable populations that have emerged in recent years and present a framework for articulating coherent and integrated research and policy agendas to address their needs. The book identifies research in progress to reflect the most up-to-date information on these issues, documents the major sources to consult on the topic, and provides recommendations regarding what still needs to be known and done to address the health and health care needs of vulnerable populations in the United States.

Houston, Texas   Lu Ann Aday
January 2001

ACKNOWLEDGMENTS

I gratefully acknowledge my colleagues who read all or part of the manuscript for the book and provided invaluable comments, all of which I took seriously in making the final revisions: Lillian Gelberg, Richard Jiménez, Judith D. Kasper, David R. Lairson, Isaac D. Montoya, Beth E. Quill, Alan Jay Richard, Carl H. Slater, and the anonymous Jossey-Bass reviewers.

Special thanks go to Anne D. Wiltshire, who helped locate and scrupulously compile the extensive literature and data on the groups that are the special focus of the book. Her hard work and careful attention to detail were immensely valuable assets.

I also gratefully acknowledge the time and effort that Regina Fisher devoted to helping prepare the manuscript for the first and second editions of the book.

I am appreciative of the supportive environment at the University of Texas School of Public Health that allowed me the flexibility to write this book. In particular I thank Stephanie Normann and the staff of the University of Texas School of Public Health Library for ordering and facilitating my access to state-of-the-art sources in this area.

My experience of writing the book was greatly enriched by the intellectual and social capital provided by this highly valued community of collaborators.

L.A.A.

THE AUTHOR

Lu Ann Aday is professor of behavioral sciences and management and policy sciences at the University of Texas School of Public Health. She received her B.S. degree from Texas Tech University in economics and her M.S. and Ph.D. degrees from Purdue University in sociology. Aday's principal research interests have focused on policy-relevant research on indicators and correlates of health services utilization and access. She has conducted major national and community surveys and evaluations of national demonstrations in this area. She is the principal author of the following books: *The Utilization of Health Services: Indices and Correlates—A Research Bibliography* (1972), *Development of Indices of Access to Medical Care* (1975), *Health Care in the United States: Equitable for Whom?* (1980), *Access to Medical Care in the U.S.: Who Has It, Who Doesn't* (1984), *Hospital-Physician Sponsored Primary Care: Marketing and Impact* (1985), and *Pediatric Home Care: Results of a National Evaluation of Programs for Ventilator Assisted Children* (1988). She is also the second coauthor of *Ambulatory Care and Insurance Coverage in an Era of Constraint* (1987, with R. M. Andersen, C. S. Lyttle, L. J. Cornelius, and M. Chen). Her most recent books, all of which have been published as second editions, are *Designing and Conducting Health Surveys: A Comprehensive Guide* (1st ed., 1989; 2nd ed., 1996); *Evaluating the Healthcare System: Effectiveness, Efficiency, and Equity* (1st ed., 1993; 2nd ed., 1998); as well as *At Risk in America: The Health and Health Care Needs of Vulnerable Populations in the United States* (1st ed. 1993). Dr. Aday is a fellow of the Association for Health Services Research and a member of the Institute of Medicine of the National Academy of Sciences.

AT RISK IN AMERICA

CHAPTER ONE

WHO ARE THE VULNERABLE?

Both the origins and remedies of vulnerability are rooted in the bonds of human communities. The parentheses that inscribe our lives (its beginnings and endings, as well as the passages within it) take form in the arms of those who care for us when we are most in need of physical help, spiritual solace, or warm companionship. Their presence supports and strengthens us, and the blessings of their caring seek to salve the wounds of body, mind, and spirit that accompany the odyssey of our lives.

To be vulnerable is to be susceptible to harm or neglect, that is, acts of commission or omission on the part of others that can wound. The word *vulnerable* is derived from the Latin verb *vulnerare* (to wound) and the noun *vulnus* (wound). To be vulnerable is to be in a position of being hurt or ignored, as well as helped, by others.

As members of human communities, we are all potentially vulnerable.

Framework for Studying Vulnerable Populations

Two different mother tongues—those of "individual rights" and the "common good"—have historically characterized American social and political discourse. The semantics of the first emphasize the meanings of autonomy, independence, and individual well-being, while the second highlights norms of reciprocity, interdependence, and the public good. Social critics have, however, observed that in contemporary American society, the first language of individualism has come to override the second mother tongue of community (Beauchamp, 1988; Bellah, Madsen, Sullivan, Swidler, & Tipton, 1985; Putnam, 1993, 1995).

James Coleman (1990), in his book *Foundations of Social Theory*, points out that to formulate meaningful theories or explanations of social phenomenon, both the macro (collective) and the micro (individual) levels of observation and analysis and their interrelationships must be examined. Focusing on individual characteristics, attitudes, or behaviors (such as violence proneness) may fail to reveal the impact that larger social influences or trends (such as media violence) have on individuals. Correspondingly, theories regarding relationships between largely collective phenomena (such as the prevalence of media violence and rates of violent crime) that fail to illuminate the dynamics of these social forces for individuals fall short of developing fully meaningful explanations of the phenomena. The measurement of collective phenomena at the individual level of analysis (methodological individualism) also tends to bias the explanations of these phenomena toward individual motivations and actions.

The approach to studying the health and health care of vulnerable populations undertaken here examines the ethical, conceptual, and political contributions of the community (macro) and individual (micro) perspectives and their interrelationships in illuminating the concept of vulnerability. Vulnerable populations are at risk of poor physical, psychological, or social health. The discussion that follows explores a framework for understanding both the community- and individual-level correlates of vulnerability to poor physical, psychological, and social health. (See Figure 1.1.)

Ethical Norms and Values

The principal ethical norms and values for guiding decision making regarding the amelioration of risk underlying an individual perspective on the origins of poor physical, psychological, or social health are personal autonomy, independence, and associated individual rights. Good health is viewed to be primarily a function of personal lifestyle choices, and poor health outcomes result because individuals fail to assume adequate personal responsibility for their health and well-being.

A community perspective on the origins of health needs focuses on the differential risks that exist for different groups as a function of the availability of opportunities and resources for maximizing their health. Norms of reciprocity, trust, and social obligation acknowledge the webs of interdependence and mutual support and caring that are essential for minimizing the risks of poor physical, psychological, or social health. Poor health results because communities fail to invest in and assume responsibility for the collective well-being of their members (Aday, Begley, Lairson, & Slater, 1998; Evans, Barer, & Marmor, 1994).

Concept: Health Status

Health is defined by the World Health Organization (WHO) as a "state of complete *physical, mental,* and *social* well-being" (World Health Organization, 1948, p. 1). Correspondingly, health can be measured along a continuum of seriousness,

FIGURE 1.1. FRAMEWORK FOR STUDYING VULNERABLE POPULATIONS.

	Policy			Level of Analysis	Ethical Norms and Values
Perspective	Social and Economic Policy	Conmmunity-Oriented Health Policy	Medical Care and Public Health Policy		

| Community | Community Resources

People
Ties between people
Neighborhood | — → | Vulnerable Populations

At risk | + ← | Community Health Needs

Physical
Psychological
Social | Statistical (Aggregate) Lives | Common good
Reciprocity
*Inter*dependence |

resource availability (+)   relative risk (+)   health status (+)   (-)

Community and Individual Well-Being

| Individual | Individual Resources

Social status
Social capital
Human capital | — → | Vulnerable Individuals

Susceptible to harm or neglect | + ← | Individual Health Needs

Physical
Psychological
Social | Individual (Identifiable) Lives | Individual rights
Autonomy
*Inde*pendence |

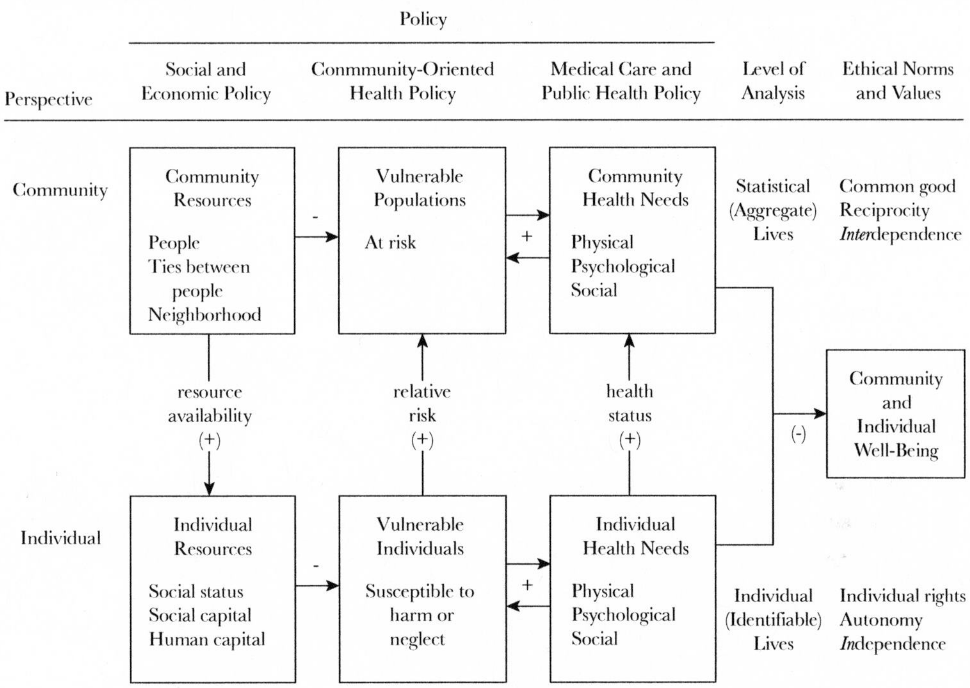

Note: A plus sign indicates a direct relationship (the likelihood of outcomes increases as the predictor increases). A minus sign indicates an inverse relationship (the likelihood of outcomes decreases as the predictor increases).

with good health being at the positive end of the continuum, defined by indicators of good health or physical development, and death at the negative end, defined by population-specific mortality (death) rates. Needs are those departures from full physical, mental, and social health that people experience in the course of their lives.

A variety of indicators of the different WHO dimensions of health (physical, mental, and social) have been developed. Generally physical health has been characterized as "the physiologic and physical status of the body" and mental or psychological health as "the state of mind, including basic intellectual functions such as memory and feelings." Physical and mental indicators tend to "end at the skin," and indicators of social health extend beyond the individual to include both the quantity and quality of social contacts with other people (Ware, 1986, pp. 205–206).

The magnitude and seriousness of individual or community needs along each of these dimensions may differ depending on how they are defined and measured. Health needs, for example, can be based on clinicians' judgments, patients' perceptions, or observed or reported levels of functioning. Clinical or diagnostic judgments of disease (such as hypertension, diabetes, and schizophrenia) are based on the administration of relevant diagnostic tests or procedures by medical or mental health professionals. Individuals' perceptions of illness are based on self-reported symptoms or their assessments of whether they think of their health as excellent, good, or poor or other aspects of their own subjective physical, mental, or social well-being. A third approach focuses on individuals' abilities to perform certain functions or activities, based on behavioral, rather than perceptual or clinical, criteria. Need characterized in this way underlies conceptions of the "sick role," a sociological concept that points out that people change their usual behavior in certain ways (go to bed, take time off from work, and so on) when they are sick. Each of these conceptualizations is used in measuring the health and health care needs of vulnerable populations (McDowell & Newell, 1996; Twaddle & Hessler, 1977).

Community health needs assessments focus on statistical indicators of the rates of prevalence or incidence of morbidity or mortality, such as infant mortality rates, human immunodeficiency virus (HIV) seroprevalence, and percentage of the elderly with limitations in activities of daily living. Individual health needs assessments measure the health status of individual community residents or patients (based on symptoms or diagnoses of illness, for example). The former has principally been the focus of public health policy and planning and the latter of personal medical care service delivery and practice.

Often anecdotes regarding identifiable individual tragedies, such as a child dying of acquired immunodeficiency syndrome (AIDS) or an infant in need of a kidney transplant, are more likely to compel policymakers' attention than do the aggregate, statistical indicators of suffering.

Concept: Relative Risk

Vulnerable populations are at risk of poor physical, psychological, or social health. Underlying this definition of vulnerability is the epidemiological concept of risk, in the sense that there is a nonzero probability that an individual will become ill within a stated period of time. Community and corresponding individual characteristics are risk factors associated with the occurrence of poor physical, psychological, or social health. Risk factors refer to attributes or exposures (smoking, drug use, and lead paint poisoning, for example) that are associated with or lead to increases in the probability of occurrence of health-related outcomes.

Relative risk refers to the ratio of the risk of poor health among groups that are exposed to the risk factors versus those that are not (Last et al., 1995). Relative risk reflects the differential vulnerability of different groups to poor health. The "differential vulnerability hypothesis" argues that negative or stressful life events (such as unemployment, divorce, or death of a loved one) hurt some people more than others. Findings based on this hypothesis show that the mental health and well-being of low socioeconomic status (SES) groups tend to be more adversely affected by stressful or negative events than is the case for those with higher SES and that historical and current social status differences help to explain these differences (Hamilton, Broman, Hoffman, & Renner, 1990; McLeod & Kessler, 1990).

The concept of risk assumes that there is always a chance that an adverse health-related outcome will occur. We are all potentially at risk of poor physical, psychological, and social health. People may, however, be more or less at risk of poor health at different times in their lives, and some individuals and groups are likely to be more at risk than others at any given point in time, as documented in actuarial tables.

Being in poor physical health (such as having a debilitating chronic illness) may also make one more vulnerable to (at risk of) poor psychological health (such as depression) or social health (few supportive social contacts). The risk of harm or neglect is increased for those who are in poor health and have few material (economic) and nonmaterial (psychological or social) resources to assist them in coping with illness.

Concept: Resource Availability

The beginning point for understanding the factors that increase the risk of poor health originates in a macrolevel look at the availability and distribution of community resources (see Figure 1.1). Individual risks vary as a function of the opportunities and material and nonmaterial resources associated with the social characteristics (age, gender, and race and ethnicity) of the individuals themselves, the nature of the ties between them (family members, friends, and neighbors, for example), and the schools, jobs, incomes, and housing that characterize the neighborhoods in which they live. The corresponding rewards and resources available to individuals as a function of these social arrangements are social status (prestige and power), social capital (social support), and human capital (productive potential). These factors, and associated cultural beliefs and contexts, may be viewed as the fundamental social causes that shape differential environmental and behavioral exposures to health risks between groups (Link & Phelan, 1995; Taylor, Repetti, & Seeman, 1997; Williams & Collins, 1995).

Social status is associated with positions that individuals occupy in society as a function of age, sex, or race and ethnicity, and the corollary socially defined opportunities and rewards, such as prestige and power, they have as a result. The prevalence of certain types of illness and the need to depend on others for assistance due to poor health differ at different stages of life (infancy, adolescence, adulthood, and old age). Socially defined roles characterizing individuals at different stages of the life cycle—the dependency of infants and the elderly on others, risk-taking behavior on the part of adolescents, and occupation-related exposures among working-age adults—can, for example, lead to differential exposures to health risks. Women report higher rates of many types of illness than men, which has been variously attributed to their differing health needs, the stress associated with the complex of deferential and demanding roles women play, as well as to the fact that it is more socially acceptable for women to admit their vulnerability. Men may be placed at greater risk of poor health outcomes as a function of working in hazardous jobs or being influenced by societal gender role expectations regarding heavy drinking or the use of violence to settle disputes. Minorities often have poorer health and fewer material and nonmaterial resources to meet their needs, associated with historical and contemporary patterns of discrimination and related residential or occupational segregation, more limited economic or educational opportunities, and the disproportionate exposure to environmental risks in predominantly minority neighborhoods. Individuals with a combination of statuses (poor, minority elderly women or young males) that put them at a high risk of having both poor health and few material and nonmaterial resources are in a highly vulnerable position (Kennedy, Kawachi, Lochner, Jones, & Prothrow-Stith, 1997; Williams & Collins, 1995).

Social capital resides in the quantity and quality of interpersonal ties among people. Social networks provide social capital to members in the form of social support and associated feelings of belonging, psychological well-being, and self-esteem. The value of social capital to individuals (for example, single mothers) is that it provides resources (such as having someone to count on for child care) they can use to achieve other interests (such as going to school or working). Social support is an important resource for individuals in coping with and minimizing the impact of negative life events or adversity on their physical and mental health. Physical, psychological, and social well-being are directly enhanced for people who have supportive social networks. Communities constitute the reservoir in which social capital resources are both generated and drawn on by individual community members. Those who are likely to have the least social capital (or the fewest social ties to count on) are people living alone or those in female-headed families, those who are not married or in an otherwise committed intimate relationship, people who do not belong to any voluntary organizations (such as churches or volunteer interest groups), and those who have weak or nonexistent social networks of family or friends (Coleman, 1988, 1990, 1993; Portes, 1998; Putnam, 1993, 1995).

Human capital refers to investments in people's skills and capabilities (such as vocational or public education) that enable them to act in new ways (master a trade) or enhance their contributions to society (enter the labor force). Neighborhoods that have poor schools, high rates of unemployment, and substandard housing reflect low levels of investments in the human capital (or productive potential) of the people who live there. Similarly, individuals who are poorly educated, unemployed, and poorly housed are likely to have the fewest resources for coping with illness or other personal or economic adversities. Higher levels of education are associated with better overall health. Extensive research, especially in Great Britain, has documented that workers in higher-status occupations have lower rates of morbidity and mortality than those in lower-status jobs. Large relative income inequalities between groups, as well as sustained economic deprivation over the life course, produce large health inequalities. The lack of adequate or safe housing can also exacerbate exposure to health risks (Coleman, 1990; Folland, Goodman, & Stano, 1997; Fullilove & Fullilove, 1999; Kawachi & Kennedy, 1997; Lynch, Kaplan, & Shema, 1997; Whiteis, 1998; Wilkinson, 1996).

The relative importance and relationship of predictors of risk of poor physical, psychological, or social health are summarized in Figure 1.2.

Social status differences for different age, gender, or racial and ethnic subgroups are made manifest in the differential availability of personal and political power and associated human and social capital resources to different subgroups. These disparities are reinforced either informally through socially defined norms and behavioral expectations or formally through legally sanctioned differences in access to human resources (such as schools, jobs, income, or housing)—for children versus adults; men versus women; or majority versus minority racial and ethnic groups, for example. The purposive blocking of access to resources for

FIGURE 1.2. PREDICTORS OF POPULATIONS AT RISK.

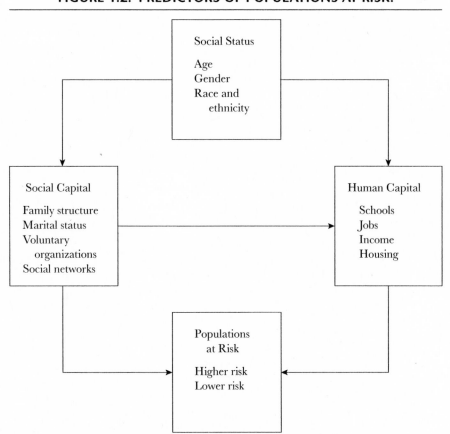

certain groups relative to others on the basis of these ascribed characteristics is defining of the discrimination associated with age, gender, and race in U.S. society.

The webs of mutual dependencies defining of the social life of families, friendship networks, churches, volunteer service organizations, self-help groups, neighborhood or civic organizations, and related community groups are generative of the social capital or support that can be both invested in and drawn on to achieve individuals' personal and purposive aims, enhancing feelings of self-esteem or a sense of belonging, creating child care alternatives, or calling on others for assistance when ill, for example.

The social status and social capital resources of individuals and groups in a community influence the level of investments that are likely to be made in the schools, jobs, housing, and associated earning potential of the families and individuals living within it. Social capital can enhance the generation of human capital through family and community support for students to stay in school. When neighborhood residents come together and seek or are invited to become empowered to work toward shared interests and goals, the prospect for social and human capital formation within the community is enhanced, and the corollary vulnerability of individual members within it diminished.

Table 1.1 summarizes different groups' risk of poor physical, psychological, and social health based on the availability of community and associated individual resources. In the chapters that follow, these hypothesized differences in risk will be analyzed based on subgroup variation in the incidence or prevalence of poor health among the vulnerable populations being examined.

Policy

To begin to envision and attend to the dimensions and scope of the problem of vulnerability to poor physical, psychological, and social health in the United States, policymakers must come to draw on the language of community and the normative compass it provides.

The final chapter of the book outlines the elements of a community-oriented health policy to address the health and health care needs of vulnerable populations. This perspective acknowledges the essential social origins and consequences of vulnerability to poor physical, psychological, and social functioning. It encourages, invests in, and empowers U.S. families and communities to be full participants in shaping their collective health and well-being. A community-oriented point of view seeks to produce networks of cooperation and support rather than wedges of bureaucratic division and indifference between individuals and institutions, to form communities of caring for the vulnerable. And finally, community-oriented health policy integrates rather than reinforces distinct policymaking domains, in exploring the roles that both social and economic, as well as medical care and public health, policies play in ameliorating the health risks and consequences of vulnerability.

TABLE 1.1. COMPARISONS OF RELATIVE RISK.

Community and Individual Resources	Relative Risk	
	Higher Risk	Lower Risk
The people: Social status		
Age	Infants Children Adolescents Elderly	Working-age adults
Gender	Females	Males
Race and ethnicity	African Americans Hispanics Native Americans Asian Americans	Whites
The ties between people: Social capital		
Family structure	Living alone Female head	Extended families Two-parent families
Marital status	Single Separated Divorced Widowed	Married, mingles
Voluntary organizations	Nonmember	Member
Social networks	Weak	Strong
The neighborhood: Human capital		
Schools	Less than high school	High school or beyond
Jobs	Unemployed Blue collar	White collar
Income	Poor Low income	Middle income High income
Housing	Substandard	Adequate or better

Note: The terms to designate the race and ethnicity categories in this table will be used in discussing these groups in general. When presenting specific data in the text on these groups, the designation (such as black or Asian) in the original source from which the data were derived will generally be used. *Mingles* refers to individuals who are not married but are living with a sexual partner. *Voluntary organizations* include churches, volunteer interest groups, and civic and neighborhood organizations.

Health Needs of Vulnerable Populations

The vulnerable populations that are the primary focus of this book are high-risk mothers and infants, those who are chronically ill and disabled, persons living with HIV/AIDS, those who are mentally ill and disabled, alcohol or substance abusers, those who are suicide or homicide prone, abusing families, homeless persons, and immigrants and refugees. These groups are arrayed in Table 1.2, based on their principal health needs. The impact of the availability of material and nonmaterial resources in contributing to their vulnerability to (risk of) poor health, as well as the consequences of their poor health for the prospect of vulnerability to subsequent harm or neglect, will be explored.

There are a number of reasons for choosing to focus on these groups in examining the health and health care needs of vulnerable populations:

- These groups' needs are serious and in many cases debilitating or life-threatening ones.
- They require an extensive or intensive set of medical and nonmedical services.
- The growth in their number and the seriousness of their needs are placing increasing demands on the medical care, public health, and related service delivery sectors.
- Their complex and multifaceted needs are not adequately met through existing financing or service delivery arrangements.
- Federal, state, and local policymakers increasingly are concerned about how to deal with the demands they place on existing systems of care, as well as how to ameliorate the prospect they appear to represent of a growing number of Americans at risk of serious physical, psychological, and social health problems.

Other groups may well be considered to be vulnerable populations—for example, incarcerated populations, selected immigrant groups, or the multiproblem homeless. Furthermore, poor health along one dimension (say, physical) is quite likely to be compounded with poor health along others (psychological or social, for example). Comorbidities and the associated cumulative risks of illness are greatest for those who have problems along more than one of these

TABLE 1.2. PRINCIPAL HEALTH NEEDS OF VULNERABLE POPULATIONS.

Physical	Psychological	Social
High-risk mothers and infants	Mentally ill and disabled	Abusing families
Chronically ill and disabled	Alcohol or substance abusers	Homeless persons
Persons living with HIV/AIDS	Suicide or homicide prone	Immigrants and refugees

dimensions. A categorization of groups, based on their cross-cutting needs, appears in Table 1.3. This categorization is intended to illuminate the overlapping, multifaceted nature of needs that many of the most vulnerable experience. The principal groups examined here are meant to be illustrative, but not exhaustive, of what may be identified as vulnerable populations, both now and in the future.

Alternative theoretical perspectives on the origins of vulnerability may focus more on genetic or biological determinants of poor physical, mental, or social health and well-being. The framework introduced here, however, is intended to provide a set of lenses and guide for identifying the social determinants of health and illness and thereby develop a more broad-gauged policy agenda, incorporating medical care, public health, and social and economic policy as essential partners in ultimately mitigating both the foundational and immediate causes of vulnerability to poor physical, psychological, and social health.

Topics in Studying Vulnerability

The framework introduced here (see Figure 1.1) provides a conceptual, empirical, and normative point of reference for understanding the origins and consequences of poor health that can guide the development of coherent and relevant research and policy agendas to address the health and health care needs of what appear to be a growing number of vulnerable populations. The major topics regarding these groups that will be addressed in the chapters that follow and the relationships among them are summarized in Figure 1.3.

The assumption underlying the framework (Figure 1.1) and the approach to these topics (Figure 1.3) is that social and economic, as well as medical care and public health, programs and policies are intended to address the health and health care needs of vulnerable populations and the availability of community and individual resources to meet them. As implied in Figure 1.3, policies that establish programs and payers of services influence the resources that are available to vulnerable populations to address their needs. In the chapters that follow, the characteristics of existing programs and services and how they are financed are described, and their current success is evaluated in terms of organizational and financial barriers to access; the overall costs and cost benefit or cost-effectiveness; and the structure, process, and outcome measures of the effectiveness of these programs and services. The content addressed in the respective chapters identified in Figure 1.3 will provide a knowledge base for recommendations regarding how better to design programs and policies to address the needs of vulnerable populations and to improve on the access, cost, and effectiveness of their care.

TABLE 1.3.   CROSS-CUTTING HEALTH NEEDS OF
VULNERABLE POPULATIONS.

	Vulnerable Populations			
Vulnerable Populations	**High-Risk Mothers and Infants**	**Chronically Ill and Disabled**	**Persons Living with HIV/AIDS**	**Mentally Ill and Disabled**
High-Risk Mothers and Infants	**X**	Chronically ill/ technology-assisted children	Pediatric AIDS cases	Developmentally disabled infants
Chronically Ill and Disabled	Chronically ill/ technology-assisted children	**X**	HIV-positive individuals	Chronically mentally ill
Persons Living with HIV/AIDS	Pediatric AIDS cases	HIV-positive individuals	**X**	Central nervous system– impaired persons with AIDS
Mentally Ill and Disabled	Developmentally disabled infants	Chronically mentally ill	Central nervous system– impaired persons with AIDS	**X**
Alcohol or Substance Abusers	Fetal alcohol syndrome/ crack babies	Chronic alcoholics/ drug addicts	IV drug user/ persons with AIDS	Mentally ill substance abusers
Suicide or Homicide Prone	Child homicides	Suicidal long-term care patients	Suicidal persons with AIDS/ prisoners with AIDS	Suicidal/ criminally insane
Abusing Families	Battered pregnant women and infants	Abused disabled or elderly	Homophobic families/AIDS boarder babies	Dysfunctional families
Homeless Persons	Pregnant homeless women	Homeless persons with chronic disease	Homeless adults, runaways with AIDS	Homeless mentally ill
Immigrants and Refugees	Pregnant refugee women	Refugees with chronic disease	Refugees with AIDS	Refugees with posttraumatic distress

Alcohol or Substance Abusers	Suicide or Homicide Prone	Abusing Families	Homeless Persons	Immigrants and Refugees
Fetal alcohol syndrome/ crack babies	Child homicides	Battered pregnant women and infants	Pregnant homeless women	Pregnant refugee women
Chronic alcoholics/ drug addicts	Suicidal long-term care patients	Abused disabled or elderly	Homeless persons with chronic disease	Refugees with chronic disease
IV drug user/ persons with AIDS	Suicidal persons with AIDS/prisoners with AIDS	Homophobic families/AIDS boarder babies	Homeless adults, runaways with AIDS	Refugees with AIDS
Mentally ill substance abusers	Suicidal/ criminally insane	Dysfunctional families	Homeless mentally ill	Refugees with posttraumatic distress
X	Alcohol/drug-related suicides or homicides	Addictive families	Alcoholic/drug-abusing homeless persons	Alcoholic/ drug-abusing refugees
Alcohol/drug-related suicides or homicides	X	Violent families	Suicidal/ violence-prone homeless persons	Suicidal/ violence-prone refugees
Addictive families	Violent families	X	Runaways	Maltreated refugee children
Alcoholic/ drug-abusing homeless persons	Suicidal/ violence-prone homeless persons	Runaways	X	Political detainees
Alcoholic/ drug abusing refugees	Suicidal/ violence-prone refugees	Maltreated refugee children	Political detainees	X

FIGURE 1.3. TOPICS IN STUDYING VULNERABLE POPULATIONS.

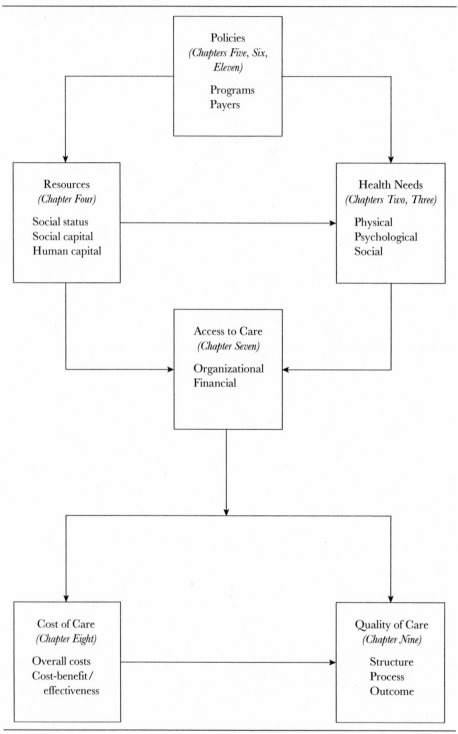

Note: Chapter Ten reviews the research on these and related topics.

Conclusion

This chapter has provided a definition of vulnerable populations—populations at risk of poor physical, psychological, or social health—and a framework for examining the social determinants of vulnerability. The vulnerable populations that are the primary focus of this book are high-risk mothers and infants, those who are chronically ill and disabled, persons living with HIV/AIDS, those who are mentally ill and disabled, alcohol or substance abusers, those who are suicide or homicide prone, abusing families, homeless persons, and immigrants and refugees. In each of the chapters that follow, a summary of common themes across groups precedes a detailed review of the evidence presented separately for each group. This approach is intended to apply and verify the utility of the framework for organizing and interpreting the array of disparate evidence on the health and health care needs of vulnerable populations—both those examined here in detail, as well as others that may subsequently trouble our national conscience.

CHAPTER TWO

HOW MANY ARE VULNERABLE?

Vulnerable populations are an immediate and visible reality of the experiences that touch our lives. Homeless persons reach out to us at the intersections near our homes and in front of the neighborhood stores from which we emerge with our abundance. Persons living with HIV/AIDS are the youngsters who sit next to our children in school, the coworkers with whom we have shared coffee and committee assignments, as well as the friend's son who has come home to die. Alcohol, substance, and other abuse emerge as a part of our, not just others', experiences when we seek to illuminate and speak the secrets our families have sought to keep. Chronic illness takes on a painful, personal reality with the news that an elderly parent or a beloved partner has Alzheimer's disease or cancer. The experience of vulnerability is or can be a part of all of our lives.

This chapter sets out the aggregate statistical data on the number and growth of the vulnerable populations that are a focus of this book. These data provide a look at the national level regarding how many Americans are at risk of poor physical, psychological, and social health, and whether their numbers have increased over time. An inventory of the major national data sources available on these populations is provided at the end of the book.

Many of the groups described here (such as high-risk mothers and infants, those who are chronically ill and disabled, and persons living with HIV/AIDS) have been the focus of the Year 2000 and 2010 Public Health Service Objectives for improving the nation's health formulated by the public health community to serve as national benchmarks of progress (Public Health Service, 1990; U.S. Department of Health and Human Services, 1998).

Cross-Cutting Issues

This chapter presents data on the prevalence and trends in the number of individuals in the following groups: high-risk mothers and infants, the chronically ill and disabled, persons living with HIV/AIDS, the mentally ill and disabled, alcohol or substance abusers, suicide or homicide prone, abusing families, homeless persons, and immigrant and refugee populations. These and other vulnerable populations are at risk of poor physical, psychological, and social health, which may be measured in a variety of ways.

Prevalence

Two main problems in estimating the number of people who are vulnerable are that the quality and completeness of the data for identifying them are limited, and the categories of vulnerable populations for which data are reported are not mutually exclusive but overlapping; many experience problems in more than one area of functioning. Vulnerable populations, as conveyed in Table 1.3, are more likely to experience a number of comorbidities.

The data sources used for identifying the groups examined here are clinical diagnoses of disease, patient self-reports of illness, vital statistics inventories on births and deaths, and health and social service agency records on clients. These different sources tend to yield varying estimates of those in need within a particular group, which also makes direct comparisons of the magnitude of need across groups problematic. Different universes (or groups) of individuals are used as the basis for different estimates. Further, estimates based on survey data (such as the prevalence of alcohol or substance abuse or family violence) may also have systematic biases resulting when only selected groups or individuals are included in or respond to the survey, as well as variable (standard) errors associated with the size and complexity of the sample design. Between-group and over-time differences for which explicit standard errors or tests of statistical significance are not reported should be interpreted with caution. Trend data that document increases in certain types of problems (such as child abuse and neglect) are also confounded by the increased visibility and likelihood of reporting these types of events. Methodological limitations underlying estimates of the number and growth of vulnerable populations are discussed in Chapter Ten and noted in the tables presented in this and the next chapter.

A variety of indicators of need, based on clinical diagnoses, subjective perceptions of illness, and behavioral limitations, are available. The most direct indicators of the need for assistance with functioning are those measuring limitations in activities of daily living among the chronically physically ill. The most immediate evidence of direct neglect or injury consists of case reports and rates of family abuse or violence. For other major categories of the vulnerable examined here, vulnerability is mirrored in other indicators of poor physical, psychological, and social health or functioning (for example, low birthweight; deaths due to HIV/AIDS, drug-related causes, suicide, or homicide; and homelessness).

Many people have more than one type of health problem. Low birthweight babies may have congenital defects or other adverse outcomes associated with prematurity that result in long-term physical or mental impairment. High-risk categories of mothers and infants include those in which the mother or her sex partner uses drugs or are HIV positive. Pregnant women with abusive partners or those who are homeless or fleeing political persecution are particularly at risk of poor outcomes for themselves and their unborn children. Accurate national estimates on the number of these and other groups with a multiplicity of cross-cutting needs are not readily available. An examination of data for discrete sub-categories should not obscure this mosaic of physical, psychological, and social needs that characterize the lives of many of the vulnerable.

Trends

The variety of indicators of vulnerable populations examined here indicate that during the 1990s, the incidence of serious physical, psychological, and social needs was exacerbated (at worst) and unameliorated (in some cases) for millions of Americans.

The HIV/AIDS epidemic grew from a handful of gay males in the San Francisco area in the early 1980s identified by the Centers for Disease Control and Prevention (CDC) and experiencing what the media called "Gay-Related Immune Disorder" to, over the ensuing decades, hundreds of thousands of Americans having either died from or currently living with HIV/AIDS. The number of homeless persons has increased an average of 15 percent a year, with estimates now ranging up to 1 million men, women, or children homeless on any given night to twice that number who may be homeless at some time during the year. Around 8 million people immigrated to the United States during the 1990s, a large proportion of whom are refugees carrying with them the physical, psychological, and social wounds of war. The number of children abused by family members or other intimates has burgeoned to an estimated 2 million children, and with the greater use of firearms, intentional acts of violence toward oneself or others are becoming increasingly deadly in their consequences.

Although fewer Americans smoke, drink, or use illicit drugs in general than was the case in the 1980s, the use of cocaine (and particularly crack) among hard-core addicts has resulted in increases in the numbers of drug-related deaths. Previously favorable trends in reducing the numbers or rates of high-risk mothers and newborns slowed during the 1990s, and the dependency needs of the chronically physically and mentally ill are becoming more, not less, visible, as the number of infants, adults, and elderly experiencing these conditions continues to increase.

Population-Specific Overview

In the discussion that follows, data are presented on the trends in the growth of an array of vulnerable populations.

High-Risk Mothers and Infants

High-risk childbearing is signaled by high rates of teenage pregnancies, prospective mothers' failing to receive adequate prenatal care, infants who are premature or underweight at birth, as well as by mothers and babies who die at a time when the beginning rather than the end of life is promised.

The trends during the 1990s reflect a troublesome slowdown or in some cases reversal of previously favorable progress in reducing the numbers of vulnerable mothers and newborns. The current reality falls short of the Year 2000 Public Health Service Objectives for these groups, and the trends portend, at best, slow progress toward and, at worst, a retreat from moving toward those goals. (See Table 2.1.)

Low Birthweight. Between 1970 and 1985, the proportion of live births that were low birthweight (LBW) infants (less than 2,500 grams, or 5.5 pounds) declined from 7.93 percent to a low of 6.75 percent. By 1997, however, the rate had increased to 7.51 percent. A corresponding trend can be observed for very low birthweight (VLBW) infants (less than 1,500 grams, or 3.3 pounds). The VLBW rate declined from 1.17 percent in 1970 to 1.15 percent in 1980, but by 1997 it had risen to 1.42 percent. The changes in the rates of LBW and VLBW infants from the lowest rates in the early to mid-1980s represented an 11 percent and 23 percent increase, respectively. An important factor contributing to the high level of low birthweight is the incidence of preterm births (those born before thirty-seven completed weeks of gestation). The preterm birthrate rose from 11.0 percent in 1996 to 11.4 percent in 1997. The proportion of preterm births has risen 8 percent since 1990 (from 10.6 percent) and more than 20 percent since 1981 (from 9.4 percent) (National Center for Health Statistics, 1999a).

The Year 2000 Objectives for the nation provided for no more than 5 percent of all live births being a LBW infant and no more than 1 percent VLBW. The 1997 rates of 7.51 percent and 1.42 percent, respectively, are higher than the national objectives and appear to be increasing rather than declining.

Infant Mortality. Low birthweight is one of the leading correlates of infant death. Infant mortality rates have, however, declined steadily over the past twenty to thirty years, due primarily to the technologies and procedures for saving LBW and VLBW infants. The total number of infant deaths per 1,000 live births in 1997 (7.2) was less than one-third of the 1970 totals (20.0). Similarly, the neonatal mortality rate (deaths of infants under twenty-eight days) was 4.8 in

TABLE 2.1. INDICATORS OF HIGH-RISK MOTHERS AND INFANTS.

Indicators	Year															
	1970	1975	1980	1985	1986	1987	1988	1989	1990	1991	1992	1993	1994	1995	1996	1997
Low birthweight[1]																
Percentage of live births less than 2,500 grams	7.93	7.38	6.84	6.75	6.81	6.90	6.93	7.05	6.97	7.12	7.08	7.22	7.28	7.32	7.39	7.51
Percentage of live births less than 1,500 grams	1.17	1.16	1.15	1.21	1.21	1.24	1.24	1.28	1.27	1.29	1.29	1.33	1.33	1.35	1.37	1.42
Infant mortality[2]																
Total	20.0	16.1	12.6	10.6	10.4	10.1	10.0	9.8	9.2	8.9	8.5	8.4	8.0	7.6	7.3	7.2
Neonatal	15.1	11.6	8.5	7.0	6.7	6.5	6.3	6.2	5.8	5.6	5.4	5.3	5.1	4.9	4.8	4.8
Postneonatal	4.9	4.5	4.1	3.7	3.6	3.6	3.6	3.6	3.4	3.4	3.1	3.1	2.9	2.7	2.5	2.5
Prenatal care[3]																
Percentage of mothers who received prenatal care in the third trimester or no prenatal care	7.9	6.0	5.1	5.7	6.0	6.1	6.1	6.4	6.1	5.8	5.2	4.8	4.4	4.2	4.0	3.9
Teen births[4]																
Live births per 1,000 females																
10–14 years	1.2	1.3	1.1	1.2	1.3	1.3	1.3	1.4	1.4	1.4	1.4	1.4	1.4	1.3	1.2	1.1
15–17 years	38.8	36.1	32.5	31.0	30.5	31.7	33.6	36.4	37.5	38.7	37.8	37.8	37.6	36.0	33.8	32.1
18–19 years	114.7	85.0	82.1	79.6	79.6	78.5	79.9	84.2	88.6	94.4	94.5	92.1	91.5	89.1	86.0	83.6
Maternal mortality[5]																
Deaths per 100,000 live births all ages, age-adjusted	21.5	*12.8	9.4	7.6	7.0	6.1	8.0	7.3	7.6	7.2	7.3	6.7	7.9	6.3	6.4	7.6

Note: An asterisk indicates that the figure is not age adjusted.

Sources: National Center for Health Statistics reports. See Resource B for specific references to table items marked with superscript numerals.

1997 compared to 15.1 in 1970, and the postneonatal mortality rate (deaths of infants ages twenty-eight days up to one year) was 2.5 in 1997 relative to 4.9 in 1970. The rates at the end of the 1990s were moving toward the Year 2000 Objectives of no more than 7.0 total infant deaths, 4.5 neonatal deaths, and 2.5 postneonatal deaths per 1,000 live births. As will be discussed in Chapter Three, however, substantial disparities in the rates of infant mortality continue to persist between racial and ethnic subgroups.

Prenatal Care. Obtaining no or inadequate prenatal care puts mothers and infants at a considerably higher risk of adverse pregnancy outcomes (Institute of Medicine, 1988d). The percentage of women who had no prenatal care or did not seek care until the last trimester of their pregnancy declined from 7.9 percent in 1970 to 5.1 percent in 1980. The rate increased to 6.4 percent in 1989, but subsequently it declined to a low of 3.9 percent in 1997. The percentage of women seeking prenatal care in the first trimester of their pregnancy has increased steadily over the past three decades, from 76.3 percent in 1980 to 82.5 percent in 1997, but still fell short of the Year 2000 goal of 90 percent (National Center for Health Statistics, 1999d).

Teen Births. The rates of births per 1,000 for very young mothers ten to fourteen years of age have remained relatively stable since 1970 (1.1 to 1.4 per 1,000 females). The birthrates for teenage mothers fifteen to seventeen years of age declined from 1970 to the mid-1980s, but then began to increase. The 1997 rates for mothers fifteen to seventeen years old (32.1) and eighteen to nineteen years old (83.6) mothers evidenced a decline once again.

Maternal Mortality. The number of women who died of pregnancy or birth-related complications per 100,000 live births declined from 21.5 in 1970 to 6.1 in 1987. In 1988, the rate rose sharply to 8.0, 31 percent higher than the rate in the previous year. Data for 1995 show that the rate declined to 6.3 but rose sharply again in 1997 to 7.6. This figure remains more than twice that of the Year 2000 Objective of a maximum of 3.3 maternal deaths per 100,000 live births.

Chronically Ill and Disabled

The impact of long-term chronic disease (such as heart disease, cancer, and stroke) is reflected in reports of how many people are living with these problems, how seriously they are limited in their abilities to go about their normal daily activities as a result, and ultimately how many die from these illnesses and associated complications.

Deaths due to major chronic illness have declined significantly over the past twenty years for some conditions (such as heart disease and stroke) but not for others (chronic obstructive pulmonary disease, cancer, and diabetes). Estimates of the number of Americans who have to limit their usual daily activities in some way due to chronic illness range as high as 38 million. (See Table 2.2.)

TABLE 2.2. INDICATORS OF CHRONICALLY ILL AND DISABLED.

Year

Indicators	1970	1975	1980	1985	1986	1987	1988	1989	1990	1991	1992	1993	1994	1995	1996	1997
Age-adjusted death rates for selected chronic diseases per 100,000 persons[1]																
Heart disease	253.6	217.8	202.0	181.4	176.0	170.8	167.7	157.5	152.0	148.2	144.3	145.3	140.4	138.3	134.5	130.5
Stroke	66.3	53.7	40.8	32.5	31.1	30.4	29.9	28.3	27.7	26.8	26.2	26.5	26.5	26.7	26.4	25.9
Cancer	129.8	129.4	132.8	134.4	134.1	134.0	134.0	134.5	135.0	134.5	133.1	132.6	131.5	129.9	127.9	125.6
Chronic obstructive pulmonary disease	13.2	*	15.9	18.8	18.9	18.9	19.6	19.6	19.7	20.1	19.9	21.4	21.0	20.8	21.0	21.1
Cirrhosis	14.7	13.7	12.2	9.7	9.3	9.2	9.1	9.0	8.6	8.3	8.0	7.9	7.9	7.6	7.5	7.4
Diabetes	14.1	11.4	10.1	9.7	9.7	9.8	10.2	11.6	11.7	11.8	11.9	12.4	12.9	13.3	13.6	13.5

Indicators	1985	1986	1987	1988	1989	1990	1991	1992	1993	1994	1995	1996
Number of selected chronic conditions per 1,000 persons (self-reported)[2]												
Heart disease	82.6	78.1	82.4	84.1	75.9	78.5	82.6	85.8	83.6	85.8	80.6	78.2
Hypertension	125.1	122.6	118.6	121.5	113.6	110.2	111.8	110.6	108.3	108.8	114.4	107.1
Stroke	11.6	11.9	11.4	10.4	10.8	11.7	11.5	13.0	13.2	11.5	12.7	11.3
Visual impairment	36.4	35.3	33.3	34.7	32.4	30.6	32.1	35.7	36.6	33.1	32.5	31.3
Hearing impairment	90.7	87.7	88.0	90.8	83.1	94.7	91.2	94.6	95.0	86.3	85.8	83.4
Arthritis	128.6	130.8	131.8	129.9	127.3	125.3	125.2	132.5	128.4	128.8	124.7	127.3
Emphysema	8.9	8.5	8.5	7.9	8.2	8.2	6.6	7.6	7.6	7.8	7.1	6.9
Asthma	36.8	41.0	40.1	41.2	47.7	41.9	47.2	49.2	51.4	56.1	56.8	55.2
Diabetes	26.2	27.9	27.8	25.8	26.6	25.3	29.0	29.5	30.7	29.9	33.2	28.9

Indicators	1975	1980	1985	1986	1987	1988	1989	1990	1991	1992	1993	1994	1995	1996
Age-adjusted degree of activity limitation due to chronic conditions, percent[3]														
Limited but not in major activity	3.5	3.4	4.2	4.2	4.0	4.0	4.1	4.1	4.3	4.3	4.4	4.4	4.3	4.1
Limited in amount or kind of major activity	7.2	6.9	5.5	5.4	5.2	5.3	5.2	5.0	5.2	5.5	5.9	5.6	5.3	5.2
Unable to carry on major activity	3.3	3.5	3.7	3.7	3.7	3.8	3.9	3.9	4.0	4.3	4.3	4.4	4.3	4.4
Total with activity limitation	13.9	13.7	13.4	13.3	12.9	13.1	13.4	12.9	13.5	14.2	14.6	14.3	13.9	13.6

Indicators	1975	1980	1985	1986	1987	1988	1989	1990	1991	1992	1993	1994
Limitation in selected activities of daily living (ADLs) or instrumental activities of daily living (IADLs), 15+ years of age living in the community[4][@]												
Number in thousands (and percent) with at least one ADL (personal care activities)									7,854 (4.0)			8,195 (4.1)

	1991	1994
Number of ADLs		
1	3,292 (1.7)	3,602 (1.8)
2–3	2,309 (1.2)	2,547 (1.3)
4 or more	2,253 (1.2)	2,046 (1.0)
Number (percent) with at least one IADL (home management activities)	11,623 (6.0)	11,998 (5.9)
Number of IADLs		
1	4,987 (2.6)	5,382 (2.7)
2–3	4,445 (2.3)	4,623 (2.3)
4 or more	2,190 (1.1)	1,992 (1.0)
Percent with at least one ADL or IADL	13,392 (6.9)	13,854 (6.8)

Indicators	1977	1985	1986	1987	1988	1989	1990	1991	1992	1993	1994	1995
Limitation in selected activities of daily living (ADLs) or instrumental activities of daily living (IADLs), living in nursing homes[5#]												
Percent with at least one ADL (personal care activities)	88.7	90.2										96.9
Number of ADLs												
1	14.5	11.2										7.2
2–3	22.5	17.9										45.2
4 or more	51.6	61.1										43.9
Percent with at least one IADL (home management activities)		84.8										88.4
Number of IADLs												
1		6.9										8.4
2–3		22.5										31.0
4 or more		55.3										49.1

* Chronic obstructive pulmonary disease was not coded in the same way in 1975.

@ ADLs include bathing, dressing, eating, transferring, and toileting. IADLs include use of telephone, handling money, getting around outside the home, preparing meals, and doing light housework.

ADLs include bathing, dressing, eating, transferring, toileting, and continence. IADLs include use of telephone, handling money, securing personal items, and care of personal possessions.

Source: NCHS reports; McNeil (1999a, 1999b). See Resource B for specific references to table items marked with superscript numerals.

Death Rates for Chronic Diseases. Heart disease has been the leading cause of death over the past twenty years, followed by cancer and stroke. The number of deaths due to heart disease declined 48 percent from 253.6 per 100,000 in 1970 to 130.5 in 1997. Although still short of the Year 2000 Objective of 20.0, the rate for strokes had declined over 60 percent to 25.9 by 1997, compared to 66.3 in 1970. The death rates for cirrhosis of the liver also decreased over this same period, from 14.7 to 7.4. Cancer death rates increased between 1970 (129.8) and 1990 (135.0), but declined to below 1970 levels (to 125.6) by 1997. After a fifteen-year decrease in death rates from diabetes from 1970 (14.1) to 1986 (9.7), the rates began to climb once again, reaching 13.5 in 1997. The death rates for chronic obstructive pulmonary disease increased substantially from 13.2 in 1970 to 21.1 in 1997.

Prevalence of Chronic Conditions. Hypertension and arthritis are the most frequently reported chronic conditions among the noninstitutionalized population. The prevalence of these conditions has declined somewhat since 1985. The rates for hypertension declined from 125.1 in 1985 to 107.1 per 1,000 persons in 1996. For arthritis, the corresponding rates were 128.6 and 127.3. On the other hand, the prevalence of asthma increased substantially between 1985 (36.8) and 1996 (55.2). The 1996 rates for diabetes (28.9) were also higher than the 1985 estimates (26.2). The numbers of conditions per 1,000 persons in 1996 for other conditions were as follows: hearing impairment (83.4), heart disease (78.2), visual impairment (31.3), stroke (11.3), and emphysema (6.9). The basic rank ordering of the prevalence of major chronic conditions has not changed substantially since 1985.

Limitation in Major Activity Due to Chronic Conditions. The percentage of the U.S. noninstitutionalized population who limit their major daily activities due to chronic illness has remained approximately 13 percent to 14 percent since the 1970s. Based on the National Center for Health Statistics National Health Interview Survey, the usual activities for the respective age groups are as follows: play for children less than five; going to school for children ages six to seventeen; working for adults ages eighteen to sixty-four; and managing self-care activities for elderly age sixty-five and over. The distribution of severity of activity limitation has remained relatively stable over this time period. In 1996, the distribution of types of limitation was as follows: limited but not in major activity (4.1 percent), limited in amount or kind of major activity (5.2 percent), and unable to carry on major activity (4.4 percent). This amounts to over 38 million people who had some activity limitation and over 26 million who were limited in or unable to carry out their major activity.

Limitation in Activities of Daily Living (ADL) and Instrumental Activities of Daily Living (IADL). Surveys of the functional impact of illness, particularly for the elderly, have focused on estimates of the numbers of individuals who are unable to carry on basic personal care activities (such as bathing, transferring to a bed or chair, dressing, toileting, feeding, and walking—also referred to as activities of daily living or ADLs) or home management activities (such as using a telephone, handling money, shopping, and preparing meals—instrumental activities of daily living, or IADLs). The questions asked to obtain this information and the types of activities inventoried vary across studies, so comprehensive trend data on ADLs and IADLs are not available.

According to the Survey of Income and Program Participation, around 4 percent of adults fifteen years of age and older living in the community had limitations in personal care activities (ADLs), and around 6 percent had IADL limitations. About 7 percent of community-dwelling adults reported having at least one type of activity limitation (ADL or IADL).

The prevalence of activity limitation is much higher among the institutionalized nursing home population. Based on the 1995 National Nursing Home Survey, almost all nursing home residents (96.9 percent) had at least one ADL, and 88.4 percent had one or more IADLs. Persons living in nursing homes in 1995 were less likely to have four ADL or IADL limitations than was the case among those in residence in 1985. Data from the 1982–1994 National Long-Term Care Surveys documented an accelerating decline in disability among the U.S. elderly population, related to increases in educational levels and reductions in risk factors among the elderly over time (Manton, Stallard, & Corder, 1998; Singer & Manton, 1998).

Estimates of the number of children, working-age adults, and elderly living in the community with substantial limitations in function have also been derived from the Survey of Income and Program Participation (SIPP). The percentages of children with any physical or mental limitation in 1994–1995 were as follows: 2.6 percent for those up to two years of age, 5.2 percent for those three to five years old, 12.7 percent for those age six to fourteen, and 12.1 percent for young people fifteen to twenty-one. Individuals age fifteen and over were identified as having a serious disability if they were unable to perform one or more functional activities (seeing, hearing, speaking, lifting or carrying, using stairs, or walking); needed personal assistance with an ADL or IADL; used a wheelchair; were a long-term user of a cane, crutches, or a walker; had a developmental disability or Alzheimer's disease; were unable to do housework; were receiving federal disability benefits; or were sixteen to sixty-seven years old and unable to work at a job or business. The prevalence of serious disablement increased steadily with age: ages fifteen to twenty-one, 3.2 percent; ages twenty-two to forty-four, 6.4 percent; ages forty-five to fifty-four, 11.5 percent; ages fifty-five to sixty-four, 21.9 percent; ages sixty-five to seventy-nine, 27.8 percent; age eighty and up, 53.5 percent (McNeil, 1997). The prevalence of serious disability in the United States is then likely to increase as the proportion of elderly in the U.S. population increases.

Persons Living with HIV/AIDS

AIDS emerged on the public health landscape early in the 1980s in the United States, mysterious in its origins and debilitating and seemingly universally fatal in its consequences. Although in Africa AIDS has primarily been a disease of heterosexuals, in the United States its afflictions were first felt within the confines of the gay community (as Gay-Related Immune Disorder, or GRID). Over time in the United States, however, its ravages have extended to heterosexuals, particularly those who use illicit drugs and their children.

Public health prevention efforts and new antiretroviral therapies for delaying the progression from HIV to AIDS or to inhibit its transmission from mother to child (nucleoside analogs, such as zidovudine [ZDV], which is also referred to as azidothymidine [AZT]; nonnucleosides; and protease inhibitors, among others) have led to positive shifts in the trends in AIDS incidence and prevalence and deaths due to AIDS. Attention has correspondingly turned to monitoring the prevalence of HIV infection, in tracing the likely future course of the epidemic. (See Table 2.3.)

HIV Prevalence. In 1999, over 100,000 people in the United States were estimated to be living with the HIV virus that had not yet progressed to AIDS (Centers for Disease Control and Prevention, 1999a). Based on provisional data for 1994–1997 in twenty-five reporting states examining the relative distribution of cases in which HIV infection versus AIDS was the initial diagnosis, 72 percent were diagnosed with HIV compared to 28 percent for whom AIDS was the initial diagnosis. Although the vast majority of individuals are being diagnosed earlier in the course of the disease than in the past, the proportion of newly diagnosed persons with HIV remained relatively stable over this period, signaling that there have not been significant declines in the number of individuals newly at risk for AIDS. Studies in selected sites participating in CDC–sponsored HIV seroprevalence surveys documented that in 1997, the average prevalence rates among clients seen at participating sites were relatively high (for example, 14.8 percent in drug treatment centers and 3.9 percent in sexually transmitted disease clinics).

AIDS Cases. Prior to 1983, there were fewer than eight hundred reported cases of AIDS. However, in 1983 alone, over two thousand new cases were reported. The number of cases continued to increase throughout the 1980s and into the 1990s. A difficulty in tracing trends in the AIDS epidemic is that the definition of AIDS cases has been changed three times (in 1985, 1987, and 1993) to capture the complex of conditions characterizing HIV/AIDS. The large increase from 1992 to 1993 shown in Table 2.3 largely stems from the change in case definition in 1993. Since that time, the number of new AIDS cases has declined, reflecting the earlier diagnosis and more effective treatment of HIV. As of June 1999, 711,344 cumulative cases of AIDS had been reported in the United States, and

288,000 individuals in the United States were estimated to be living with AIDS (Centers for Disease Control and Prevention, 1999a).

The principal mode of HIV transmission among children is perinatally through their HIV-infected mother. In the early years of the AIDS epidemic, the principal mode of transmission for adults was through male homosexual or bisexual contact. More recently transmission through intravenous drug use and heterosexual sexual contacts has increased.

HIV/AIDS-Related Deaths. As with the reporting of AIDS cases, trends in death rates due to HIV/AIDs are troublesome to trace precisely due to changes in case definitions. However, since 1995 there is evidence that death rates have declined, reflecting the prolongation of life for many persons living with HIV/AIDS.

Mentally Ill and Disabled

The mentally ill and disabled include individuals who experience neuroses and psychoses, as well as those with mental retardation or other cognitive impairments. Sources of data to estimate the magnitude of mental illness in the United States include surveys that ask people whether they have had certain mental health problems, as well as patient census or visit data obtained from institutions that care for the mentally ill.

Data on the prevalence of mental illness in the United States indicate that almost 50 percent of Americans have experienced a mental health problem at some time in their life, and more than half that number (30 percent) reported having a problem in the last year. (See Table 2.4.) From 7 to 10 million Americans have been estimated to have serious mental illness, that is, emotional disorders that seriously interfere with their ability to function in the primary activities of daily life (such as self-care, interpersonal relationships, working, or going to school) and require prolonged mental health care as a result.

Community Prevalence Rates. The Epidemiological Catchment Area (ECA) surveys conducted during the early 1980s in five U.S. cities (New Haven, Connecticut; Baltimore, Maryland; St. Louis, Missouri; Durham, North Carolina; and Los Angeles) represented one of the first major epidemiological studies to estimate the prevalence of mental illness among general community populations (Robins & Regier, 1991). The ECA was, however, criticized for not being a nationally representative sample of the U.S. population. The National Comorbidity Survey (NCS), conducted between 1990 and 1992, attempted to address this and other limitations of the earlier ECA surveys. The NCS, a nationally representative survey of persons aged fifteen to fifty-four in the noninstitutionalized population in the United States, included an expanded set of questions and criteria for identifying various categories of mental illness; and whereas the ECA was primarily designed as an incidence and prevalence study, the NCS also included an examination of the predictors of mental illness and related comorbidities (Kessler, 1994, 1995; Kessler et al., 1994). Beginning in 1994, the National Household

TABLE 2.3.   INDICATORS OF PERSONS LIVING WITH HIV/AIDS.

Indicators						*Year*
	1985	1986	1987	1988	1989	1990
HIV diagnoses[1]						
Number (percent) of persons initially diagnosed with HIV infection, not AIDS, age 13+						
Number (percent) of persons initially diagnosed with HIV infection, not AIDS, age 13+, by transmission category						
Men who have sex with men						
Injecting drug use						
Men who have sex with men and inject drugs						
Heterosexual contact						
Other/risk not reported or identified						

	1985	1986	1987	1988	1989	1990
Median (range) percent positive HIV prevalence[2]@@						
Sexually transmitted disease clinics					2.2 (0.0–38.5)	2.1 (0.0–39.0)
Drug treatment centers					4.1 (0.0–48.2)	3.9 (0.0–49.3)
Women's health clinics					0.2 (0.0–2.6)	0.2 (0.0–2.5)
Tuberculosis clinics					3.4 (0.0–46.3)	5.9 (0.0–58.3)
Childbearing women					0.15 (0.0–0.58)	0.15 (0.0–0.66)
Civilian applicants for military service					0.12	0.12
Blood donors					0.0084	0.0051
Job Corps entrants					0.36	0.34
Sentinel hospital patients					0.9 (0.1–7.7)	0.9 (0.1–7.6)
National Clinical Laboratory Survey					0.89	
Ambulatory Sentinel Practice Network						0.2

	1985	1986	1987	1988	1989	1990
AIDS cases[3]#						
Total number	8,161	13,147	21,088	30,719	33,595	41,569
Under 13	128	183	322	571	596	723
13+	8,033	12,964	20,766	30,148	32,999	40,846
Number by transmission category, 13+ (percent distribution)						
Men who have sex with men	5,357 (66.7)	8,542 (67.0)	13,550 (66.1)	17,860 (60.0)	19,688 (60.3)	23,826 (58.3)
Injecting drug use	1,387 (17.3)	2,244 (17.6)	3,548 (17.3)	6,926 (23.3)	7,212 (22.1)	9,280 (22.7)

1991	1992	1993	1994	1995	1996	January–June 1997	Cumulative Total
			15,571 (71)	14,895 (72)	14,652 (74)	7,571 (74)	52,690 (72)
							17,098 (66)
							9,671 (71)
							2,088 (71)
							9,279 (79)
							14,552 (78)

1991	1992	1993	1994	1995	1996	1997
	1.6 (0.1–25.1)	3.0 (0.3–12.2)				3.9 (0.5–11.4)
	7.5 (0.6–52.9)	5.4 (0.8–48.4)				14.8 (0.0–37.7)
	0.2 (0.0–3.3)					
	1.0 (0.1–5.8)					

1991	1992	1993	1994	1995	1996	1997	1998	Cumulative Total (as of December 1998)
43,701	45,771	102,211	77,237	71,039	66,659	58,254	48,269	688,200
667	749	871	972	747	656	448	382	8,461
43,034	45,022	101,340	76,265	70,292	66,003	57,806	47,887	679,739
23,872 (56.1)	24,467 (54.3)	49,600 (48.9)	35,291 (46.3)	30,939 (44.0)	27,316 (41.4)	21,163 (36.6)	16,642 (34.8)	326,051 (48.0)
10,347 (24.3)	11,003 (24.4)	28,124 (27.8)	21,054 (27.6)	18,583 (26.4)	16,405 (24.9)	14,110 (24.4)	11,070 (23.1)	173,693 (25.6)

(*Continued on page 30*)

TABLE 2.3.   (*Continued*)

Indicators	1985	1986	1987	1988	1989	1990
						Year
AIDS cases[3]# (continued)						
Men who have sex with men and inject drugs	655	989	1,551	2,037	2,189	2,804
	(8.2)	(7.8)	(7.6)	(6.8)	(6.7)	(6.9)
Hemophilia/coagulation disorder	71	122	206	297	285	348
	(0.9)	(1.0)	(1.0)	(1.0)	(0.9)	(0.9)
Heterosexual contact	151	341	647	1,187	1,507	2,261
	(1.9)	(2.7)	(3.2)	(4.0)	(4.6)	(5.5)
Sex with injecting drug user	*107*	*237*	*444*	*862*	*1,063*	*1,495*
Receipt of blood transfusion, blood components, or tissue	166	298	616	810	722	788
	(2.1)	(2.3)	(3.0)	(2.7)	(2.2)	(1.9)
Other/risk not reported or identified	246	212	387	661	1,030	1,539
	(3.1)	(1.7)	(1.9)	(2.2)	(3.2)	(3.8)
	1985	**1986**	**1987**	**1988**	**1989**	**1990**
Deaths of persons with AIDS[4]						
Counts of deaths in persons with HIV/AIDS*	6,972	12,110	16,412	21,119	27,791	31,538
Estimated deaths of persons with AIDS@						
Under 13						
13+						
Number by transmission category, 13+ (percent distribution)						
Men who have sex with men						
Injecting drug use						
Men who have sex with men and inject drugs						
Hemophilia/coagulation disorder						
Heterosexual contact						
Receipt of blood transfusion, blood components, or tissue						
Other/risk not reported or identified						
			1987	**1988**	**1989**	**1990**
Death rates for HIV infection, age-adjusted per 100,000 persons[5]						
			5.5	6.7	8.7	9.8

Note: The AIDS case reporting definitions were revised in 1985, 1987, and 1993.

@@ Data are from standardized unlinked seroprevalence surveys for which there is variability in the number and types of sites reporting across time periods.

Data from different periods should be compared with caution. Data are regularly adjusted for reporting delays, and delays in investigation of modes of exposure result in underestimation in some risk categories.

1991	1992	1993	1994	1995	1996	1997	1998	Cumulative Total (as of December 1998)
2,454	3,168	7,210	4,443	3,742	3,044	2,357	1,984	43,640
(5.8)	(7.0)	(7.1)	(5.8)	(5.3)	(4.6)	(4.1)	(4.1)	(6.4)
311	334	1,080	505	443	321	206	162	4,911
(0.7)	(0.7)	(1.1)	(0.7)	(0.6)	(0.5)	(0.4)	(0.3)	(0.7)
2,707	3,523	9,054	8,240	8,112	8,609	7,869	6,736	66,490
(6.4)	(7.8)	(8.9)	(10.8)	(11.5)	(13.0)	(13.6)	(14.1)	(9.8)
1,681	*1,942*	*3,938*	*2,944*	*2,738*	*2,647*	*2,180*	*1,843*	*26,246*
663	602	1,097	688	622	548	393	293	8,382
(1.6)	(1.3)	(1.1)	(0.9)	(0.9)	(0.8)	(0.7)	(0.6)	(1.2)
2,188	1,925	5,175	6,044	7,851	9,760	11,708	11,000	56,572
(5.1)	(4.3)	(5.1)	(7.9)	(11.2)	(14.8)	(20.3)	(23.0)	(8.3)

1991	**1992**	**1993**	**1994**	**1995**	**1996**	**1997**	**1998**	
36,616	41,094	44,636	48,663	48,371	34,947	14,338	—	
		44,991	49,442	49,895	37,221	21,445	17,171	
		539	578	537	426	218	121	
		44,452	48,864	49,358	36,795	21,227	17,050	
		23,674	24,973	24,356	16,436	8,401	6,467	
		(53.3)	(51.1)	(49.3)	(44.7)	(39.6)	(37.9)	
		12,325	13,956	14,431	11,661	7,352	6,019	
		(27.7)	(28.6)	(29.2)	(31.7)	(34.6)	(35.3)	
		3,117	3,426	3,332	2,504	1,365	1,142	
		(7.0)	(7.0)	(6.8)	(6.8)	(6.4)	(6.7)	
		369	372	355	268	156	110	
		(0.8)	(0.8)	(0.7)	(0.7)	(0.7)	(0.6)	
		4,189	5,414	6,242	5,447	3,678	3,114	
		(9.4)	(11.1)	(12.6)	(14.8)	(17.3)	(18.3)	
		550	526	485	387	208	154	
		(1.2)	(1.1)	(1.0)	(1.1)	(1.0)	(0.9)	
		229	197	156	94	67	43	
		(0.5)	(0.4)	(0.3)	(0.3)	(0.3)	(0.3)	

1991	**1992**	**1993**	**1994**	**1995**	**1996**	**1997**		
11.3	12.6	13.8	15.4	15.6	11.1	5.8		

* Reported numbers of deaths among persons diagnosed with AIDS. These deaths are not necessarily caused by HIV-related disease.

@ These numbers do not represent actual deaths. They are point estimates adjusted for delays in the reporting of deaths and for the redistribution of cases initially reported with no identified risk.

Sources: CDC and NCHS reports. See Resource B for specific references to table items marked with superscript numerals.

TABLE 2.4. INDICATORS OF MENTALLY ILL AND DISABLED: COMMUNITY PREVALENCE RATES.

Indicators	1990	1991	1992	1993	1994	1995	1996	1997
Prevalence of mental disorders, percent[1]								
Any NCS disorder								
Lifetime		48.0						
12 month		29.5						
Substance use disorders								
Alcohol abuse without dependence								
Lifetime		9.4						
12 month		2.5						
Alcohol dependence								
Lifetime		14.1						
12 month		7.2						
Drug abuse without dependence								
Lifetime		4.4						
12 month		0.8						
Drug dependence								
Lifetime		7.5						
12 month		2.8						
Any substance abuse/ dependence								
Lifetime		26.6						
12 month		11.3						
Affective disorders								
Major depressive episode								
Lifetime		17.1						
12 month		10.3			7.6		6.3	7.9
Manic episode								
Lifetime		1.6						
12 month		1.3						
Dysthymia								
Lifetime		6.4						
12 month		2.5						
Any affective disorder								
Lifetime		19.3						
12 month		11.3						
Anxiety disorder								
Panic disorder								
Lifetime		3.5						
12 month		2.3			2.5		2.9	2.9
Agoraphobia without panic disorder								
Lifetime		5.3						
12 month		2.8			2.0		1.6	1.8
Social phobia								
Lifetime		13.3						
12 month		7.9						
Simple phobia								
Lifetime		11.3						
12 month		8.8						

TABLE 2.4.   (*Continued*)

Indicators	Year							
	1990	1991	1992	1993	1994	1995	1996	1997
Prevalence of mental disorders, percent[1]								
Generalized anxiety disorder								
Lifetime		5.1						
12 month		3.1			2.1		2.0	2.1
Any anxiety disorder								
Lifetime		24.9						
12 month		17.2						
Other disorders								
Antisocial personality								
Lifetime		3.5						
12 month		—						
Nonaffective psychosis@								
Lifetime		0.7						
12 month		0.5						

Note: The National Comorbidity Study (NCS) was conducted from 1990 to 1992 and covered persons fifteen to fifty-four years of age. The National Household Survey on Drug Abuse (NHSDA), conducted in 1994, 1996, and 1997, covered persons twelve years of age and older. This difference in the population studied may have contributed to differences in estimates from the NCS and NHSDA. Furthermore, although the screening scales used for the NHSDA are based on questions used in the NCS, the changes, together with differences in the way the surveys were administered, may also have affected the comparability of results.

@Nonaffective psychosis includes schizophrenia, schizophreniform disorder, schizoaffective disorder, delusional disorder, and atypical psychosis.

Sources: Kessler et al. (1998) and Substance Abuse and Mental Health Services Administration reports. See Resource B for specific references to table items marked with superscript numerals.

Survey on Drug Abuse (NHSDA) added and adopted questions from the NCS to screen for major depressive episodes, generalized anxiety disorder, panic attack, and agoraphobia. Although these questions are not entirely comparable to the NCS questions, their inclusion in the NHSDA permits ongoing monitoring of the prevalence of these conditions in the U.S. population and by selected subgroups (Substance Abuse and Mental Health Services Administration, 1996).

Based on the 1990–1992 NCS, almost half (48 percent) of the U.S. population was estimated to have experienced a mental disorder sometime in their life, and around 30 percent (29.5 percent) experienced an episode within the past twelve months. The most common psychiatric disorders were major depression and alcohol dependence. Seventeen percent had experienced a major depressive episode (MDE) sometime in their life, and one out of ten (10.3 percent) experienced such an episode within the past year. About 14 percent of respondents had a history of alcohol dependence, and 7.2 percent were characterized as experiencing alcohol dependence within the past year. The next most common disorders were social and simple phobias, with lifetime prevalences of 13.3 percent and 11.3 percent, respectively, and twelve-month prevalences of 7.9 percent and

8.8 percent, respectively. Considering the presence of any of the major groups of disorders, substance abuse disorders were more likely to have been a problem at some point in one's lifetime (26.6 percent), followed by anxiety disorders (24.9 percent) and affective disorders (19.3 percent). People were more likely to have experienced some type of anxiety disorder within the previous twelve months (17.2 percent), relative to the occurrence of affective (11.3 percent) or substance abuse (11.3 percent) disorders.

Among respondents who reported some type of disorder in their lifetime, 21 percent had experienced only one such disorder, 13 percent had two, and 14 percent had three or more disorders. The co-occurrence of severe twelve-month disorders was also highly concentrated (89.5 percent) among those who had three or more lifetime disorders. The NCS data then suggest that while a history of psychiatric disorder is common among persons fifteen to fifty-four years of age in the United States, the major burden of mental illness is borne disproportionately by about one-sixth of the U.S. population, who experience an array of disorders (Kessler et al., 1994).

Estimates of the prevalence of selected disorders (major depressive episode, generalized anxiety disorder, agoraphobia, and panic attack), based on the 1994, 1996, and 1997 NHSDA, confirmed that around one out of ten Americans had experienced at least one of these syndromes during the previous year. Although the precise estimates fluctuate in the respective years, the NHSDA documented that from 6 to 8 percent of Americans experienced a major depressive episode, and around 2 to 3 percent experienced an anxiety disorder within the past year.

The national prevalence of serious mental illness, such as schizophrenia and other psychoses, has been estimated to range from 4.5 to 6.3 percent, representing 7 to 10 million individuals who experience a mental illness that seriously interferes with daily living skills, such as eating or bathing; instrumental living skills including maintaining a household, managing money, and taking prescribed medication; or functioning adequately in social, family or vocational or educational contexts (Kessler et al., 1998; Willis, Willis, Manderscheid, Male, and Henderson, 1998).

Treated Rates: Mental Health Facilities. Persons with mental illness are treated in a variety of care settings, including twenty-four-hour hospitals, twenty-four-hour residential care facilities, and less-than-twenty-four-hour mental health care outpatient settings. (See Table 2.5.) Patients with different types of diagnoses are seen within these respective settings. Based on 1994 data, clients with schizophrenia and other psychoses were more likely to be treated in twenty-four-hour care settings, particularly hospitals. Patients with mood disorders and other mental health diagnoses were more likely to be seen in out-of-hospital settings, especially less-than-twenty-four-hour facilities.

Treated Rates: Nursing Homes. Findings from the 1995 National Nursing Home Survey revealed that over half (58.6 percent) of nursing home residents had at least one mental disorder. (See Table 2.6.) The most prevalent disorder

TABLE 2.5. INDICATORS OF MENTALLY ILL AND DISABLED: TREATED RATES, MENTAL HEALTH FACILITIES.

	Major Diagnostic Group			
Indicators	Schizophrenia and Other Psychoses	Mood Disorders	Other Mental Health Disorders	Total
Number (percent) of clients receiving mental health treatment, 1994[1]				
24-hour hospital	63,769 (49)	39,836 (31)	25,920 (20)	129,525 (100)
24-hour residential	24,496 (39)	18,738 (25)	27,366 (36)	75,600 (100)
Less-than-24-hour hospital	786,550 (26)	1,038,809 (34)	1,250,793 (40)	3,076,152 (100)

Source: Rouse (1998). See Resource B for specific references to table items marked with superscript numerals.

TABLE 2.6. INDICATORS OF MENTALLY ILL AND DISABLED: TREATED RATES, NURSING HOMES.

	Year	
Indicators	1985	1995
Number (percent) of nursing home residents with mental disorders[1]@		
Total (percent) with any mental disorder	697,000 (46.7)	907,000 (58.6)
Mental retardation	50,600 (7.3)	31,400 (3.5)
Alcohol and drug abuse	24,700 (3.5)	21,200 (2.3)
Organic brain syndromes (including Alzheimer's disease)	488,100 (70.0)	726,800 (80.1)
Depressive disorders	48,000 (6.9)	154,900 (17.1)
Schizophrenia and other psychoses	162,400 (23.3)	149,100 (16.4)
Anxiety disorders	22,000 (3.2)	57,800 (6.4)
Other mental illnesses	*16,500 (2.4)	41,500 (4.6)

@ The percentage with any mental disorder is based on all nursing home residents. The percentage with a specific mental disorder is based on nursing home residents who had any mental disorder. Subgroups add to more than the total because residents with multiple disorders are counted more than once. Numbers may not add to totals because of rounding. Percentages are based on unrounded numbers.

* Data should not be assumed to be reliable because the sample size is between 30 and 59 or the sample is greater than 59 but has a relative standard error over 30 percent.

Source: NCHS data. See Resource B for specific references to table items marked with superscript numerals.

was organic brain syndrome (OBS), including Alzheimer's disease. Among residents identified as having a mental disorder, 80.1 percent were diagnosed with OBS, an increase from 70.0 percent in 1985. Around one in six had schizophrenia and other psychoses (16.4 percent) or depressive disorders (17.1 percent), and 6.4 percent had anxiety disorders. Mental retardation (3.5 percent), alcohol and drug abuse (2.3 percent), and other mental illnesses (4.6 percent) accounted for the remainder of the diagnoses among mentally ill nursing home residents.

Alcohol or Substance Abusers

Alcohol and substance users differ from abusers in that the latter have developed a long-term physical or psychological dependency on (or addiction to) drugs, alcohol, or tobacco. National surveys of households and high school seniors provide data on those who have used or are currently using (and may be abusing) these substances. Vital statistics and emergency room and medical examiner data on alcohol or drug-related medical emergencies or deaths more directly reflect the life-threatening consequences for those who routinely or seriously abuse these substances.

The percentage of the U.S. population reported to use illicit drugs declined from the late 1970s to the early 1990s. Since 1993, there is evidence that use has increased, especially among those twelve to seventeen years old. The number of adults experiencing medical emergencies or dying from the effects of cocaine has increased, confirming a growth in a subgroup of users who are seriously addicted to this particular drug. Users of cocaine may also use other drugs, such as heroin, which could result in multidrug interactions and overdose. (See Table 2.7.)

Household Population, Twelve Years Old and Up. Based on the NHSDA, which covers the population age twelve and older living in households in the contiguous United States, since 1979 a relatively steady percentage (around one-third) of the U.S. population is estimated to have ever used illicit drugs (Substance Abuse and Mental Health Services Administration, 1999c). The proportion reporting drug use in the past year during the 1990s (10 to 11 percent) was significantly lower than the 1979 rates of 17.5 percent, one of the periods of highest drug use in the United States, as was the case for drug use in the past month: 14.1 percent in 1979 compared to 6 to 7 percent in the 1990s. The lifetime, past-year, and past-month rates of use of marijuana, the most commonly used illicit drug, have declined since the period of their peak prevalence during the late 1970s. These trends do not apply across all age groups of the U.S. population. Lifetime, annual, and past-month rates of any illicit drug use, as well as marijuana and cocaine use, among youths twelve to seventeen years of age have increased since 1992 (Substance Abuse and Mental Health Services Administration, 1999c).

In 1998 almost 81 percent of the U.S. population (about 177 million persons) were estimated to have had a drink of alcohol at least once in their life. Nearly as many people (69.7 percent or 152 million) had ever tried cigarettes at least once in their life. Based on 1998 data, around two-thirds of the U.S. population (64 percent) had consumed alcohol, and about one-third (30.6 percent) had smoked cigarettes in the past year. The percentages using alcohol and cigarettes in the past month were 51.7 percent and 27.7 percent, respectively. Past-year and past-month rates of alcohol use and smoking have declined significantly since 1985 (Substance Abuse and Mental Health Services Administration, 1999c).

High School Seniors. Although the proportion of all high school seniors who said they had used an illicit drug at least once during the past month in 1998 (25.6 percent) was much lower than a high of 38.9 percent in 1978 and 1979, this percentage represents an increase from a low of 14.4 percent in 1992. Marijuana was and continues to be the most frequently used illicit drug. The annual and thirty-day (reflecting the more current) prevalence of marijuana use declined from the early 1980s through 1992, but has increased, to 37.5 percent and 22.8 percent, respectively. From 1986 to 1992, both annual and monthly use of cocaine decreased. From 1992 to 1998, annual use rose significantly from 3.1 percent to 5.7 percent, and thirty-day prevalence rose modestly from 1.3 percent to 2.4 percent. The rates of crack cocaine use have increased correspondingly since 1992 (Johnston, O'Malley, & Bachman, 1999).

The percentage of high school seniors reporting they had consumed an alcoholic beverage in the past month declined from almost three-fourths of seniors in 1980 to around half in the early 1990s. From 1993 to 1997, there was a slight upward drift in high school seniors' annual alcohol use rates. In 1998, over a third (35.1 percent) of U.S. high school seniors reported having smoked cigarettes in the past month. The percentage of current smokers among high school students declined from 36.7 percent in 1975 to a low of 27.8 percent in 1992, but has tended to increase since then.

Alcohol-Related Mortality Rates. There has been no significant change in alcohol-related mortality rates in recent years. During the period from 1985 to 1995, the rates of death attributable to alcohol-related causes, including alcohol-related accidents and diseases such as cirrhosis of the liver, ranged between 6.7 and 7.3 per 100,000.

Emergency Room Drug Abuse Reports. Reports of drug-related visits to an emergency room in participating cities are reported through the Drug Abuse Warning Network (DAWN). Because of changes in the sampling frame and estimation algorithms over time, trends based on the DAWN data must be interpreted with caution. The number of drug-related emergency room visits in 1998 (542,544) represents a 46 percent increase from 1990 (371,208). The number of incidents related to cocaine more than doubled during this same period, an increase attributed to the serious health consequences that chronic drug users experience. The number of drug-related deaths, and in particular cocaine-related

TABLE 2.7.   INDICATORS OF ALCOHOL OR SUBSTANCE ABUSERS.

Indicators	Year				
	1979	1982	1985	1988	1990
Household population, age 12+, percent drug use[1]					
Any illicit drug use@					
Past year	17.5	—	16.3	12.4	11.7
Past month	14.1	—	12.1	7.7	6.7
Marijuana and hashish					
Past year	16.6	15.9	13.6	9.8	9.4
Past month	13.2	11.5	9.7	6.2	5.4
Hallucinogens*					
Past year	2.9	2.2	1.7	1.6	1.2
Past month	1.9	0.9	1.2	0.6	0.4
Cocaine (crack)*					
Past year	4.8	5.6	5.1	3.6	2.7
	(—)	(—)	(—)	(0.7)	(0.7)
Past month	2.6	2.4	3.0	1.6	0.9
	(—)	(—)	(—)	(0.3)	(0.3)
Alcohol use					
Past year	72.9	67.9	72.9	68.1	66.0
Past month	63.2	56.6	60.2	54.9	52.6
Cigarette use					
Past year	—	—	40.5	38.5	36.1
Past month	—	—	38.7	35.3	32.6
Household population, 12–17 years, percent drug use[2]					
Any illicit drug use@					
Past year	24.3	—	20.7	14.9	14.1
Past month	16.3	—	13.2	8.1	7.1
Marijuana and hashish					
Past year	21.3	17.7	16.7	10.7	9.6
Past month	14.2	9.9	10.2	5.4	4.4
Cocaine					
Past year	3.6	3.7	3.4	2.5	1.9
Past month	1.5	1.9	1.5	1.2	0.6
Alcohol use					
Past year	55.9	46.1	52.7	45.5	41.8
Past month	49.6	34.9	41.2	33.4	32.5
Cigarette use					
Past year	—	—	29.9	26.8	26.2
Past month	—	—	29.4	22.7	22.4
Household population, 18–25 years, percent drug use[2]					
Any illicit drug use@					
Past year	45.5	—	37.4	29.1	26.1
Past month	38.0	—	25.3	17.9	15.0
Marijuana and hashish					
Past year	44.2	37.4	34.0	26.1	23.0
Past month	35.6	27.2	21.7	15.3	12.7
Cocaine					
Past year	17.0	15.9	13.6	10.5	6.5
Past month	9.9	7.0	8.1	4.8	2.3

			Year				
1991	1992	1993	1994	1995	1996	1997	1998
11.1	9.7	10.3	10.8	10.7	10.8	11.2	10.6
6.6	5.8	5.9	6.0	6.1	6.1	6.4	6.2
8.9	7.9	8.5	8.5	8.4	8.6	9.0	8.6
5.1	4.7	4.6	4.8	4.7	4.7	5.1	5.0
1.3	1.2	1.2	1.3	1.6	1.7	1.9	1.6
0.5	0.4	0.4	0.5	0.7	0.6	0.8	0.7
2.6	2.1	1.9	1.7	1.7	1.9	1.9	1.7
(0.7)	(0.6)	(0.7)	(0.6)	(0.5)	(0.6)	(0.6)	(0.4)
1.0	0.7	0.7	0.7	0.7	0.8	0.7	0.8
(0.3)	(0.2)	(0.3)	(0.2)	(0.2)	(0.3)	(0.3)	(0.2)
68.1	64.7	66.5	66.9	65.4	64.9	64.1	64.0
52.2	49.0	50.8	53.9	52.2	51.0	51.4	51.7
36.2	35.2	33.2	31.7	32.0	32.3	32.7	30.6
33.0	31.9	29.6	28.6	28.8	28.9	29.6	27.7
13.1	10.4	11.9	15.5	18.0	16.7	18.8	16.4
5.8	5.3	5.7	8.2	10.9	9.0	11.4	9.9
8.5	6.9	8.5	11.4	14.2	13.0	15.8	14.1
3.6	3.4	4.0	6.0	8.2	7.1	9.4	8.3
1.3	1.0	0.7	1.1	1.7	1.4	2.2	1.7
0.4	0.3	0.4	0.3	0.8	0.6	1.0	0.8
41.2	33.3	35.9	36.2	35.1	32.7	34.0	31.8
27.0	20.9	23.9	21.6	21.1	18.8	20.5	19.1
23.7	21.4	22.5	24.5	26.6	24.2	26.4	23.8
20.9	18.4	18.5	18.9	20.2	18.3	19.9	18.2
26.6	24.1	24.2	24.6	25.5	26.8	25.3	27.4
15.4	13.1	13.6	13.3	14.2	15.6	14.7	16.1
22.9	21.2	21.4	21.8	21.8	23.8	22.3	24.1
12.9	10.9	11.1	12.1	12.0	13.2	12.8	13.8
6.7	5.5	4.4	3.6	4.3	4.7	3.9	4.7
2.2	2.0	1.6	1.2	1.3	2.0	1.2	2.0

(Continued on page 40)

TABLE 2.7. (*Continued*)

Indicators	Year				
	1979	1982	1985	1988	1990
Alcohol use					
Past year	84.6	80.6	84.2	79.6	78.1
Past month	75.1	66.6	70.1	64.7	62.8
Cigarette use					
Past year	—	—	49.9	50.9	45.1
Past month	—	—	47.4	45.6	40.9

Household population, 26–34 years, percent drug use[2]

Any illicit drug use@					
Past year	23.0	—	26.2	19.1	18.4
Past month	20.8	—	23.1	14.7	10.9
Marijuana and hashish					
Past year	20.5	21.4	20.2	14.2	14.4
Past month	19.7	19.0	19.0	11.3	9.5
Cocaine					
Past year	5.7	9.3	10.5	7.0	5.9
Past month	3.0	3.5	6.3	2.8	1.9
Alcohol use					
Past year	81.7	81.1	81.9	78.8	77.2
Past month	71.6	71.5	70.6	65.3	64.4
Cigarette use					
Past year	—	—	48.8	47.2	47.9
Past month	—	—	45.7	42.1	42.4

Household population, 35+ years, percent drug use[2]

Any illicit drug use@					
Past year	3.9	—	5.5	5.1	5.2
Past month	2.8	—	3.9	2.3	3.1
Marijuana and hashish					
Past year	4.3	6.2	4.3	3.7	4.2
Past month	2.9	3.9	2.6	1.8	2.4
Cocaine					
Past year	0.4	1.2	0.9	0.7	0.8
Past month	0.2	0.5	0.5	0.4	0.2
Alcohol use					
Past year	70.1	63.8	70.5	65.4	63.4
Past month	59.7	53.0	57.5	52.6	49.5
Cigarette use					
Past year	—	—	36.9	34.3	31.5
Past month	—	—	35.5	32.4	28.9

Indicators	1975	1980	1985	1986	1987	1988	1989
High school seniors, percent drug use[3]							
Any illicit drug use@@							
Past year	45.0	53.1	46.3	44.3	41.7	38.5	35.4
Past month	30.7	37.2	29.7	27.1	24.7	21.3	19.7
Marijuana and hashish							
Past year	40.0	48.8	40.6	38.8	36.3	33.1	29.6
Past month	27.1	33.7	25.7	23.4	21.0	18.0	16.7
Inhalants							
Past year	—	7.9	7.5	8.9	8.1	7.1	6.9
Past month	—	2.7	3.0	3.2	3.5	3.0	2.7

Year							
1991	**1992**	**1993**	**1994**	**1995**	**1996**	**1997**	**1998**
80.7	75.6	76.9	78.5	76.5	75.3	75.1	74.2
63.1	58.6	58.7	63.1	61.3	60.0	58.4	60.0
46.9	46.8	43.7	41.1	42.5	44.7	45.9	47.1
41.7	41.5	37.9	34.6	35.3	38.3	40.6	41.6
15.5	15.4	14.6	14.8	14.6	14.6	14.3	12.7
10.0	11.4	9.5	8.5	8.3	8.4	7.4	7.0
11.6	11.5	11.1	11.5	11.8	11.3	11.2	9.7
7.7	9.3	7.5	6.9	6.7	6.3	6.0	5.5
4.4	4.3	3.8	3.5	3.1	3.5	3.1	2.7
1.9	1.5	1.0	1.3	1.2	1.5	0.9	1.2
79.1	77.3	79.2	78.8	77.0	77.2	74.6	74.5
62.7	62.3	63.8	65.3	63.0	61.6	60.2	60.9
41.9	42.8	38.7	36.0	38.4	39.2	37.7	36.6
37.3	38.2	34.2	32.4	34.7	35.0	33.7	32.5
5.5	4.4	5.5	5.7	5.0	5.3	6.1	5.5
3.4	2.5	3.0	3.2	2.8	2.9	3.6	3.3
4.6	3.8	4.6	4.1	3.4	3.8	4.4	4.1
2.6	2.0	2.4	2.3	1.8	2.0	2.6	2.5
1.2	0.8	0.9	0.9	0.8	0.9	1.1	0.9
0.5	0.2	0.4	0.4	0.4	0.4	0.5	0.5
65.9	63.5	65.5	66.2	65.0	64.9	64.1	64.6
50.4	47.4	49.8	54.1	52.6	51.7	52.8	53.1
33.8	32.4	30.9	29.6	28.7	29.1	29.7	26.7
31.6	30.0	28.2	27.9	27.2	27.0	27.9	25.1

1990	**1991**	**1992**	**1993**	**1994**	**1995**	**1996**	**1997**	**1998**
32.5	29.4	27.1	31.0	35.8	39.0	40.2	42.4	41.4
17.2	16.4	14.4	18.3	21.9	23.8	24.6	26.2	25.6
27.0	23.9	21.9	26.0	30.7	34.7	35.8	38.5	37.5
14.0	13.8	11.9	15.5	19.0	21.2	21.9	23.7	22.8
7.5	6.9	6.4	7.4	8.2	8.4	8.5	7.3	7.1
2.9	2.6	2.5	2.8	2.9	3.5	2.9	2.9	3.1

(*Continued on page 42*)

TABLE 2.7.   (*Continued*)

Indicators	1975	1980	1985	1986	1987	1988	1989
Hallucinogens							
Past year	—	10.4	7.6	7.6	6.7	5.8	6.2
Past month	—	4.4	3.8	3.5	2.8	2.3	2.9
Cocaine (crack)							
Past year	5.6	12.3	13.1	12.7	10.3	7.9	6.5
				(4.1)	(3.9)	(3.1)	(3.1)
Past month	1.9	5.2	6.7	6.2	4.3	3.4	2.8
					(1.3)	(1.6)	(1.4)
Alcohol use**							
Past year	84.8	87.9	85.6	84.5	85.7	85.3	82.7
Past month	68.2	72.0	65.9	65.3	66.4	63.9	60.0
Cigarette use							
Past month	36.7	30.5	30.1	29.6	29.4	28.7	28.6
Daily use	26.9	21.3	19.5	18.7	18.7	18.1	18.9

Indicators		1985	1986	1987	1988	1989
Alcohol-related mortality rates[4]						
Age-adjusted rate per 100,000		7.0	6.7	6.8	7.1	7.3

Indicators	1985	1986	1987	1988	1989	1990
Emergency room drug abuse reports[5#]						
Total episodes	334,500	352,500	396,400	403,600	425,904	371,208
Cocaine mentions	28,800	51,700	91,800	101,600	110,013	80,355

@ Any illicit drug refers to using, at least once, any of the following: marijuana or hashish, cocaine (including crack), inhalants, hallucinogens (including PCP and LSD), heroin, or any prescription-type psychotherapeutic used nonmedically.

* The National Household Survey on Drug Abuse was revised in 1994. The estimates for hallucinogen use and for crack use prior to 1994 reported here have not been adjusted to reflect the change.

@@ "Any illicit drug use" refers to using any of the following: marijuana, LSD, other hallucinogens, crack, other cocaine, or heroin, or any use of other narcotics, amphetamines, barbiturates, methaqualone, or tranquilizers not under a doctor's orders.

deaths, did not diminish over this time period. In 1997, the overall number of deaths due to drug abuse as reported by medical examiners was 9,616, after having risen from 8,812 in 1994. The wider availability of crack cocaine (which is smoked rather than inhaled), as well as increases in the number of chronic cocaine addicts, have contributed to these higher numbers of deaths (Substance Abuse and Mental Health Services Administration, 1999b).

Suicide or Homicide Prone

The ultimate harm resulting from violent and intentional acts to injure oneself or others is reflected in suicide and homicide rates. These estimates are derived from what medical examiners report as the cause of death on victims' death

1990	1991	1992	1993	1994	1995	1996	1997	1998
6.0	6.1	6.2	7.8	7.8	9.7	10.7	10.0	9.2
2.3	2.4	2.3	3.3	3.2	4.6	3.8	4.1	4.1
5.3	3.5	3.1	3.3	3.6	4.0	4.9	5.5	5.7
(1.9)	(1.5)	(1.5)	(1.5)	(1.9)	(2.1)	(2.1)	(2.4)	(2.5)
1.9	1.4	1.3	1.3	1.5	1.8	2.0	2.3	2.4
(0.7)	(0.7)	(0.6)	(0.7)	(0.8)	(1.0)	(1.0)	(0.9)	(1.0)
80.6	77.7	76.8	76.0					
			72.7	73.0	73.7	72.5	74.8	74.3
57.1	54.0	51.3	51.0					
			48.6	50.1	51.3	50.8	52.7	52.0
29.4	28.3	27.8	29.9	31.2	33.5	34.0	36.5	35.1
19.1	18.5	17.2	19.0	19.4	21.6	22.2	24.6	22.4

1990	1991	1992	1993	1994	1995	1996	1997	1998
7.2	6.8	6.8	6.7	—	6.7			

1991	1992	1993	1994	1995	1996	1997	1998
393,968	433,493	460,910	518,521	513,633	514,347	527,058	542,544
101,189	119,843	123,423	142,878	135,801	152,433	161,087	172,014

** In 1993, the question on alcohol use was revised. The data in the upper line came from the original wording; the data on the lower line came from the newer wording.

The sampling methodology was changed in 1988. Revisions in the estimation procedure were implemented in 1993. The estimates reported here for 1985 to 1988 have been rounded to the nearest 100.

— Estimate not available.

Sources: Substance Abuse and Mental Health Services Administration reports; Johnston, O'Malley, & Bachman (1999); Indian Health Service (1998, 1999). See Resource B for specific references to table items marked with superscript numerals.

certificates, which, as discussed in Chapter Ten, are relatively accurate sources for determining suicide intent as a cause of death. Although suicide death rates did not change substantially from 1950 to 1980, the homicide rate doubled during this period and has fallen only slightly since. Firearms have become an increasingly important and deadly contributor to both suicide and homicide statistics. (See Table 2.8.)

Suicide. Suicide is the eighth leading cause of death in the United States. The 1997 age-adjusted suicide rate was 10.6 per 100,000 people, closely approximating the Year 2000 Objective of 10.5. Data from the 1990–1992 National Comorbidity Survey documented that 13.5 percent of respondents fifteen to fifty-four years of age in the United States had thought about suicide at some point in their

TABLE 2.8. INDICATORS OF SUICIDE OR HOMICIDE PRONE.

Indicators	1950	1970	1975	1980	1985	1986	1987	1988	1989	1990	1991	1992	1993	1994	1995	1996	1997
										Year							
Age-adjusted death rates per 100,000 resident population[1]																	
Suicide	*11.0	*11.8	12.6	11.4	11.5	11.9	11.7	11.4	11.3	11.5	11.4	11.1	11.3	11.2	11.2	10.8	10.6
Homicide and legal intervention	*5.4	*9.1	10.5	10.8	8.3	9.0	8.6	9.0	9.4	10.2	10.9	10.5	10.7	10.3	9.4	8.5	8.0

*Includes deaths of nonresidents of the United States.

[1]Includes deaths of nonresidents of the United States. See Resource B for specific references to table items marked with superscript numerals.

Sources: NCHS reports. See Resource B for specific references to table items marked with superscript numerals.

lives. Suicide attempts are estimated to occur eight times more often than suicide deaths, with ratios of attempts to completed suicides being much higher for females (twenty-five to one) compared to males (three to one), which is due to a large extent to the differential means used to commit suicide. Injuries from gunshots, which account for a large proportion of male suicides, result in the majority of suicidal deaths. Unsuccessful suicide attempts principally entail poisoning by pill ingestion or the infliction of minor lacerations (Kessler, Borges, & Walters, 1999; National Center for Health Statistics, 1991b; Public Health Service, 1990; Rosenberg et al., 1987).

Homicide and Legal Intervention. The Year 2000 Objective was to reduce homicides to no more than 7.2 per 100,000. In terms of this objective, homicide is defined as death due to injuries purposely inflicted by another person, not including deaths caused by law enforcement officers or legal execution (which constitute around 0.2 per 100,000 deaths). The age-adjusted rate in 1997, including those due to legal intervention, was 8.0. Since 1950 these rates have ranged from a low of 5.2 (1960) to a high of 10.9 (1991). Firearms are an increasingly important contributor to homicide-related deaths (National Center for Health Statistics, 1991b; Public Health Service, 1990).

Suicide and homicide rates differ a great deal for different age, sex, and race groups, which will be discussed in Chapter Three.

Abusing Families

Perhaps the most vulnerable individuals are those who are intentionally harmed by close family members or friends. Estimates of the number of children, elderly adults, and spouses who are abused by their family or other intimates are based on cases reported to relevant public agencies, the informed opinions of people who head these agencies, as well as what family members say about the occurrence of such incidents, which may or may not actually be reported to any official agency or authority. Reports of family abuse and neglect have increased dramatically over the past twenty years. Around 3 million children and 2 million elderly adults are estimated to have experienced physical or emotional abuse or neglect. The incidence of unreported violence may be even higher. (See Table 2.9.)

Child Abuse and Neglect Reports. The National Study on Child Neglect and Abuse Data System collects annual data on official reports of child maltreatment from state-level child protective service (CPS) programs. Some children may have been reported and counted more than once during the year due to repeated instances of maltreatment. In 1997, around 3 million children were reported to have experienced maltreatment (abuse or neglect). The rate of reporting was estimated at 42.1 per 1,000 U.S. children. This is substantially higher than the number (1,154,000) and rates (18.1) of reports of children who were abused or neglected in 1980.

TABLE 2.9. INDICATORS OF ABUSING FAMILIES.

Indicators	Year													
	1980	1985	1986	1987	1988	1989	1990	1991	1992	1993	1994	1995	1996	1997
Child abuse and neglect reports[1*]														
Number of children reported in 1,000s	1,154	1,928	2,086	2,178			2,578	2,696	2,923	2,940	2,939	2,948	3,032	2,980
Child report rate per 1,000 U.S.children	18.1	30.6	32.8	34.0			40.3	42.0	43.6	43.2	43.3	43.0	43.1	42.1
Child abuse and neglect incidence rates[2@]														
Number of children in 1,000s, harm standard (endangerment standard)	625		931 (1,424)							1,554 (2,816)				
Rate per 1,000 U.S. children, harm standard (endangerment standard)	9.8 (—)		14.8 (22.6)							23.1 (41.9)				
Domestic elder abuse[3]														
Number of reports in 1,000s			117	128	140	—	211	213	—	227	241	286	293	
Violence by intimates[4]														
Number of violent victimizations of women 12 years and older in 1,000s									952	1,072	1,003	954	838	
Number of violent victimizations of men 12 years and older in 1,000s									146	164	176	115	148	
Rate of violent victimization of women, per 1,000 women									8.8	9.8	9.1	8.6	7.5	
Rate of violent victimization of men, per 1,000 men									1.4	1.6	1.7	1.1	1.4	

*The trend data reported should be interpreted with caution. The number of states and territories participating varies in different years, local data collection protocols are not uniform, and some data include estimates rather than counts. Estimates are updated periodically, so that the rates presented here may differ from those in prior and subsequent NCANDS reports.

@The endangerment standard includes children who had actually experienced harm and adds others who have not yet been harmed by maltreatment but who experienced abuse or neglect that put them in danger of being harmed. The endangerment standard was not used in the 1980 study.

Sources: American Humane Association (1989); Administration for Children, Youth and Families, Children's Bureau (1999); Sedlak & Broadhurst (1996); Tatara & Kuzmeskus (1997); Greenfeld et al. (1998). See Resource B for specific references to table items marked with superscript numerals.

Based on 1997 data available from forty-three states, the major types of maltreatment were as follows: neglect (54 percent), physical abuse (24 percent), sexual abuse (12 percent), and emotional maltreatment (8 percent). Approximately 11 percent of victims were subjected to other types of maltreatment, such as abandonment, congenital drug addiction, or threats to harm a child. Some children experienced more than one of these types of abuse (Administration for Children, Youth and Families, Children's Bureau, 1999).

Child Abuse and Neglect Incidence Rates. Another source of child abuse and neglect rates, the Study of the National Incidence and Prevalence of Child Abuse and Neglect, differs from the National Study on Child Neglect and Abuse Reporting in the following ways: it is based on a national probability sample of community professionals in selected U.S. counties regarding cases their agencies had handled, rather than a routine reporting system; it includes CPS as well as non-CPS agencies; estimates are based on unduplicated counts of individual children; and data were collected at only three points in time (1980, 1986, and 1993).

Based on the 1980 Study of the National Incidence and Prevalence of Child Abuse and Neglect, 625,100 (or 9.8 per 1,000) children were identified as having been abused or neglected. Using the same definition, based on whether a child had actually experienced demonstrable harm (the "harm standard"), in 1986, there was a 49 percent increase in the number of children to 931,000 (14.8 per 1,000). The largest increase between 1980 and 1986 by type of abuse was in the category of sexual abuse: rates almost tripled (from 0.7 to 1.9). The 1986 study also included a broader and more inclusive definition, which reflected the incidence of children who were at risk of maltreatment but had not yet been actually harmed. Incorporating this "endangerment standard" as well, 1,424,400 (22.6 per 1,000) children had been or were at risk of abuse or neglect.

Data from the 1993 survey documented a two-thirds increase in the total number of abused and neglected children from 1986 (to 1,554,000 or 23.1 per 1,000 children), using the harm standard (had actually been harmed). Under the endangerment standard (at risk of maltreatment but not yet actually harmed), the number of abused or neglected children doubled over this same period to 2,816,000 (or 41.9 per 1,000 children). The incidence rates of abuse and neglect, respectively, in the 1993 study based on the harm standard were 11.1 and 13.1 per 1,000 children. The incidence rates of abuse and neglect abuse using the more inclusive endangerment standard in 1993 were 18.2 and 29.2 per 1,000 children, respectively. The incidences of specific types (more than one of which may have been reported for a given child), using the more inclusive definition, were as follows: physical abuse (9.1), sexual abuse (4.5), emotional abuse (7.9) (Sedlak & Broadhurst, 1996).

The Year 2000 Objectives provided that the rates of maltreatment overall and for each specific type of maltreatment fall below the rates in the 1986 Study of the National Incidence and Prevalence of Child Abuse and Neglect. The incidence rates of abuse and neglect in that study, using the more inclusive definition, were 9.4 and 14.6 per 1,000 children, respectively. The incidence of specific types of abuse (more than one of which may have been reported for a given child) were as follows: physical abuse (4.9), sexual abuse (2.1), and emotional abuse (3.0) (National Center on Child Abuse and Neglect, 1988; Public Health Service, 1990; Sedlak, 1991). Evidence from the 1993 survey documents that these rates have doubled since 1986.

Domestic Elder Abuse. The Survey of States on the Incidence of Elder Abuse is based on a structured survey form sent to state adult protective service and state units on aging in fifty-four jurisdictions. There were an estimated 293,000 reports of elder abuse, neglect, or exploitation in domestic (home or noninstitutionalized) settings identified in fiscal year (FY) 1996. Around two-thirds of these reports were substantiated. The count of elderly victims was estimated to be 17.9 percent less than the count of reports, meaning that there were approximately 241,000 elderly abuse victims in FY 1996 (Tatara & Kuzmeskus, 1997).

The number of reported cases of elder maltreatment in FY 1996 represented an increase of 150.4 percent since the time of the first survey in FY 1986. The distribution of specific types of maltreatment that occurred in forty-one states during FY 1996 was as follows: neglect (55 percent), physical abuse (14.6 percent), financial or material exploitation (12.3 percent), psychological or emotional abuse (7.7 percent), sexual abuse (0.3 percent), and other types or unknown (10.1 percent) (Tatara & Kuzmeskus, 1997). Based on an estimate by the National Aging Resource Center on Elder Abuse that only one in fourteen incidents of elder abuse are actually reported, the number of reportable cases was estimated to be much greater than the actual number of reports: 2.16 million in FY 1996 (Tatara & Kuzmeskus, 1997).

Family Violence. The National Surveys of Family Violence, conducted in 1976 and 1986, attempted to identify incidents of intrafamily violence that may not have been reported to child or adult protective services or other agencies. The 1976 study used a personal interview survey and the 1986 study a telephone interview about violent incidents that had occurred within the family during the previous year (1975 and 1985, respectively).

Methodological and societal changes make interpretations of comparisons between the 1976 and 1986 studies problematic, although both suggest that the incidents of family violence actually reported to authorities are far fewer than the number that actually occur. The rates of very severe parent-to-child violence (parent kicked, bit, or hit child with fist; beat up the child; or used a gun or knife), based on that study, were 36 per 1,000 children aged three to seventeen in 1975 and 19 per 1,000 children in 1985. The rate of very severe family violence estimated for children in 1985 (19.0 per 1,000 children), based on this survey, is twice the rate of abuse (9.4 per 1,000 children) actually reported to agencies in 1986, according to the Study of the National Incidence and Prevalence of Child Abuse and Neglect (Gelles & Straus, 1988; National Center on Child Abuse and Neglect, 1988; Straus, Gelles, & Steinmetz, 1981).

The Bureau of Justice Statistics within the U.S. Department of Justice collects data on domestic violence through its National Crime Victimization Survey, Uniform Crime Reporting Program, and related reporting systems and surveys. In 1996 there were 838,000 victimizations of women by intimates, or a rate of 7.5 per 1,000 women, reflecting a decline from a high of 9.8 women in 1993. Although less likely than males to experience violent crimes overall, women are five to eight times more likely than men to be victimized by an intimate. A number of these incidents are also likely to be related to alcohol or drug abuse.

Homeless Persons

Varying estimates of the number of homeless exist, depending on how homelessness is defined (whether doubling up with relatives in hard times counts), when the data are gathered (during the day versus at night, or in the summer versus winter months), as well as where one looks for homeless individuals (in shelters versus on the streets).

Based on data from a variety of sources, it appears that approximately 1 million men, women, and children may not have a place to call home on any given night, and two to three times as many are in this situation at some point during the year. (Estimates from different sources are reported in Table 2.10, and the methodological problems underlying these estimates are more fully discussed in Chapter Ten.)

The earliest projections of the number of homeless persons, published in 1982 and 1983 by a homeless advocacy group, the Community for Creative Non-Violence, estimated that there were 2 to 3 million homeless persons on any given night (Hombs & Snyder, 1982, 1983). In 1984 the U.S. Department of Housing and Urban Development, using several different extrapolation techniques, estimated many fewer homeless persons. Estimates ranged from 192,000 to 586,000 nationwide, with the most likely number estimated to be between 250,000 to 350,000 (U.S. Department of Housing and Urban Development, 1984).

Later studies tended to confirm estimates in the hundreds of thousands rather than the millions. In 1986, Freeman and Hall (1986), applying a street-to-shelter ratio, estimated there were some 287,000 homeless persons. Based on estimates from fifty U.S. cities, and varying the rates for large, medium, and small cities, Tucker (1987) projected 700,000 individuals to be homeless. In March 1987, using a nationally representative random sample of homeless adults who used soup kitchens and shelters in cities of 100,000 or more, the Urban Institute projected the number of homeless persons in to be 496,000 to 600,000 (Burt & Cohen, 1989).

In 1988, the National Alliance to End Homelessness recomputed the 1984 U.S. Department of Housing and Urban Development figures, applying different

TABLE 2.10. INDICATORS OF HOMELESS PERSONS.

Indicators	Year			
	1984	1987	1988	1996
Homeless				
U.S. Department of Housing and Urban Development[1]	250,000–350,000			
Urban Institute[2,3]		*496,000–600,000 ***(1+million)		****444,000–842,000 ***(2.3–3.5 million)
National Alliance to End Homelessness[4]			**736,000 ***(1.3–2.0 million)	

* Numbers refer to the count of homeless at a given time (March 1987).

** Numbers refer to a reestimated count of the homeless at a given time, using U.S. Department of Housing and Urban Development (1984) data adjusted for an estimated 20 percent average annual rate of growth in the homeless.

***Numbers in parentheses refer to the estimated number of people homeless at some time during the year.

****Numbers refer to the count of homeless at given times—respectively, October 1996 and February 1996.

*****Numbers refer to the count of homeless at a given time.

Sources: U.S. Department of Housing and Urban Development (1984); Burt & Cohen (1989); Burt & Aron (2000); National Alliance to End Homelessness (1988). See Resource B for specific references to table items marked with superscript numerals.

rates of homelessness to the city and suburbs, resulting in a revised estimate of 355,000 (rather than 250,000 to 350,000) homeless individuals in 1984. Based on reports from local officials regarding increases in the demand for shelter services, the Alliance estimated an annual growth rate of 20 percent in the number of homeless persons, yielding an estimated upper bound on the number on any given night to be 736,000 in 1988 (National Alliance to End Homelessness, 1988). Although not primarily intended to estimate the number of homeless, a 1996 study conducted by the Urban Institute under the auspices of the Interagency Council of the Homeless yielded corresponding estimates of from 444,000 to 842,000 homeless persons at selected times (Burt & Aron, 2000).

The number who experienced homelessness some time during the year is estimated to be around twice the number homeless on any given night. Based on the Urban Institute data, there were then a maximum of 1.2 million people homeless some time during 1987 (Burt & Cohen, 1989). According to the National Alliance to End Homeless projections, around 1.3 to 2.0 million people experienced homelessness during 1988 (National Alliance to End Homelessness, 1988). In 1996 the Urban Institute study estimated that 2.3 to 3.5 million individuals were homeless at some time during the year (Burt & Aron, 2000). A report from the Partnership for the Homeless, pointed out that "most attempts at estimating the homeless by cities and localities have concluded that the homeless comprise from 0.7 to 1.1 percent of their respective populations," confirming that "there may be as many as two million homeless across the nation" (Partnership for the Homeless, 1989, p. 3).

The numbers reported for different years do not necessarily accurately reflect trends in the growth of the number of homeless persons because of differences in the definitions, data gathering methods, and bases for projections used, although several studies have documented annual increases in the demands for emergency and associated homeless shelters and services in U.S. cities since 1985 (National Alliance to End Homelessness, 1988; Partnership for the Homeless, 1987, 1989; U.S. Conference of Mayors, 1999).

A random digit dialing survey of the U.S. population conducted in 1990, which asked whether respondents had "ever had a time in your life [or within the past five years] when you considered yourself homeless," yielded relatively high estimates of lifetime and five-year prevalence of all types of homelessness: 14.0 percent (26 million people) and 4.6 percent (8.5 million people), respectively. The rate of lifetime "literal" homelessness (actually sleeping in shelters, abandoned buildings, bus and train stations, and so forth) was 7.4 percent (13.5 million people) and of literal homelessness in the past five years was 3.1 percent (5.7 million people) (Link et al., 1994). These relative rates were confirmed in a 1994 follow-up study with respondents who had self-defined themselves as homeless in the 1990 study, and a stratified sample of respondents who had not so defined themselves (a control group) (Link et al., 1995). The results of these national surveys tend to suggest that point-prevalence estimates of homelessness, such as those reported in Table 2.10, may tend to underestimate the number of individuals who have experienced intermittent periods of homelessness at some time in their lives.

Immigrants and Refugees

National data on the number and characteristics of people currently living in the United States who voluntarily left their home countries, as well as those who were pushed out by political, military, or economic hardship, are available from the U.S. Immigration and Naturalization Service. Studies of the specific health and health care needs of these immigrant and refugee populations are generally local in nature or limited to subgroups of émigrés.

Around 7.6 million people legally immigrated to the United States from 1991 to 1998. A large proportion were fleeing political or military conflicts in their countries of origin, and many have experienced the death of or separation from family members, as well as serious physical or psychological problems, as a result. (See Table 2.11.)

Immigrants. Immigrants are aliens admitted for legal permanent residence in the United States. The procedures for admission depend on whether the alien is residing inside or outside the United States at the time of application for permanent residence. Eligible aliens residing outside the United States are issued immigrant visas by the U.S. Department of State. Eligible aliens residing in the United States are allowed to change their status from temporary to permanent residence by applying to the Immigration and Naturalization Service. Nonresident aliens admitted to the United States for a temporary period are considered nonimmigrants rather than immigrants.

The number of immigrants to the United States has increased steadily over the past three decades: 1961–1970, 3,321,700; 1971–1980, 4,493,300; 1981–1990, 7,338,100; and 1991–1998, 7,605,077.

Immigrants have an official and legal (documented) status: that of aliens who are admitted for the purpose of obtaining permanent residence. In addition, there were an estimated half-million persons who immigrated without applying

TABLE 2.11.   INDICATORS OF IMMIGRANTS AND REFUGEES.

Indicators	Year			
	1961–1970	1971–1980	1981–1990	1991–1998
Total number[1]				
Immigrants@	3,321,700	4,493,300	7,338,100	7,605,077
Refugees	212,843	539,447	1,013,620	914,989

@Totals for immigrants are rounded to the nearest one hundred in source tables.

Sources: U.S. Bureau of the Census reports. See Resource B for specific references to table items marked with superscript numerals.

for legal residence (undocumented persons) living in the United States in 1996, the vast majority of whom were from Mexico (U.S. Bureau of the Census, 1999e).

Refugees. Refugees are considered nonimmigrants when initially admitted into the United States. A series of congressional acts have specified the provisions (the length of time in residence, for example) required to permit certain groups of refugees to seek permanent residence (immigrant) status, such as the Cuban Refugee Act (1966), the Indochinese Refugee Act (1977), and the Refugee-Parolee Act (1978). The Refugee Act of 1980, effective April 1, 1980, provided for a uniform admission procedure for all countries, based on the United Nations's definition of refugees and asylees: "a well-founded fear of persecution." Under this act, refugees are eligible for immigrant status after one year of residence in the United States. Authorized admission ceilings are set annually by the President in consultation with the Congress.

Asylees differ from refugees, in that refugees petition for entrance from outside U.S. borders, while asylees enter the United States first, often without documentation, and then petition to remain. They may stay in the United States indefinitely in a temporary status and are entitled to work, but they are not entitled to certain benefits, such as Medicaid if they qualify, as are refugees. Up to 10,000 asylees may adjust to immigrant status each year (Immigration and Naturalization Service, 1999a).

The number of refugees, as well as the proportion they represent of the total immigrant population, has increased since the 1960s: 1961–1970, 212,843; 1971–1980, 539,447; 1981–1990, 1,013,620; and 1991–1998, 914,989. The proportions they represented of the total immigrant population for the respective time periods were 6 percent, 12 percent, 14 percent, and 12 percent.

Conclusion

Vulnerable populations are at risk of poor physical, psychological, or social health. There is universality in the notion of risk in that there is always a nonzero probability that one may contract illness at some point in their lives. Most individuals and their families have been or are quite likely to have been touched by the experiences of vulnerability identified here, such as a high-risk pregnancy, chronic illness, depression, substance abuse, or family physical or emotional abuse. As members of human families and communities, we are all potentially vulnerable. Chapters Three and Four identify who is most likely to be vulnerable to selected types of poor physical, psychological, and social health and in what stages of the life course and social circumstances.

CHAPTER THREE

WHO IS *MOST* VULNERABLE?

People are more or less vulnerable at different stages of their lives because of serious health problems that force them to turn to others for help. Infants and very young children are all potentially vulnerable because of their total dependence on parents or other caretakers to meet their most fundamental physical and psychological needs. As people age, they may require help with tasks such as shopping or keeping track of finances, as well as even more basic self-care needs, such as eating, dressing, or getting out of bed. The poor and those with less education tend to experience more health problems in general over the course of their lives, based on an array of indicators of need, than do their more socio-economically advantaged counterparts.

This chapter presents current national data on the varying health needs of people of differing age, gender, race, income, and education groups, as well as changes that have taken place over time for these groups, based on the indicators highlighted in Chapter Two. A variety of factors influence whether some groups are more vulnerable than others. (See Figure 1.2.) This chapter sheds light on who is most vulnerable, and the next chapter explores why.

Cross-Cutting Issues

Comparisons among groups focus on those characteristics for which data are available at the national level: age, gender, race and ethnicity, income, and education. These comparisons strongly confirm the predictions presented earlier (see Table 1.1) regarding which groups are most and least vulnerable. Further, the longitudinal (trend) data demonstrate that the problems of many of the most vulnerable worsened rather than diminished during the past two decades.

Age

The 1990s were particularly harsh for vulnerable newborns, especially those who had the compound disadvantage of being born in socioeconomically adverse circumstances. Very young, African American, poor, and less educated mothers were less likely to have adequate prenatal care. They were also more likely to bear low birthweight babies who had high risks of congenital physical or mental impairments, as well as perinatal drug addiction or HIV.

The number of children with developmental, emotional, and behavioral problems has been and is likely to continue to increase as the number of high-risk, impaired newborns who survive also grows. Compared to white youth, young African American women are much more likely to give birth to babies who die, and young African American males are many times more likely themselves to die a violent death. Young males, particularly Native American youth, are much more likely than other subgroups to drink, smoke, and use drugs and also to die as a result of these addictions. The number of children reported to be abused or neglected by their families has burgeoned in recent years, and the face of homeless persons is an increasingly youthful one, as the number of families with children and runaway youth living on the streets increase.

Although the prevalence of disability among the elderly has been declining, the oldest old (eighty-five years of age or older) are often plagued with chronic illness and associated impairments, which limit their ability to function independently. A higher proportion of the elderly also suffer from serious cognitive impairments, and many elderly nursing home residents have Alzheimer's or related organic brain disorders. White elderly men are significantly more likely than elderly women to take their own lives, and dependent elderly women are more likely to be abused by their caretakers than are elderly men.

Gender

In general, men are more likely to die from chronic disease than are women. Among those living with chronic illness, however, elderly women are much more likely than men to experience serious physical limitations in being able to continue to care for themselves. The prevalence of mental illness tends to be higher for women than men. However, men's mental health problems are more often manifested in substance abuse and antisocial behavior, whereas women are more likely to be depressed, anxious, or experience physical (somatic) symptoms.

Women's health and health care needs are also compounded by their childbearing and child-rearing roles. Mothers who have inadequate prenatal care or experience drug addiction, HIV/AIDS, spousal abuse, homelessness, or the fears associated with being in the country illegally are also very likely to be in a position of bearing or caring for children who are also extremely needy and vulnerable.

Race and Ethnicity

Data on the health and health care needs of Hispanics, Native Americans, and Asians are somewhat more limited than for whites and African Americans (reported as blacks in most statistical reports). However, based on the major indicators of need for which data are available, African American, Hispanic, and Native American men, women, and children are much more likely to be in poor health than are majority whites.

African American women are more likely to have high-risk pregnancies and to die in childbirth or from chronic disease or HIV/AIDS than are their white female counterparts. African American men are also more likely to be chronically ill and to be at risk of HIV/AIDS, death from intentional acts of violence, incarceration, and homelessness than are white males.

Hispanic women are less likely to have adequate prenatal care, but more likely to bear normal birthweight babies and experience fewer infant deaths, especially in contrast to African American women. On the other hand, as with African Americans, Hispanic men, women, and children are much more likely to contract HIV, and young Hispanic males are much more likely to die from homicides than are whites.

A higher proportion of Native American women have inadequate prenatal care and experience infant (particularly postneonatal) deaths than do white women. Native American youths are also much more likely to be substance users and abusers and to die violently from both suicide and homicide.

By a number of criteria for which data are available (infant mortality rates, HIV/AIDS prevalence, and substance use and abuse), Asian Americans are at much lower risk than are other minorities, although these risks differ by socioeconomic status. Socioeconomically disadvantaged Asian American populations, particularly some categories of Southeast Asian refugees, are likely to be socially isolated and in poor physical and mental health. Socioeconomically disadvantaged Asian American, as well as Hispanic, youth in some communities are more likely to participate in gangs than are white youth.

Income and Education

More years of formal schooling and higher incomes are directly associated with better health. Women with a high school education are much more likely to have adequate prenatal care and to bear normal birthweight babies who survive past infancy than are those who have not finished high school. People of lower socioeconomic status (those with less education, lower incomes, or employed in low-status jobs) are more likely to have serious chronic physical or mental health

exacerbate - to make more violent, bitter, or severe

problems. Economic factors play a major role in family abuse and neglect, and the vast majority of homeless persons are extremely poor. The problems of vulnerability to a variety of health risks appear to be exacerbated for the urban underclass: poor and poorly educated low-income individuals who live in economically depressed urban areas.

Population-Specific Overview

Variation in the prevalence of poor physical, psychological, and social health will be examined for different population subgroups.

High-Risk Mothers and Infants

Very young, African American, and poorly educated mothers are much less likely to have adequate prenatal care and more likely to bear low birthweight or very low birthweight infants. The rates of teenage pregnancy, preterm and low birthweight babies, inadequate prenatal care, and infant and maternal mortality are two to three times higher among African American women compared to white women. This racial disparity shows no signs of diminishing and may in fact be widening (see Table 3.1).

Low Birthweight. The percentages of low birthweight (LBW) or very low birthweight (VLBW) infants are higher among very young mothers and older mothers, that is, mothers less than fifteen years of age and those forty-five years of age or older. The percentages of LBW and VLBW infants to mothers less than fifteen years of age in 1997—respectively, 13.6 percent and 3.1 percent—were around twice the national average of 7.5 percent and 1.4 percent, respectively.

Although differences have narrowed since 1985, based on 1997 data, black mothers were twice as likely to give birth to LBW infants (13.01 percent) than were white mothers (which includes Hispanic mothers) (6.46 percent). Comparable patterns were observed for VLBW infants: 3.04 percent for blacks compared to 1.13 percent for whites. The percentage of other racial and ethnic groups with LBW/VLBW infants was more similar to that of whites: Hispanics (6.42/1.13) and Native Americans (6.75/1.19).

Mothers with a high school or college education are less likely to have LBW or VLBW infants, compared to those who have less than a high school education, which may also account for the higher rates of LBW infants among teenage mothers (National Center for Health Statistics, 1999a).

Infant Mortality. The total infant, neonatal, and postneonatal mortality rates for blacks have been around twice that of whites, and this disparity appears to be widening rather than diminishing. In 1985 the total black infant mortality rate (19.0) was 2.1 times that of the white rate (9.2). By 1997, although both

TABLE 3.1. INDICATORS OF HIGH-RISK MOTHERS AND INFANTS, BY DEMOGRAPHIC SUBGROUPS.

Indicators		Mother's Age								Mother's Race			
		<15	15–19	20–24	25–29	30–34	35–39	40–44	#45–49	White	Black	Hispanic	Native American
Low birthweight[1]													
Percentage of live births less than 2,500 grams	1985	12.9	9.3	6.9	5.9	6.0	6.9	8.3	10.3	5.65	12.65	6.16	5.86
	1997	13.6	9.5	7.4	6.6	6.9	8.3	9.7	17.4	6.46	13.01	6.42	6.75
Percentage of live births less than 1,500 grams	1985	3.2	1.8	1.2	1.0	1.1	1.3	1.5	1.8	0.94	2.71	1.01	1.01
	1997	3.1	1.8	1.4	1.2	1.3	1.6	1.9	3.9	1.13	3.04	1.13	1.19

		Mother's Age							Mother's Race			
		<15	15–19	20–24	25–29	30–34	35–39	40+	White	Black	Hispanic	Native American
Infant mortality												
Deaths per 1,000 live births[2]## Total	1985								9.2	19.0	—	11.1
	1997								6.0	14.2	5.9	7.6
Neonatal	1985								6.0	12.6	—	5.0
	1997								4.0	9.4	3.8	3.6
Postneonatal	1985								3.2	6.4	—	6.0
	1997								2.0	4.8	2.1	4.0

Prenatal care[3]

Percentage of mothers who received prenatal care in the third trimester or no prenatal care

1985	20.5	12.0	6.9	3.7	3.2	4.1	7.3	4.8	10.2	12.4	12.9
1997	16.4	7.2	5.0	3.1	2.5	2.7	3.7	3.2	7.3	6.2	8.6

Teen births[4]@

Live births per 1,000 females 10–14 years											
1985								0.6	4.5	—	1.7
1997								0.7	3.3	2.3	1.7

Live births per 1,000 females 15–17 years											
1985								24.4	69.3	—	47.7
1997								27.1	60.8	66.3	45.3

Live births per 1,000 females 18–19 years											
1985								70.4	132.4	—	124.1
1997								75.9	130.1	144.3	117.6

Maternal mortality[5]*

Deaths per 100,000 live births all ages, age-adjusted											
1985								4.9	22.1	7.1	4.5
1997								5.2	20.1	7.6	6.1

In 1997, this age group was forty-five to fifty-four years old.

No infant mortality rates for Hispanics are available for 1985. The 1997 neonatal and postneonatal mortality rates for Hispanics are actually rates for 1996. For Native Americans, 1985 rates are actually three-year rates (1984–1986) centered in 1985. Rates listed for 1997 are actually three-year rates (1994–1996) centered in 1995.

@ No teen birth rates for Hispanics are available for 1985.

* Native American rates for 1985 are actually three-year rates (1984–1986) centered in 1985. Native American rates listed for 1997 are actually three-year rates (1994–1996) centered in 1995.

Sources: NCHS and IHS reports; see Resource B for specific references to table items marked with superscript numerals.

the black and white rates had declined, the black rate (14.2) was 2.4 times the rate for whites (6.0). The black neonatal mortality rate in 1985 (12.6) was 2.1 times the white rate (6.0). In 1997, the black rate (9.4) was 2.3 times that of whites (4.0). Postneonatal rates for blacks were also correspondingly higher compared to whites in both 1985 (6.4 versus 3.2) and 1997 (4.8 versus 2.0). The infant mortality rate for Native Americans (7.6) was higher than that for whites, while the rate for Hispanics (5.9) was similar (National Center for Health Statistics, 1999c).

Analyses of linked birth and death records for 1997 showed that the infant mortality rate was higher for mothers with fewer than twelve years of schooling and lowest for those with sixteen years or more of schooling (National Center for Health Statistics, 1999e).

Prenatal Care. Although the proportion of very young teens with late or no prenatal care declined from 1985 (20.5 percent) to 1997 (16.4 percent), teenage mothers remained over four times more likely not to seek prenatal care or to wait until the last trimester to do so, compared to the national average (3.9 percent).

The percentage of women who had inadequate care in each of the racial and ethnic groups has also declined since 1985. Nonetheless, based on 1997 data, the percentage of black (7.3 percent), Hispanic (6.2 percent), and Native American (8.6 percent) women not having adequate prenatal care remained two to three times that of whites (3.2 percent). Rates of inadequate prenatal care are highest for women with the least education (Centers for Disease Control and Prevention, 1999d).

Teen Births. The 1997 birthrate per 1,000 women rates had declined to below 1985 levels for black but not for white teenagers. Nonetheless, in both 1985 and 1997, the birthrates for blacks remained around two to three times those of whites among teens age fifteen or older, but the black-white disparities for very young teens (ten to fourteen years of age) were even greater. Compared to blacks, birthrates in 1997 were higher for Hispanic teenagers age fifteen or older but lower for younger Hispanic women (ten to fourteen years of age). Birthrates for Native American teenagers tended to be higher than the rates for whites but lower than for black and Hispanic teenagers.

Maternal Mortality. Black mothers are four to five times more likely to die in childbirth than are white mothers, a differential that has persisted for decades. The number of maternal deaths per 100,000 live births in 1997 was 20.1 for blacks compared to 5.2 for whites. Maternal death rates for Hispanics (7.6) and Native Americans (6.1) were also higher compared to whites, although the rates more closely approximated the rates for white mothers.

Chronically Ill and Disabled   men / Elderly

The prevalence and the magnitude of limitation in daily activities, as well as deaths, due to chronic disease increase steadily with age. Men are more likely to die from major chronic illnesses such as heart disease, stroke, and cancer than women at any age, although among those living with chronic illness, elderly women have more problems in being able to carry out their normal daily routines. African Americans, and particularly African American men, are more likely to experience serious disabilities as well as die from chronic illness than are either white men or women (see Table 3.2).

Death Rates for Chronic Diseases. Heart disease has been and remains the major cause of death due to chronic illness among both infants and the elderly. Cancer is the principal cause of death for people of other ages. The age-adjusted death rates for heart disease, stroke, and cancer are highest among black men and lowest for Hispanic women. White men had the highest death rate due to chronic obstructive pulmonary disease (26.5).

Prevalence of Chronic Conditions. In 1996 the most prevalent chronic condition among people under forty-five years of age was asthma (58.9 per 1,000). The rates were highest for those under age eighteen (62.0), females (68.1), and blacks (76.6). The rates for all groups have increased since 1985. The prevalence of hypertension was also much higher among blacks in this age group (47.5) compared to whites (27.6).

For adults forty-five to sixty-four years old, the most common chronic conditions were arthritis (240.1 per 1,000) and hypertension (214.1). Arthritis was most prevalent among blacks (256.5) and women (284.0), although the rates for both groups have declined substantially since 1985. The prevalence of hypertension among adults forty-five to sixty-four years old remained significantly higher for blacks (375.7) compared to whites (200.4).

Among the elderly, the most common conditions were arthritis (482.7 per 1,000), hypertension (363.5), hearing impairments (303.4), and heart disease (268.7). The rates of hypertension and arthritis were generally higher among elderly women and blacks. Heart disease and hearing impairments were more common among elderly men and whites.

The prevalence of asthma and diabetes increased across all age, gender, and racial groups over the period from 1985 to 1996. Rates of diabetes are particularly high for blacks compared to non-Hispanic whites.

Limitation in Major Activity Due to Chronic Conditions. The proportion of people who must limit their major activities in some way due to a chronic health problem increases with age. In 1996 the percentage of different age groups who were limited to some extent were as follows: less than five years of age (2.6 percent),

TABLE 3.2. INDICATORS OF CHRONICALLY ILL AND DISABLED, BY DEMOGRAPHIC SUBGROUPS.

Indicators					Age				
	<1	1–4	5–14	15–24	25–34	35–44	45–54	55–64	65–74
Age-adjusted death rates for selected chronic diseases per 100,000 persons[1]									
Heart disease									
1985	25.0	2.2	1.0	2.8	8.3	38.1	153.8	443.0	1089.8
1997	16.4	1.4	0.8	3.0	8.3	30.1	104.9	302.4	753.7
Stroke									
1985	3.7	0.3	0.2	0.8	2.2	7.2	21.3	54.8	172.8
1997	7.0	0.4	0.2	0.5	1.7	6.3	16.9	44.4	134.8
Cancer									
1985	3.1	3.8	3.5	5.4	13.2	45.9	170.1	454.6	845.5
1997	2.4	2.9	2.7	4.5	11.6	38.9	135.1	395.7	847.3
Chronic obstructive pulmonary disease									
1985	1.4	0.3	0.3	0.5	0.6	1.6	10.2	47.9	149.2
1997	1.3	0.3	0.3	0.5	0.9	2.0	8.4	46.3	165.3

			Age by Sex, Race					
			Under 45					
	<18	18–44	Male	Female	White	Black	Total	Male
Number of selected chronic conditions per 1,000 persons (self-reported)[2]								
Heart disease								
1985	21.2	40.1	28.4	37.1	34.6	23.0	32.8	137.8
1996	23.6	39.3	30.7	35.5	34.4	35.0	33.1	133.5
Hypertension								
1985	*2.3	64.1	45.5	34.9	38.0	58.8	40.2	253.8
1996	*0.5	49.6	30.0	30.1	27.6	47.5	30.1	214.8
Stroke								
1985	*0.9	*1.9	*1.6	*1.4	*1.4	*2.6	1.5	20.3
1996	*0.4	*2.0	*1.3	*1.5	*1.4	*1.9	*1.4	16.3
Visual impairment								
1985	10.8	32.8	36.1	12.7	25.1	21.6	24.3	62.1
1996	6.3	24.0	21.7	12.2	17.0	20.1	17.0	61.0
Hearing impairment								
1985	19.2	49.8	45.5	30.5	41.3	18.1	38.0	208.0
1996	12.6	41.9	34.0	26.4	33.1	19.0	30.2	183.4
Arthritis								
1985	*2.2	52.1	21.6	43.9	34.6	28.0	32.8	205.9
1996	*1.9	50.1	26.1	35.8	30.7	37.5	30.9	193.0
Emphysema								
1985	*—	*1.6	*0.8	*1.2	*1.0	*0.4	*1.0	23.5
1996	*—	*0.8	*1.0	*—	*0.4	*—	*0.5	16.5
Asthma								
1985	47.8	33.4	35.9	42.0	39.6	42.5	39.0	27.4
1996	62.0	56.9	49.8	68.1	56.9	76.6	58.9	30.4
Diabetes								
1985	*1.9	9.1	5.9	6.6	6.5	*6.5	6.3	52.4
1996	*1.2	11.8	6.1	9.0	7.5	*8.4	7.6	56.9

			Age				Sex
	<5	5–14	15–44	45–64	65–74	75+	Male
Age-adjusted degree of activity limitation due to chronic conditions, percent[3]							
Limited but not in major activity							
1985	0.6	1.6	2.7	5.9	14.0	17.9	3.8
1996	0.6	1.9	2.7	5.5	12.0	18.7	4.0
Limited in amount or kind of major activity							
1985	1.1	4.2	3.6	8.8	11.5	17.3	5.1
1996	1.5	4.9	3.7	7.2	9.2	13.5	5.0
Unable to carry on major activity							
1985	0.5	0.4	1.9	8.7	11.2	9.1	4.7
1996	0.5	0.5	3.2	9.4	10.1	10.9	4.7
Total with activity limitation							
1985	2.2	6.2	8.3	23.4	36.7	44.3	13.6
1996	2.6	7.3	9.6	22.0	31.4	43.1	13.7

		Race by Sex							
		White		Black		Hispanic		Native American	
75–84	85+	M	F	M	F	M	F	M	F
2693.1	7384.1	246.2	121.7	310.8	188.3	152.3	86.5	162.2	83.7
1943.6	6198.9	168.7	90.4	236.2	147.6	113.4	64.7	136.5	73.9
601.5	1865.1	33.0	27.9	62.7	50.6	27.7	20.6	24.9	20.6
462.0	1584.6	25.7	22.5	48.6	37.9	22.1	17.0	20.1	19.9
1271.8	1615.4	160.4	110.5	239.9	131.8	92.1	64.1	87.1	60.5
1335.2	1805.0	145.9	106.0	214.8	131.2	91.4	65.4	104.0	72.8
289.5	365.4	28.7	12.9	24.8	8.8	11.8	5.7	14.1	6.5
359.6	561.9	26.5	18.5	24.5	12.7	11.5	6.7	20.3	11.4

Age by Sex, Race								
45–64				65+				
Female	White	Black	Total	Male	Female	White	Black	Total
120.9	131.0	137.0	129.0	328.8	288.1	315.2	198.7	304.5
100.3	117.4	129.4	116.4	311.3	238.0	278.2	*150.5	268.7
263.5	247.2	368.5	258.9	351.4	458.4	407.2	496.5	414.5
213.3	200.4	375.7	214.1	298.0	410.8	348.1	487.0	363.5
15.8	15.9	*37.2	17.9	76.7	50.3	60.9	*68.6	61.2
*9.6	11.6	*24.9	12.8	93.8	44.4	65.1	*70.8	65.1
27.0	43.6	*44.9	43.7	103.6	91.5	96.0	94.2	96.5
36.4	47.8	*63.1	48.3	103.8	70.0	86.1	*81.9	84.2
114.3	163.3	128.4	159.0	364.2	245.9	299.6	252.2	294.4
82.9	139.0	77.0	131.5	386.8	243.2	320.3	155.4	303.4
325.4	264.4	331.9	268.5	361.5	550.5	468.2	579.6	472.8
284.0	244.6	256.5	240.1	411.2	534.5	477.6	536.4	482.7
*7.6	16.0	*11.3	15.2	80.1	21.9	48.3	*24.8	45.8
*10.1	13.6	*14.6	13.2	33.2	31.9	35.2	*10.0	32.4
28.9	28.7	*27.5	28.2	35.5	40.3	38.1	*37.2	38.3
65.5	47.4	*50.7	48.6	37.5	51.3	45.3	*41.7	45.5
51.4	45.6	112.1	51.9	101.1	105.5	97.2	165.5	103.8
59.4	44.7	149.5	58.2	121.8	84.3	87.5	199.1	100.0

	Race		Family Income#				
Female	White	Black	<$14,000	$14,000–$24,999	$25,000–$34,999	$35,000–$45,999	$50,000+
4.5	4.3	3.9	5.6	4.3	3.7	3.8	3.2
4.2	4.1	4.0	5.8	4.2	4.3	3.8	3.5
5.8	5.5	6.1	8.5	6.3	5.2	4.6	3.7
5.2	5.0	6.5	8.8	6.3	5.0	4.1	3.4
2.9	3.4	6.4	8.3	4.5	3.1	2.4	1.8
4.1	4.0	7.0	11.8	5.2	3.8	2.6	1.6
13.2	13.1	16.3	22.4	15.0	12.0	10.7	8.8
13.5	13.1	17.6	26.4	15.7	13.2	10.6	8.5

(Continued on page 64)

TABLE 3.2. (*Continued*)

		Age		Sex		Race		
		15–64	65+	Male	Female	White	Black	Hispanic

Limitation in selected activities of daily living (ADLs) or instrumental activities of daily living (IADLs), age 15+ living in the community[4][@@]

		15–64	65+	Male	Female	White	Black	Hispanic
Percent with at least one ADL								
	1991–1992	2.1	14.5	3.2	4.6	4.0	5.5	3.2
	1994–1995	2.2	14.2	3.2	4.9	4.1	5.4	2.8
Number of ADLs								
1	1991–1992	1.0	5.6	1.5	1.9	1.7	2.1	1.4
	1994–1995	1.1	5.7	1.5	2.1	1.9	2.0	1.2
2–3	1991–1992	0.7	4.0	0.9	1.5	1.2	1.7	1.2
	1994–1995	0.7	4.5	0.9	1.6	1.2	1.9	0.8
4 or more	1991–1992	0.5	5.0	0.9	1.4	1.2	1.7	0.6
	1994–1995	0.5	4.0	0.8	1.2	1.0	1.5	0.8
Percent with at least one IADL								
	1991–1992	3.1	21.5	4.9	7.0	5.9	8.1	5.3
	1994–1995	3.3	20.5	4.8	7.0	5.9	7.7	4.6
Number of IADLs								
1	1991–1992	1.5	8.1	2.3	2.8	2.6	3.2	2.3
	1994–1995	1.7	8.2	2.3	3.0	2.7	3.2	2.1
2–3	1991–1992	1.2	8.3	1.7	2.8	2.2	3.1	2.1
	1994–1995	1.2	8.1	1.6	2.9	2.3	3.0	1.7
4 or more	1991–1992	0.4	5.2	1.0	1.3	1.1	1.8	0.9
	1994–1995	0.4	4.3	0.8	1.1	1.0	1.6	0.7
Percent with at least one ADL or IADL								
	1991–1992	3.7	23.8	5.7	7.9	6.8	9.2	5.9
	1994–1995	3.9	22.9	5.7	8.0	6.9	8.7	5.3

		Age				Sex		Race	
		<65	65–74	75–84	85+	Male	Female	White	Black

Limitation in selected activities of daily living (ADLs) or instrumental activities of daily living (IADLs), living in nursing homes[5][##]

		<65	65–74	75–84	85+	Male	Female	White	Black
Percent with at least one ADL									
	1985	73.5	86.8	91.4	95.2	84.0	92.7	90.1	92.4
	1995	@89.6	95.8	97.5	98.1	94.8	97.7	97.0	@96.2
Number of ADLs									
1	1985	11.7	14.0	11.6	9.6	12.3	10.7	11.5	7.3
	1995	9.6	9.0	7.6	6.0	8.1	6.8	7.4	@5.2
2–3	1985	19.7	18.5	18.3	16.8	18.8	17.6	17.8	19.9
	1995	50.2	48.8	46.5	43.7	47.1	45.2	45.0	53.3
4 or more	1985	42.1	54.3	61.4	68.8	53.0	64.7	60.9	65.2
	1995	@26.3	38.0	43.4	48.5	39.6	45.5	44.7	@37.9
Percent with at least one IADL									
	1985	75.0	81.4	84.4	89.0	79.6	86.8	84.6	@87.6
	1995	87.3	86.8	88.1	89.2	87.6	88.7	88.2	90.0
Number of IADLs									
1	1985	@10.1	7.8	6.6	6.0	8.5	6.3	6.9	@
	1995	8.9	9.1	7.8	8.6	7.8	8.7	8.9	@5.0
2–3	1985	@23.7	22.6	21.0	23.5	20.8	23.0	22.9	@13.8
	1995	32.3	30.1	31.4	30.6	31.3	30.8	31.5	@25.5
4 or more	1985	41.2	51.1	56.8	59.6	50.4	57.3	54.9	61.3
	1995	46.0	47.6	48.9	50.0	48.5	49.3	47.8	59.5

* Figure does not meet standard of reliability or precision.

*- Figure does not meet standard of reliability or precision and quantity zero.

In 1996, the two lowest income categories are less than $16,000 and $16,000 to $24,999.

@@ADLs include bathing, dressing, eating, transferring, and toileting. IADLs include use of telephone, handling money, getting around outside the home, preparing meals, and doing light housework.

@ Data do not meet standard of reliability or precision.

##ADLs include bathing, dressing, eating, transferring, toileting, and continence. IADLs include use of telephone, handling money, securing personal items, and care of personal possessions.

Sources: NCHS reports; McNeil (1999a, 1999b). See Resource B for specific references to table items marked with superscript numerals.

five to fourteen years old (7.3 percent), fifteen to forty-four years old (9.6 percent), forty-five to sixty-four years old (22.0 percent), sixty-five to seventy-four years old (31.4 percent), and seventy-five years and older (43.1 percent). Men were somewhat more likely to be unable to carry on their major activity (4.7 percent) than were women (4.1 percent).

Rates of activity limitation were higher for blacks (17.6 percent) than whites (13.1 percent). Blacks (7.0 percent) were almost twice as likely as whites (4.0 percent) to be unable to carry on their major activities. People in families with incomes under $14,000 were most likely (26.4 percent) and those in families with incomes of $50,000 or greater least likely to have to limit what they did because of a chronic illness (8.5 percent).

Limitation in Activities of Daily Living (ADL) and Instrumental Activities of Daily Living (IADL).

In 1994–1995, 22.9 percent of the elderly people living in the community had at least one ADL or IADL limitation. Around 14 percent had at least one ADL, and 20.5 percent had at least one IADL. The prevalence of both types of limitations was highest among women and blacks. For the elderly living in nursing homes, the oldest old and women were most likely to experience ADL or IADL limitations, although the disparities were less dramatic than among the community-dwelling elderly.

Persons Living with HIV/AIDS

In the 1980s, early in the AIDS epidemic, homosexual or bisexual males were most likely to be affected. In recent years, more and more mothers and children are at risk. Higher proportions of African Americans and Hispanics, compared to whites, are likely to be HIV positive, to develop and die of AIDS, and to have contracted the disease through drug use or sexual contact with drug users (see Table 3.3).

HIV Prevalence.

As of June 1999, around 103,000 adults and 1,800 children under thirteen years of age were living with HIV infection that had not yet progressed to AIDS. Males and blacks represent the largest numbers of those who were HIV infected (Centers for Disease Control and Prevention, 1999a). The proportion of new cases of HIV infection that had not progressed to AIDS in the twenty-five states reporting during 1994–1997 was highest among younger age groups and females (Centers for Disease Control and Prevention, 1998a).

Seroprevalence surveys, for which data by race are available, consistently show that the prevalence of HIV infection is greatest among blacks. The median clinic prevalence rate among patients seen at reporting sexually transmitted disease clinics in 1997 among men who have sex with men was twice as high for black compared to white men. Among clients seen at drug treatment centers during 1997, the prevalence rates were highest among black intravenous drug users.

TABLE 3.3. INDICATORS OF PERSONS LIVING WITH HIV/AIDS, BY DEMOGRAPHIC SUBGROUPS.

Indicators	Age				
	13–24	25–29	30–34	35–39	40+
HIV diagnoses[1]					
Number (percent) of persons initially diagnosed with HIV infection, not AIDS, age 13+	7,200 (92)	9,384 (81)	11,916 (73)	10,030 (69)	14,159 (63)

	Age <13						
	Sex		Race				
	Male	Female	White	Black	Hispanic	Native American	Asian or Pacific Islander
AIDS cases, July 1998–June 1999[2]@							
Total number (percent)	156 (48.4)	166 (51.6)	36 (11.3)	202 (63.1)	80 (25.0)	1 (0.3)	1 (0.3)
Men who have sex with men							
Injecting drug use							
Men who have sex with men and inject drugs							
Hemophilia/coagulation disorder	1 (0.6)	0	0	0	1 (1.3)	0	0
Heterosexual contact							
Sex with an injecting drug user							
Sex with bisexual male							
Sex with person with hemophilia							
Sex with transfusion recipient with HIV infection							
Sex with HIV-infected person, risk not specified							
Recipient of blood transfusion, blood components or tissue	0	0	0	0	0	0	0
Other/risk not reported or identified	14 (9.0)	10 (6.0)	3 (8.3)	14 (6.9)	7 (8.8)	0	0
Mother with/at risk for HIV infection	141 (90.4)	156 (94.0)	33 (91.7)	188 (93.1)	72 (90.0)	1 (100.0)	1 (100.0)
Injecting drug user	38	37	7	44	23	1	0
Sex with an injecting drug user	27	15	6	23	12	0	1
Sex with bisexual male	3	1	1	1	1	0	0
Sex with person with hemophilia	0	0	0	0	0	0	0
Sex with transfusion recipient with HIV infection	0	1	0	0	1	0	0
Sex with HIV-infected person, risk not specified	28	45	7	51	15	0	0
Receipt of blood transfusion, blood components or tissue	1	1	0	2	0	0	0
Has HIV infection, risk not specified	44	56	12	67	20	0	0

Sex		Race			
Male	Female	White	Black	Hispanic	Other or Unknown
37,996 (69)	14,689 (81)	17,989 (66)	30,229 (77)	3,581 (68)	949 (79)

Age 13+

Sex		Race				
Male	Female	White	Black	Hispanic	Native American	Asian or Pacific Islander
35,918 (76.8)	10,841 (23.2)	15,407 (33.0)	21,526 (46.2)	9,175 (19.7)	171 (0.4)	344 (0.7)
15,999 (44.5)		8,575 (55.7)	4,497 (20.9)	2,653 (28.9)	64 (37.4)	168 (48.8)
7,493 (20.9)	3,043 (28.1)	2,233 (14.5)	5,691 (26.4)	2,526 (27.5)	35 (20.5)	23 (6.7)
1,940 (5.4)		909 (5.9)	712 (3.3)	296 (3.2)	14 (8.2)	6 (1.7)
150 (0.4)	21 (0.2)	113 (0.7)	31 (0.1)	23 (0.3)	1 (0.6)	2 (0.6)
2,754 (7.7)	4,296 (39.6)	1,287 (8.4)	4,125 (19.2)	1,573 (17.1)	12 (7.0)	45 (13.1)
604	*1,208*	*389*	*995*	*409*	*6*	*11*
	200	*77*	*86*	*35*	*0*	*2*
7	*27*	*18*	*8*	*7*	*0*	*1*
20	*18*	*10*	*16*	*9*	*1*	*2*
2,123	*2,843*	*793*	*3,020*	*1,113*	*3*	*29*
146 (0.4)	120 (1.1)	100 (0.6)	118 (0.5)	41 (0.4)	1 (0.6)	6 (1.7)
7,436 (20.7)	3,361 (31.0)	2,190 (14.2)	6,352 (29.5)	2,063 (22.5)	44 (25.7)	94 (27.3)

(*Continued on page 68*)

TABLE 3.3.   (*Continued*)

			Age at Death		
<15	15–24	25–34	35–44	45–54	55+

Cumulative total (percent distribution) of deaths of persons with AIDS, through June 1999[3]

<15	15–24	25–34	35–44	45–54	55+
4,975	8,508	126,162	173,926	74,008	32,229
(1.2)	(2.0)	(30.1)	(41.4)	(17.6)	(7.7)

				Age				
<1	1–4	5–14	15–24	25–34	35–44	45–54	55–64	65–74

Death rates for HIV infection per 100,000 persons[4]

	<1	1–4	5–14	15–24	25–34	35–44	45–54	55–64	65–74
1987	2.3	0.7	0.1	1.3	11.7	14.0	8.0	3.5	1.3
1997	#	0.4	0.3	0.8	10.1	16.1	10.4	4.9	1.8

Note: The AIDS case reporting definitions were revised in 1985, 1987, and 1993.

@ Delays in the investigation of modes of exposure result in underestimation in some risk categories.

Based on fewer than twenty deaths.

Sources: CDC and NCHS reports. See Resource B for specific references to table items marked with superscript numerals.

Comparable racial disparities were observed among Job Corps entrants and applicants for military service (Centers for Disease Control and Prevention, 1998b).

AIDS Cases. Around 285,000 U.S. adults and over 3,500 children were living with AIDS as of June 1999. The percentage distribution of blacks and Hispanics among the 711,344 cumulative cases of AIDS that had occurred in the United States (37 percent and 18 percent of all cases, respectively) is substantially greater than the proportion they represent in the U.S. population as a whole (12.7 percent and 11 percent), respectively (Centers for Disease Control and Prevention, 1999a).

The disproportionate concentration of AIDS in minority populations (around eight out of ten) is particularly significant for children. The vast majority of children contracted the disease perinatally from their HIV-infected mother. Among mothers for whom the mode of AIDS transmission was known, IV drug use or sexual contact with an HIV-infected person were the main reasons the vast majority of mothers were at risk.

About eight of ten adult cases of AIDS are men. The number of women with AIDS has increased steadily, however, corresponding to the progression of the disease to the heterosexual and bisexual populations, particularly among drug users and their sexual partners. The vast majority of the cases of AIDS among

Sex		Race				
Male	Female	White	Black	Hispanic	Native American	Asian or Pacific Islander
359,902 (85.6)	60,299 (14.0)	197,394 (47.0)	146,010 (34.8)	72,604 (17.3)	1,067 (0.3)	2,858 (0.7)

		Race by Sex									
		Sex		White		Black		Hispanic		Native American	
75–84	85+	M	F	M	F	M	F	M	F	M	F
0.8	#	10.0	1.1	8.4	0.6	25.4	4.7	17.8	2.1	#	#
0.6	#	9.1	2.6	5.6	1.0	38.5	13.3	13.1	3.3	3.6	#

women are due to intravenous drug use (28.1 percent) or through heterosexual contact (39.6 percent), especially with injecting drug users. Around 45 percent of the cases among males were in men who had sex with men, 21 percent were through intravenous drug use, and 5.4 percent through a combination of these methods of transmission.

The mode of transmission varies considerably among racial and ethnic group. Minority women are much more likely than white women to have contracted HIV/AIDS through drug-related activity. Around twice as many blacks (26.4 percent) and Hispanics (27.5 percent), compared to whites (14.5 percent), contracted HIV/AIDS through intravenous drug use. Native Americans (20.5 percent) were also substantially more likely to contract the illness in this way.

HIV/AIDS-Related Deaths. HIV/AIDS deaths have been greatest among persons twenty-five to forty-four years of age. It is, in fact, one of the major causes of death among this age group. The vast majority of those who have died of AIDS are men, although the death rates for women have increased over time as more women have contracted HIV infection.

The 1997 death rates due to HIV infection for black males (38.5) were very high compared to other groups. Although the short-term survival rates for AIDS have increased overall, blacks continue to have lower survival rates than whites, which could relate to the stage at which care is sought, as well as the accessibility of antiretroviral therapies or related medical care.

Mentally Ill and Disabled

The prevalence of different types of mental disorders, as well as where people get treatment for them, varies for age, gender, and race groups. Children are more likely to have developmental or behavioral problems. Substance abuse, schizophrenia, affective disorders, and anxiety disorders are more prevalent among adults under sixty-five years of age. Relative to younger adults, the elderly are much more likely to have organic brain syndrome (including Alzheimer's). Although the prevalence of mental illness in general is greater for women, substance abuse and antisocial personality disorders are much more prevalent among men. Minorities living in the community report lower rates of serious mental illness, but higher rates of frequent mental distress than do whites. Minorities are, however, disproportionately represented among those with serious mental illness receiving care in twenty-four-hour hospital or residential settings (see Table 3.4).

Community Prevalence Rates. Both the Epidemiological Catchment Area and National Comorbidity Surveys (NCS) confirmed that women were more likely to have affective and anxiety disorders, while men had higher rates of alcohol abuse, drug abuse and antisocial personality disorders. The NCS documented that young adults twenty-five to thirty-four years of age were most likely to have ever experienced a mental disorder, and the youngest cohort in that study (fifteen to twenty-four years) had the highest rates of disorders within the past twelve months. Of increasing concern is the large number of children who have emotional or other problems that warrant mental health treatment, including developmental, behavior, emotional, psychophysiological, or adjustment disorders. The percentage of children nine to seventeen years of age with extreme functional impairment has been estimated to range from 5 to 9 percent (or 1.7 to 3 million children) (Friedman, Katz-Leavy, Manderscheid, & Sondheimer, 1998).

Consistent with other research, rates of almost all disorders in the NCS declined monotonically with higher income and educational levels. Blacks in the NCS had significantly lower prevalences of affective disorders, substance abuse disorders, and lifetime comorbidity than whites. There were no statistically significant differences in the occurrence of disorders among Hispanics compared to non-Hispanic whites (Kessler et al., 1994).

Estimates from the 1997 National Household Survey on Drug Abuse in general confirmed the subgroup differences documented in the NCS (see Table 3.4). The prevalence of the four affective and anxiety disorders examined in that study, especially the occurrence of a major depressive episode, was higher for women compared to men. The likelihood of having experienced one of these disorders in the past year was highest among those eighteen to twenty-five years old and lowest for older adults (fifty years of age or older). The prevalence of these disorders, especially the occurrence of a major depressive episode, was reportedly higher for non-Hispanic whites than for blacks or Hispanics and among those with less than a high school education, especially compared to college graduates.

TABLE 3.4. INDICATORS OF MENTALLY ILL AND DISABLED, BY DEMOGRAPHIC SUBGROUPS: COMMUNITY PREVALENCE RATES.

Indicators	Sex		Age				Race			Education			
	Male	Female	18–25	26–34	35–49	50+	White	Black	Hispanic	Less Than High School	High School Graduate	Some College	College Graduate
Prevalence of mental disorders, percent, National Household Survey on Drug Abuse, 1997[1]													
Any of four mental syndromes	8.3	13.6	13.3	10.8	13.1	8.5	11.9	9.6	7.9	13.6	11.3	12.0	7.7
Major depressive episode	5.9	9.7	9.4	7.3	9.6	6.1	8.8	5.3	5.6	10.2	7.5	8.7	5.9
Generalized anxiety disorder	1.6	2.6	1.9	2.6	2.3	1.7	2.2	1.6	2.0	3.7	1.7	1.8	1.6
Agoraphobia	1.2	2.4	1.9	1.9	2.7	0.9	1.7	3.0	1.2	2.8	2.4	1.6	0.4
Panic attack	2.3	3.6	3.6	3.2	3.7	1.9	3.3	2.2	1.7	3.1	3.0	3.8	1.8

Source: Substance Abuse and Mental Health Services Administration report. See Resource B for specific references to table items marked with superscript numerals.

In contrast to findings from the NCS and National Household Survey on Drug Abuse (NHSDA) studies, which examined relatively serious mental disorders, the 1993–1996 statewide Behavioral Risk Factor Surveillance System (BRFSS) found a higher prevalence of self-reported frequent mental distress (FMD) among American Indians/Alaskan Natives (12.9 percent), Hispanics (10.3 percent), and non-Hispanic blacks (9.7 percent), compared to non-Hispanic whites (8.3 percent) (Centers for Disease Control and Prevention, 1998e). An Office of Technology Assessment report synthesizing existing research on the mental health of Native American adolescents indicated that they have more serious psychological and behavioral problems than all other racial groups in the following areas: developmental disabilities, depression, suicide, anxiety, alcohol and substance abuse, self-esteem, running away and school dropout rates (Office of Technology Assessment, 1990).

Treated Rates, Mental Health Facilities. Based on the 1994 inventory of mental health organizations and hospitals, the largest age group receiving mental health treatment in any type of setting was between thirty-five and sixty-four years of age (see Table 3.5). Clients thirteen to seventeen years of age were most likely to be treated in a twenty-four-hour residential setting. Proportionately more adults thirty-five to sixty-four years of age were treated in twenty-four-hour hospital settings, as were the elderly. Of the 3.9 million persons seen in mental health organization and hospital psychiatric settings in 1994, 52 percent were male, and 48 percent were female. Proportionately more males than females were treated in twenty-four-hour hospital or residential settings. About 9 percent of patients

TABLE 3.5. INDICATORS OF MENTALLY ILL AND DISABLED, BY DEMOGRAPHIC SUBGROUPS: TREATED RATES, MENTAL HEALTH FACILITIES.

Indicators	Age						Total
	<13	13–17	18–34	35–64	65–74	75+	
Number (percent) of clients receiving mental health treatment, 1994[1]							
24-hour hospital	5,434 (4)	10,829 (7)	34,854 (24)	71,627 (49)	13,892 (10)	8,828 (6)	145,464
24-hour residential	10,656 (12)	26,459 (29)	19,611 (21)	29,590 (32)	4,182 (5)	1,195 (1.3)	91,693
Less-than-24-hour hospital	435,339 (12)	388,201 (11)	1,005,444 (27)	1,503,570 (41)	248,035 (7)	99,312 (2)	3,679,901

Note: The percentage Hispanic is based on a separate classification of clients as Hispanic or non-Hispanic.

Source: Rouse (1998). See Resource B for specific references to table items marked with superscript numerals.

receiving care in twenty-four-hour treatment settings were Hispanic. A somewhat higher proportion of Hispanics (12 percent) were seen in less-than-twenty-four-hour facilities. There were proportionately more blacks receiving care in twenty-four-hour (24 to 25 percent), relative to less-than-twenty-four-hour (18 percent) settings. Native Americans and Asians and Pacific Islanders composed only 1 to 2 percent of the clients seen in any of these mental health treatment facilities.

Treated Rates, Nursing Homes. Based on the 1995 National Nursing Home Survey, around half (55.0 percent) of nursing home residents less than sixty-five years of age had a mental impairment compared to 58.9 percent of the elderly (see Table 3.6). This represents an increase in the proportion of the elderly residents of nursing homes with a mental disorder compared to the 1985 National Nursing Home Survey (44.9 percent). In both years, among those less than sixty-five, schizophrenia and other psychoses, mental retardation, and organic brain syndrome were the major psychiatric diagnoses. Around half of the elderly (49.3 percent) in nursing homes in 1995 and about a third in 1985 (35.3 percent) had organic brain syndrome. Over half of both men and women residents had some type of a mental disorder. Men were more likely to have a diagnosis of mental retardation or alcohol and drug abuse, and women more often had organic brain syndrome. The distribution of disorders did not differ substantially by race.

Alcohol or Substance Abusers

Young adults in their late teens and early twenties, particularly men, are more likely to smoke, drink, and use illicit drugs than their younger or older counterparts. Native American youth are much more likely to use alcohol, drugs, and

Sex		Race				
Male	Female	White	Black	Hispanic	Native American	Asian American
87,430	58,034	106,081	36,277	13,283	1,265	1,841
(60)	(40)	(73)	(25)	(9)	(1)	(1)
56,589	35,104	67,024	22,206	7,894	1,569	894
(62)	(38)	(73)	(24)	(9)	(2)	(1)
1,889,123	1,790,778	2,893,136	676,346	429,886	50,409	60,010
(51)	(49)	(79)	(18)	(12)	(1)	(2)

TABLE 3.6. INDICATORS OF MENTALLY ILL AND DISABLED, BY DEMOGRAPHIC SUBGROUPS: TREATED RATES, NURSING HOMES.

	Age@		Sex		Race		
Indicators	<65	65+	Male	Female	White	Black	Hispanic
Percent of nursing home residents with mental disorders[1]							
Total							
1985	60.9	44.9	46.2	46.9	46.8	46.4	46.3
1995	55.0	58.9	57.5	59.0	59.0	55.5	55.9
Mental retardation							
1985	17.3	1.6	5.3	2.6	3.5	*	*
1995	11.2	1.2	3.9	1.3	2.1	*	*
Alcohol and drug abuse							
1985	*	*1.3	4.6	*	1.6	*	*
1995	*5.2	1.0	3.6	*0.5	1.2	*	*
Organic brain syndromes (including Alzheimer's disease)							
1985	13.4	35.3	26.8	35.1	32.8	33.5	32.4
1995	19.9	49.3	42.5	48.6	47.4	43.7	48.6
Depressive disorders							
1985	*	3.2	*	3.8	3.3	*	*
1995	*8.6	10.1	8.8	10.5	10.7	*	*
Schizophrenia and other psychoses							
1985	28.3	8.6	12.8	10.1	10.7	*13.6	*
1995	22.4	8.5	10.0	9.5	9.3	12.7	*
Anxiety disorders							
1985	*	*1.2	*	*1.4	1.5	*	*
1995	*	3.7	2.7	4.1	3.9	*	*
Other mental illnesses							
1985	*	*0.8	*	*	*1.1	*	*
1995	*	2.6	3.4	2.4	2.8	*	*

@ Excludes age unknown.

*Data do not meet standard of reliability or precision (sample size fewer than thirty) and are therefore not reported; or where reported data should not be assumed to be reliable because the sample size is between thirty and fifty-nine, or the sample is greater than fifty-nine but the relative standard error is over 30 percent.

Source: NCHS data. See Resource B for specific references to table items marked with superscript numerals.

cigarettes than are either white or other minority youth. Minority users are also more likely to develop life-threatening patterns of abuse, as evidenced by higher rates of addiction-related deaths. Death rates for cirrhosis of the liver and other alcohol-related causes are greater among Native Americans. Minorities (particularly African Americans) constitute a disproportionate number of medical emergencies and deaths due to cocaine abuse. (See Tables 2.7 and 3.7.)

Household Population, Twelve Years and Older. As documented in Table 2.7, the highest rates of any illicit drug use within the past month or year, especially marijuana, were among young adults eighteen to twenty-five years of age, and the lowest rates were for those thirty-five years of age or older. The prevalence of alcohol and cigarette use was also highest among eighteen to twenty-five year olds, and the lowest among those under age eighteen. As documented in Chapter Two, however, the rates of illicit drug use and cigarette smoking have increased among children and adolescents twelve to seventeen years of age since the early 1990s.

In 1998, the rates of illicit drug use were substantially higher for men compared to women—both over the past year (13.1 versus 8.2 percent) and the past month (8.1 versus 4.5 percent). (See Table 3.7.) The prevalence of current cocaine use among men (1.1 percent) was twice that of women (0.5 percent). Larger percentages of men (58.7 percent) had used alcohol in the past month compared to women (45.1 percent). Although the differences were not as dramatic, more men (29.7 percent) than women (25.7 percent) had smoked cigarettes during that period.

In 1998, the monthly prevalence of illicit drug use overall was somewhat higher for blacks (8.2 percent) compared to whites (6.1 percent) and Hispanics (6.1 percent). Marijuana use was slightly higher among blacks than Hispanics. Monthly alcohol use was higher among whites (55.3 percent), compared to Hispanics (45.4 percent) or blacks (39.8 percent). The percentage that had smoked in the past month was somewhat higher for whites (27.9 percent) and blacks (29.4 percent) compared to Hispanics (25.8 percent). Rates of substance abuse tend to be high among Native American populations. Based on combined estimates from the 1991–1993 National Household Survey on Drug Abuse, the percentage of Native Americans twelve years of age and older who experienced various types of substance abuse (compared to the U.S. population) was as follows: had used an illicit drug in the past year, 19.8 percent (versus 11.9 percent); used cigarettes in the past year, 52.7 percent (versus 30.9 percent); and were dependent on alcohol, 5.6 percent (versus 3.5 percent) (Substance Abuse and Mental Health Services Administration, 1998d).

The prevalence of illicit drug and alcohol use was lowest for college graduates. The highest percentages of current smokers were among those with a high school education (34.3 percent) or less (36.9 percent), and the lowest percentage (15.2 percent) was for those with a college education.

TABLE 3.7. INDICATORS OF ALCOHOL OR SUBSTANCE ABUSERS, BY DEMOGRAPHIC SUBGROUPS.

Indicators	Sex		Race			Adult Education			
	Male	Female	White	Black	Hispanic	Less Than High School	High School Graduate	Some College	College Graduate
Household population 12+ years, percent drug use[1][@@]									
Any illicit drug use[@]									
Past year									
1985	19.7	13.3	—	—	—	—	—	—	—
1998	13.1	8.2	10.4	13.0	10.5	—	—	—	—
Past month									
1985	14.9	9.5	12.3	12.7	8.9	—	—	—	—
1998	8.1	4.5	6.1	8.2	6.1	6.5	6.2	6.9	3.7
Marijuana and hashish									
Past year									
1985	17.2	10.2	—	—	—	—	—	—	—
1998	10.8	6.5	8.4	10.6	8.2	—	—	—	—
Past month									
1985	12.6	7.1	10.0	9.9	6.4	—	—	—	—
1998	6.7	3.5	5.0	6.6	4.5	4.8	5.3	5.3	3.1
Hallucinogens									
Past year									
1985	—	—	—	—	—	—	—	—	—
1998	2.0	1.3	1.8	0.4	1.6	—	—	—	—
Past month									
1985	—	—	—	—	—	—	—	—	—
1998	0.8	0.6	0.8	0.2	0.7	—	—	—	—

Household population 12+ years, percent drug use[1]

	1	2	3	4	5	6	7	8	9
Cocaine (crack)									
Past year									
1985	6.8(—)	3.6(—)	—(—)	—(—)	—(—)	—(—)	—(—)	—(—)	—(—)
1998	2.3(0.6)	1.2(0.3)	1.7(0.3)	1.9(1.3)	2.3(0.7)	—(—)	—(—)	—(—)	—(—)
Past month									
1985	3.9	2.1	3.0	3.4	2.5	1.4(—)	0.8(—)	0.7(—)	0.5(—)
1998	1.1(0.2)	0.5(0.2)	0.7(0.1)	1.3(0.9)	1.3(0.3)				
Alcohol use									
Past year									
1985	78.0	68.2	—	—	—	—	—	—	—
1998	68.3	60.0	67.8	50.4	58.5	—	—	—	—
Past month									
1985	69.2	52.0	62.8	50.6	49.3	40.4	52.3	60.1	65.5
1998	58.7	45.1	55.3	39.8	45.4				
Cigarette use									
Past month									
1985	45.3	36.2	—	—	—	—	—	—	—
1998	32.8	28.4	30.8	31.2	29.6	—	—	—	—
Daily use									
1985	43.4	34.5	38.9	38.0	40.0	36.9	34.3	29.2	15.2
1998	29.7	25.7	27.9	29.4	25.8				

(Continued on page 78)

TABLE 3.7. (Continued)

Indicators	Sex		Race		
	Male	Female	White	Black	Hispanic
High school seniors, percent drug use[2##]					
Any illicit drug use[#]					
Past year					
1985	48.3	43.8	47.6	35.9	43.9
1998	45.2	37.2	44.0	32.3	41.9
Marijuana and hashish					
Past year					
1985	43.1	37.8	41.6	33.4	37.8
1998	41.7	33.0	39.9	30.0	37.2
Past month					
1985	—	—	—	—	—
1998	26.5	18.8	24.4	18.3	31.6
Inhalants					
Past year					
1985	6.9	4.5	5.9	2.0	6.5
1998	7.5	5.1	7.9	1.7	4.5
Past month					
1985	—	—	—	—	—
1998	2.9	1.7	2.8	0.9	1.8
Hallucinogens					
Past year					
1985	8.1	4.4	7.0	1.2	5.7
1998	11.0	6.8	11.3	1.4	6.8
Past month					
1985	—	—	—	—	—
1998	5.1	2.3	4.5	0.7	2.8

High school seniors, percent drug use[2]

Cocaine (crack)					
Past year					
1985	14.8	11.2	13.0	5.3	16.3
1998	6.8 (3.1)	4.5 (2.0)	6.3 (2.6)	0.9 (0.3)	6.7 (3.9)
Past month					
1985	—	—	—	—	—
1998	3.0 (1.4)	1.7 (0.6)	2.5 (1.0)	0.6 (0.2)	2.7 (1.4)
Alcohol use					
Past year					
1985	—	—	—	—	—
1998	76.1	72.6	78.5	59.7	74.3
Past month					
1985	69.8	62.1	71.2	42.8	58.1
1998	57.3	46.9	57.7	33.3	49.8
Cigarette use					
Past month					
1985	28.2	31.4	31.3	18.1	25.5
1998	36.3	33.3	41.7	14.9	26.6
Daily use					
1985	17.8	20.6	20.4	9.9	11.8
1998	22.7	21.5	28.3	7.4	13.6

(Continued on page 80)

TABLE 3.7. (Continued)

Indicators	Age								Race	
	15–24	25–34	35–44	45–54	55–64	65–74	75–84	85+	Native American	All Races
Alcohol-related mortality rates, 1992–1994[3]										
Age-adjusted rate per 100,000	0.3	2.4	10.1	16.9	22.2	18.8	11.1	4.6	45.5	6.7

	Age				Sex		Race			
	12–17	18–25	26–34	35+	Male	Female	White	Black	Hispanic	Other
Emergency room drug abuse reports, 1998, percent[4]										
Total episodes	10.9	19.1	25.5	44.1	51.9	47.2	54.5	25.2	10.5	1.0
Cocaine mentions	2.5	14.2	34.3	48.7	65.3	33.8	30.8	49.2	12.3	0.5

@@ A new version of the NHSDA instrument was fielded for the first time in 1994. Rates reported here for 1985 have been adjusted to improve their comparability with estimates based on the revised instrument.

—Not Reported.

@ "Any illicit drug" refers to using, at least once, any of the following: marijuana or hashish, cocaine (including crack), inhalants, hallucinogens (including PCP and LSD), heroin, or any prescription-type psychotherapeutic used nonmedically.

No data on use of drugs in the past month by race were reported prior to 1991 in the annual reports. Percentages for racial subgroups for 1998 are based on combined data for 1997 and 1998. Crack use was not reported prior to 1986. Questions on alcohol use were revised in 1993 and 1994. The data for alcohol use in 1985 have not been adjusted to reflect this change.

"Any illicit drug use" refers to using any of the following: marijuana, LSD, other hallucinogens, crack, other cocaine, or heroin, or any use of other narcotics, amphetamines, barbiturates, methaqualone, or tranquilizers not under a doctor's orders.

Sources: Substance Abuse and Mental Health Services Administration reports; Johnston, O'Malley, & Bachman (1999); Indian Health Service (1998). See Resource B for specific references to table items marked with superscript numerals.

High School Seniors. Based on 1998 data, U.S. female high school seniors were less likely to have used drugs than males. Females were also less likely to use alcohol, but the percentages of those smoking cigarettes daily were similar for males and females. Black high school seniors consistently reported lower rates of illicit drug, alcohol, and cigarette use than whites, and Hispanic youths tended to have intermediate rates between those of blacks and whites.

Alcohol-Related Mortality Rates. The number of deaths due to alcohol-related causes per 100,000 deaths was highest for adults fifty-five to sixty-four years old (22.2). The overall rate for Native Americans (45.5) was more than six times that of all other races combined (6.7).

Emergency Room Drug Abuse Reports. The majority of people seen in an emergency room for drug-induced emergencies were thirty-five years of age or older (44.1 percent). Somewhat more men (51.9 percent) than women (47.2 percent) and more whites (54.5 percent) than blacks (25.2 percent) were seen. However, many more men (65.3 percent) than women (33.8 percent) and more blacks (49.2 percent) than whites (30.8 percent) were seen for cocaine-related emergencies. (Note that these estimates here and in Table 3.7 do not add up to 100 percent due to missing data on these variables.)

Suicide or Homicide Prone

Of those who die from intentional acts of violence, elderly white men and young Native American men are most likely to kill themselves. Young African American, Native American, and Hispanic men are most likely to be killed at the hand of others. The violence-related death rates for these groups have increased dramatically in recent years, primarily due to the greater use of deadly weapons, particularly firearms, in these encounters (see Table 3.8).

Suicide. Although the overall suicide rate did not change significantly from 1950 to 1980, suicide rates among young persons, particularly young white men, increased dramatically. From 1950 to 1980, the rates among white males fifteen to twenty-four years of age increased 324 percent, from 6.6 per 100,000 to 21.4 per 100,000. The number of suicides among white males and females fifteen to nineteen years of age in which firearms were used doubled between 1968 and 1980 (Fingerhut & Kleinman, 1989; NCHS, 1991b).

Based on 1997 data, death rates due to suicide were much higher for white males (18.4) compared to black males (11.2), white females (4.4), or black females (1.9). Rates were dramatically higher for elderly white males seventy-five to eighty-four years of age and eighty-five or older.

Compared to whites as a whole, suicide rates tend to be lower for Hispanics and higher for Native Americans. As with whites, males are more at risk of

TABLE 3.8. INDICATORS OF SUICIDE OR HOMICIDE PRONE, BY DEMOGRAPHIC SUBGROUPS.

	Age								
Indicators	<1	1–4	5–14	15–24	25–34	35–44	45–54	55–64	65–74
Age-adjusted death rates per 100,000 resident population[1]									
Suicide									
1985	—	—	0.8	12.8	15.3	14.6	15.7	16.8	18.7
1997	—	—	0.8	11.4	14.3	15.3	14.7	13.5	14.4
Homicide and legal intervention									
1985	5.4	2.5	1.2	11.9	14.8	11.3	8.1	5.7	4.3
1997	8.3	2.4	1.2	16.8	12.8	8.4	5.6	3.9	2.9

Source: NCHS report. See Resource B for specific references to table items marked with superscript numerals.

committing suicide. The suicide rate for Native American males in 1997 (21.3) was essentially twice the national average (10.6).

Year 2000 Objectives for lowering suicide rates were targeted toward at-risk age, gender, and race and ethnicity groups: youth aged fifteen to nineteen (8.2), men aged twenty to thirty-four (21.4), white men aged sixty-five and older (39.2), and American Indians and Alaskan Natives (12.8) (Public Health Service, 1990). The 1997 rates for all of these groups, particularly elderly males, fell short of these objectives.

Homicide and Legal Intervention. While white males are most at risk of death due to suicide, black males are most at risk of a homicide-related death. Based on 1997 data, the disparity between homicide rates per 100,000 for black males (48.3), compared to black females (9.3), white males (7.0), and white females (2.3), was significant. The rate for black males twenty-five to forty-four years old was 113.3 (National Center for Health Statistics, 1999d).

Compared to whites, rates of homicide are higher for both Hispanics and Native Americans. Although the disparities have narrowed since the 1950s, the 1997 homicide rate for Native American (16.7) and Hispanic (18.2) males was two to three times the national average (8.0). As with suicide rates, the rates of homicide-related deaths are highest for young Native American and Hispanic males fifteen to twenty-four years old (27.7 and 42.7, respectively) (National Center for Health Statistics, 1999d).

The 1997 homicide rates exceeded the Year 2000 Objectives for American Indians and Alaskan Natives (11.3), young Hispanic men ages fifteen to thirty-four (42.5), and particularly at-risk young black men ages fifteen to thirty-four (72.4) (Public Health Service, 1990).

Age		Race by Sex							
		White		Black		Hispanic		Native American	
75–84	85+	Male	Female	Male	Female	Male	Female	Male	Female
23.9	19.4	19.9	5.3	11.5	2.1	10.4	1.8	19.9	4.4
19.3	20.8	18.4	4.4	11.2	1.9	10.4	1.7	21.3	4.4
4.3	4.2	8.1	2.9	50.2	10.9	26.7	4.2	20.0	4.8
2.9	3.8	7.0	2.3	48.3	9.3	18.2	3.1	16.7	5.2

Abusing Families

Unemployment + economic Hardship [handwritten margin note]

Unemployment and associated economic hardship play a major role in cases of maltreatment, and particularly neglect, within families (see Table 3.9).

Child Abuse and Neglect Reports. The age distribution of children for which maltreatment was reported in 1997 is as follows: birth to two years (19.3 percent), three to five years (20.0 percent), six to eight years (20.0 percent), nine to eleven years (16.2 percent), twelve to fourteen years (14.7 percent), and fifteen to seventeen years (10.2 percent). The rate of victims of neglect and medical neglect generally decreased with the child's age, while the rates of physical, sexual, and emotional maltreatment increased with age. Slightly more than half (52.3 percent) of maltreated children were female.

In 1997 the racial and ethnic distribution of maltreated children was as follows: white (66.7 percent), black (29.5 percent), Hispanic (13.3 percent), and Native American (2.5 percent). The percentage distribution of African American and Native American victims of child abuse was almost twice the representation of children in these racial and ethnic groups in the U.S. population as a whole. White and Asian and Pacific Islander children who experienced maltreatment represented a somewhat lower relative distribution (Administration for Children, Youth and Families, Children's Bureau, 1999).

Child Abuse and Neglect Incidence Rates. Older children are more likely to be victims of abuse or neglect than are very young children. However, children are consistently vulnerable to sexual abuse from age three on. Girls were three times as likely to be sexually abused as were boys, whereas boys had a greater risk of emotional neglect and serious injury. Children living in single-parent families or

TABLE 3.9. INDICATORS OF ABUSING FAMILIES, BY DEMOGRAPHIC SUBGROUPS.

Indicators	Age						Sex	
	0–2	3–5	6–8	9–11	12–14	15–17	Male	Female
Child abuse and neglect reports[1]								
Number of children reported in 1,000s (percent), 1997*	124 (19.3)	128 (20.0)	129 (20.0)	105 (16.2)	95 (14.7)	66 (10.2)	317 (47.4)	350 (52.3)
Child abuse and neglect incidence rates, 1993[2]@								
Number of children in 1,000s, harm standard (endangerment standard)	122 (317)	205 (444)	364 (661)	294 (527)	319 (479)	230 (306)	748 (1,378)	802 (1,382)
Rate per 1,000 U.S. children, harm standard (endangerment standard)	10.0 (26.0)	17.8 (38.6)	33.1 (60.2)	25.9 (46.4)	29.6 (44.4)	22.4 (29.7)	21.7 (40.0)	24.5 (42.3)

	Age					
	60–64	65–69	70–74	75–79	80–84	85+
Domestic elder abuse[3]						
Victims of domestic elder abuse, percent, 1996	9.2	11.4	17.2	18.3	19.1	21.4

	Age							Race	
	12–15	16–19	20–24	25–34	35–49	50–64	65+	White	Black
Violence by intimates, 1992–1996[4]									
Rate of violent victimization of women, per 1,000 women	2.6	20.1	20.7	16.5	7.2	1.3	0.2	8.2	11.7
Rate of violent victimization of men, per 1,000 men								1.4	2.1

*The number of states reporting varies for different categories, and some data include estimates. Percentage breakdowns by race exclude victims classified as "other" or "unknown."

@ The endangerment standard includes children who had actually experienced harm and adds others who have not yet been harmed by maltreatment but who experienced abuse or neglect that put them in danger of being harmed.

Sources: Administration for Children, Youth and Families, Children's Bureau (1999); Sedlak, Hantman, & Schultz (1997); Tatara & Kuzmeskus (1997); Greenfeld et al. (1998). See Resource B for specific references to table items marked with superscript numerals.

	Race			Annual Family Income			Family Structure		
White	Black	Hispanic	Native American	Less Than $15,000	$15,000–29,999	$30,000 or More	Both Parents	Mother or Father	Neither Parent
391 (66.7)	173 (29.5)	70 (13.3)	14 (2.5)	—	—	—	—	—	—
1,125 (2,205)	315 (547)	— (—)	— (—)	636 (1,297)	296 (491)	83 (147)	721 (1,248)	491 (934)	62 (106)
20.8 (37.4)	31.6 (55.0)	— (—)	— (—)	47.0 (95.9)	20.0 (33.1)	2.1 (3.8)	15.5 (26.9)	27.3 (52.0)	22.9) (39.3)

Sex		Race				
Male	Female	White	Black	Hispanic	Native American	Other or Unknown
32.4	67.3	66.4	18.7	10.4	0.7	3.8

		Annual Household Income						
Hispanic	Other	Less Than $7,500	$7,500–14,999	$15,000–24,999	$25,000–34,999	$35,000–49,999	$50,000–74,999	$75,000 or More
7.2	5.6	21.3	12.3	10.4	7.2	5.8	4.4	2.7
1.3	0.5	2.7	1.4	1.8	1.8	1.1	1.5	0.5

in families with annual incomes below $15,000 were much more likely to be subject to actual or potential maltreatment than were children living with both parents, or in families with annual incomes of $30,000 or greater, respectively (Sedlak & Broadhurst, 1996).

Domestic Elder Abuse. The prevalence of domestic elder abuse increases with increasing age. The elderly victims of domestic abuse are more often women (67.3 percent). Around two-thirds of elder abuse victims are white, with 18.7 percent black, 10.4 percent Hispanic, 0.7 percent Native American, and 3.8 percent other races. The major perpetrators of domestic elder abuse were adult children (36.7 percent), spouse (12.6 percent), other relatives (10.8 percent), grandchildren (7.7 percent), service provider (3.5 percent), friend or neighbor (3.2 percent), unrelated caregiver (4.3 percent), sibling (2.7 percent), and all others or unknown perpetrators (18.5 percent) (Tatara & Kuzmeskus, 1997).

Family Violence. During 1992–1996, the highest rates of violent victimization of women by their intimates occurred among young women sixteen to twenty-four years of age. Rates were higher for black women (11.7 per 1,000 women), compared to whites (8.2), Hispanics (7.2), and those of other races (5.6). Women whose annual family incomes were under $7,500 were at substantially greater risk than women in higher income families.

Findings from the National Surveys of Family Violence confirm that "economic adversity and worries about money pervade the typical violent home" (Gelles & Straus, 1988, p. 84). According to these investigators, the prototypical abusive parent was single, under thirty years old, married less than ten years, had his or her first child before the age of eighteen, and was unemployed, or if employed, worked part-time in a manual labor job. There were no differences between blacks and whites in the rates of abusive violence toward children.

The typical "wife beater," according to the same study, experienced status inconsistency—that is, a man's educational background was higher than his occupational attainment, or his neighbor's or wife's occupational attainments were greater than his own. He was young (eighteen to twenty-four years old), married less than ten years, employed part-time or not at all, and was dissatisfied with his economic security, although many individual abusers were quite affluent. The authors concluded, "Perhaps the most telling of all attributes of the battering man is that he feels inadequate and sees violence as a culturally acceptable way to be both dominant and powerful" (Gelles & Straus, 1988, p. 89). Although the rates of wives' battering husbands were also high, three-fourths of the violence committed by women was hypothesized to be in self-defense (Gelles & Straus, 1988, p. 90).

Homeless Persons

The precise composition of the homeless varies in different cities and localities. Nonetheless, a profile of homeless persons emerges from the array of national and local studies.

A twenty-six-city survey conducted in 1999 by the U.S. Conference of Mayors showed the following characteristics of the homeless population in the cities studied: single men (43 percent), families with children (37 percent), single women (13 percent), and unaccompanied youth (7 percent). Around a fourth (27 percent) of homeless persons were children. Data from this and other sources demonstrated a decline from 1985 to 1999 in the proportion of homeless persons who were single men (from 60 percent to 43 percent) and an increase in the proportion that were families with children (from 27 percent to 37 percent). The racial and ethnic composition of homeless persons was 50 percent black, 31 percent white, 13 percent Hispanic, 4 percent Native American, and 2 percent Asian. The U.S. Conference of Mayors study also documented that only 21 percent of homeless persons were employed in full- or part-time jobs, 14 percent were veterans, 19 percent were mentally ill, and 31 percent were alcohol or substance abusers (U.S. Conference of Mayors, 1999).

These findings bear out the profile of homeless persons found in other studies. In general, they are relatively young adults: the median age is from the late twenties to late thirties. The average age of homeless women is generally younger than that of men, and a relatively small percentage are sixty-five or over, compared to the general U.S. population. Traditionally more men than women have been homeless, although the proportion of women among homeless persons has increased in recent years to an estimated 20 to 35 percent. Minorities are over-represented among homeless persons in most cities. Adults are much less likely to have a high school education and to be employed compared to the U.S. population as a whole. Homeless persons have extremely low incomes—generally much lower than the U.S. poverty level. The majority have physical health problems, an estimated 25 to 40 percent have mental health problems, and a comparable proportion have alcohol or substance abuse problems. The majority of homeless clients (71 percent) are in central cities, 21 percent are in the suburbs and urban fringe areas, and 9 percent are in rural areas. This contrasts with the distribution of the U.S. population in poverty of 43, 34, and 23 percent, respectively (Burt et al., 1999).

Data from the 1996 Urban Institute study of clients of homeless assistance programs documented differences in the characteristics of single homeless clients and those in homeless families (see Table 3.10). Single homeless clients were predominantly male, while the vast majority of clients in homeless families included women and children. Single homeless clients were less likely to have ever been or currently married and were more likely to have a high school education and to be veterans. Families with children are much more likely to have

TABLE 3.10. INDICATORS OF HOMELESS PERSONS, BY DEMOGRAPHIC SUBGROUPS.

	Sex		Race				
Indicators	Male	Female	White	Black	Hispanic	Native American	Other
Characteristics of homeless, percent, 1996							
Urban Institute[1]							
All homeless clients	68	32	41	40	11	8	1
Clients in homeless families	16	84	38	43	15	3	1
Single homeless clients	77	23	41	40	10	8	1

*Percentage less than 0.5 but greater than 0.
Source: Burt et al. (1999). See Resource B for specific references to table items marked with superscript numerals.

been homeless for relatively short periods of time (less than three months) than have single homeless clients (Burt et al., 1999).

Immigrants and Refugees

During the 1960s, the largest number of immigrants came from Europe and North America, particularly Mexico. In the 1970s, there was a substantial increase in immigrants from Asia, reflecting the out-migration subsequent to the Vietnam War. Refugees were a substantial proportion of the Asian immigrants during this period. The estimated number of documented and undocumented persons from Central and South America who fled in response to the warfare in those areas increased substantially during the 1980s. The increased numbers of refugees from Europe and Africa in the 1990s mirror the effects of civil war within countries on those continents. Around two-thirds of those submitting claims for asylum in 1997 were from Mexico, El Salvador, Guatemala, Haiti, India, People's Republic of China, or Iraq. The vast majority of refugees were from the former Soviet Union, Bosnia-Herzegovina, Vietnam, and Somalia (Immigration and Naturalization Service, 1999a, 1999c). The demographic and socioeconomic profiles of different immigrant and refugee groups vary a great deal (see Table 3.11).

Compared to documented Mexican immigrants, undocumented Mexican immigrants are likely to be younger, have been in the United States a shorter period of time, have fewer years of education, are less likely to read and write English, and have lower incomes (Rumbaut, Chavez, Moser, Pickwell, & Wishik, 1988).

Age			Educational Attainment		
			Less Than High School	High School Graduate/General Equivalency Diploma	More Than High School
17–24	25–54	55+			
12	80	8	38	34	28
26	75	*	53	21	27
10	81	9	37	36	28

The characteristics of different subgroups of Indochinese refugees (such as Chinese, Vietnamese, Hmong, Khmer, and Lao) also differ. The fertility of Hmong women (number of children under five years of age per 1,000 women of childbearing age) has been found to be much higher than the other Asian subgroups, for example. Literacy rates in terms of the ability to read or speak English are low, particularly for Indochinese refugee women. The vast majority of Indochinese refugees have incomes below the poverty level. Those most disadvantaged have been in the United States the shortest period of time.

Those who have been here the longest, particularly the Vietnamese refugees, appear to have fared better than the other groups in terms of finding employment and earning incomes sufficient to elevate them above the poverty level. The first wave of refugees (almost all Vietnamese), admitted to the United States during 1975–1976, were better educated and came under more favorable economic conditions than did larger waves of refugees who arrived after 1979 (Haines, 1989; Rumbaut, Chavez, Moser, Pickwell, & Wishik, 1988).

The earlier waves of refugees from Cuba in the late 1950s and 1960s were of a much higher socioeconomic status, compared to those who came later, particularly the approximately 125,000 people who were admitted to the United States as a part of the Mariel boat lift of 1980. A number of former prisoners and others deemed "undesirable" by the Cuban regime entered the United States under this arrangement.

The Central American population, many of whom do not have official legal status in the United States, tend to be composed of a larger proportion of males, particularly young males. Literacy rates and rates of employment are low. As with many of the Indochinese refugee population, those who do work are employed in very low-paying service jobs (Urrutia-Rojas & Aday, 1991).

TABLE 3.11. INDICATORS OF IMMIGRANTS AND REFUGEES, BY DEMOGRAPHIC SUBGROUPS.

	Continent of Birth					
Indicators	Europe	Asia	North America	South America	Africa	Other*
Total Number[1]						
Immigrants@						
1961–1970	1,238,600	445,300	1,351,100	228,300	39,300	19,100
1971–1980	801,300	1,633,800	1,645,000	284,400	91,500	37,300
1981–1990	705,600	2,817,400	3,125,000	455,900	192,300	41,900
1991–1996	875,600	1,941,800	2,740,600	344,000	213,200	31,000
Refugees						
1961–1970	55,235	19,895	132,068	123	5,486	36
1971–1980	71,858	210,683	252,633	1,244	2,991	38
1981–1990	155,512	712,092	121,840	1,976	22,149	51
1991–1996	312,815	286,125	111,744	3,025	34,224	189

@ Totals for immigrants are rounded to the nearest one hundred in source tables.

*Other includes Oceania and country of origin unknown.

Sources: U.S. Bureau of the Census reports. See Resource B for specific references to table items marked with superscript numerals.

Conclusion

The evidence presented here clearly documents the role of social and economic status on the prevalence and incidence of poor physical, psychological, and social health along a number of different dimensions and strongly confirms the predictions presented earlier (see Table 1.1) regarding which groups are most and least vulnerable. Furthermore, the longitudinal data demonstrate that the problems of many of the most vulnerable worsened rather than diminished during the past two decades. The next chapter explores the social, political, and economic conditions and trends that give rise to greater vulnerability to poor health.

CHAPTER FOUR

WHY ARE THEY VULNERABLE?

no education
single
unemployed

This chapter addresses the question of why some groups are more vulnerable than others. The current and changing profile of the American people, the ties between and among them, and the neighborhoods in which they live are examined in the context of whether some groups are more at risk of poor physical, psychological, and social health as a result of the more limited availability of community and associated individual resources (social status, social capital, and human capital). (See Figures 1.1 and 1.2 and Table 1.1.)

National Profile and Trends

The current and changing profiles of the American people, in general, and those most at risk, in particular, are highlighted.

The People

Trends at the beginning of the twenty-first century point to older Americans living longer and families on average having fewer children. As a result of these and other demographic changes, such as the aging of the baby boom generation, the elderly are becoming an increasing proportion of the U.S. population.

The number of Americans age sixty-five and over nearly doubled between 1960 and 1998, from 16.7 million to 34 million or from 9.2 percent to 12.7 percent of the population. The number of elderly is expected to increase to nearly 40 million or almost 14 percent by the year 2010, and a growing proportion of the elderly will be among the oldest old (eighty-five years of age or older).

On the other hand, although the number of children under age eighteen in 1998 (76 million) is greater than that in 1960 (64 million), the proportion that children represent of the U.S. population has declined sharply over that same period, from 36 percent in 1960 to 28 percent in 1998. By 2010, the proportion of children is expected to be around 24 percent (U.S. Bureau of the Census, 1991, 1999e).

Minorities, including African Americans, Hispanics, Native Americans, and Asian Americans, now make up a larger proportion of the U.S. population than in the past. From 1980 to 1998, the Asian and Pacific Islander population more than doubled, from approximately 3.7 million (1.6 percent) to 10.5 million (3.9 percent). The Hispanic population also doubled, from 14.6 million (6.4 percent) to 30.2 million (11.2 percent), and the Alaskan Indian, Eskimo, and Aleut population increased over 70 percent, from 1.4 million (0.6 percent) to 2.4 million (0.9 percent). The growth of the Hispanic population has been due to both immigration and natural increase, while the rapid growth of the Asian population has been due largely to immigration. Around four out of ten of the legal immigrants to the United States since 1980 were from Asia (U.S. Bureau of the Census, 1999e).

The number and percentage of African Americans also increased, from 26.7 million (11.8 percent) in 1980 to 34.4 million (12.7 percent) in 1998. Although the actual number of whites increased from 1980 (194.7 million) to 1998 (223.0 million), the percentage they represented of the total U.S. population declined (from 85.9 percent to 82.5 percent). The rate of growth in the number of minority children in particular has been and is expected to continue to be greater than for white children over the coming decade (U.S. Bureau of the Census, 1999e).

Overall, U.S. baby boomer adults are an increasingly graying population, while new and newborn Americans increasingly reflect a rainbow of racial and ethnic diversity.

Ties Between People

The average number of people living in the same household has diminished steadily over time. The average number per household was 2.62 in 1998, down from 3.14 in 1970. Around 26 million people—one-quarter of U.S. households—live alone. This estimate represents an increase of around 8 million people since 1980 and more than a doubling of those living alone since 1970. This increase in one-person households reflects a combination of major social trends: more elderly widows, more young people delaying marriage, and lowered overall birthrates.

In 1998, 53 percent of U.S. households consisted of married-couple families, down from 61 percent in 1980 and 71 percent in 1970. The number and proportion of children living in single-parent families has also increased. In 1998, 32 percent of families with children under age eighteen were one-parent families, compared to 22 percent in 1980. Divorce and separation are the major causes of single parenthood. About half of U.S. marriages can be expected to end in divorce, and the majority involve children. The other major cause of single parenthood is out-of-wedlock births. In 1970 approximately 11 percent of all births in the United States were to unmarried mothers; by 1998 about a third were (U.S. Bureau of the Census, 1991, 1999e).

Although African American children are more likely to live with one parent than are white or other minority children, the growth in single parenthood was substantial for all racial and ethnic groups over the past three decades. Furthermore, although for whites the increase in the number of children living in single-parent families with their mother is primarily due to divorce and separation, the number of births among young, unmarried white women has also increased substantially over this period. Taken together, these trends suggest that more than half of all white children and three-fourths of African American children are likely to live some portion of their childhood in single-parent (largely female-head) families (National Commission on Children, 1991; U.S. Bureau of the Census, 1999e).

Around three out of ten of the elderly live alone, and the likelihood of living alone increases with age. Women outnumber men among all age categories of the elderly and account for the vast majority of the elderly living alone. Men, regardless of age, are much more likely to be living with a spouse. Most elderly women living by themselves are widows, although many may have contact with children or other relatives (Commonwealth Fund Commission on Elderly People Living Alone, 1988; U.S. Bureau of the Census, 1999e).

In summary, an increasing number of young as well as elderly U.S. adults are living by themselves, and more and more U.S. children are growing up in families with one, rather than two, parents at home to care for them.

The Neighborhood

Social and economic trends indicate a declining level of material and nonmaterial investments in U.S. neighborhoods and associated human capital resources (schools, jobs, family incomes, and housing).

The federal commitment to providing funds for education has declined since the 1970s. The proportion of total expenditures for elementary and secondary education provided by the federal government was 7.4 percent in 1970, rose to 9.1 percent in 1980, and then declined to 5.6 percent by 1990. This decline places greater demands on the state and local financing of public education. Considerable disparities exist within and across states in the level of investments in primary and secondary education, however. Equity in the financing of schools across well-to-do and poor districts has been a major political and legal controversy in many states and localities (Children's Defense Fund, 1990; U.S. Bureau of the Census, 1991, 1999e).

Since 1980 the number of high-paying jobs in manufacturing has decreased. Many of the new jobs that have been created are in the lower-paying service sector, such as the fast food industry and building and hotel maintenance and housekeeping sectors. Furthermore, despite generally more favorable economic trends, wages in the service sector have not increased as much as have those of managerial, professional, or technical workers. A contributor to the increasing disparity in wages between the lowest- and highest-paying sectors is the fact that between 1981 and 1990, the federal minimum wage remained constant at $3.35 per hour until 1990, when it was increased to $3.80, and then to $4.25 in 1991. By 1997 it had increased to $5.15 per hour. Even with this increase in the federal minimum wage, however, a parent working full time throughout the year at the minimum wage would still earn only around 80 percent of the poverty-level income for a family of three (Children's Defense Fund, 1998).

Trends in employment and associated wages during the previous decade, as well as changes in the tax laws during this same period, have contributed to increasing disparities in the distribution of family income in the United States. For example, in 1980 14.6 percent of the income overall was received by the U.S. families in the top 5 percent of the income categories; by 1998 their share had increased to 21.4 percent. A similar trend was observed for those who were in the top 20 percent income categories, whose share of income increased from 41.1 percent to 49.2 percent over the same period. For all other income tiers, the percentage share of income declined—and at progressively higher rates, the lower their family incomes. These trends are related to the fact that lower-wage salaries as well as welfare benefits have not kept pace with inflation. The number and percentage of Americans who have incomes below federal poverty-level standards declined substantially from 1960 (39.9 million, 22.2 percent) to 1979 (26.1 million, 11.7 percent), and then began to climb to between 13 and 15 percent during the 1980s and 1990s. In 1998, 12.7 percent or 34.5 million Americans were below the poverty level (U.S. Bureau of the Census, 1991, 1999c, 1999d, 1999e).

The number of affordable housing units for low-income families and individuals has sharply diminished since the late 1970s. Overall, assistance provided by the Department of Housing and Urban Development to add new units to the stock of low-income housing declined from about $32 billion in 1978 to about $10 billion in 1989, a reduction of over 80 percent adjusted for inflation. While spending for low-income housing has sharply declined, the federal government provides billions annually in indirect tax subsidies to homeowners through allowing them to deduct mortgage interest and property taxes for federal income tax purposes (Levitan, 1990). The lack of affordable housing is one of the major factors contributing to the increased number of homelessness since the early 1980s.

The impact of these economic and social trends has been greatest for vulnerable subgroups of the U.S. population.

Despite the overall growth in the economy, the percentage of children in poverty increased from 14.9 percent in 1970 to about 20 percent in the 1980s and 1990s. In 1997, 13.4 million (19.2 percent of) children were living in poverty. The percentage of poor children was much greater for African American (36.8 percent) and Hispanic (36.4 percent) compared to white (15.4 percent) children. Nonetheless, in absolute numbers, white children comprise the vast majority of poor children (U.S. Bureau of the Census, 1999e).

Families headed by women, high school dropouts, or persons younger than age twenty-five still face the greatest risks of living in poverty. Employment opportunities and earning potential during the previous decade have been most sharply reduced for young workers, particularly males, those with less than a high school education, and minorities. Young men between the ages of twenty and twenty-nine who cannot earn enough to support a family are three to four times less likely to marry than those with adequate earnings. Among those who are married, the man's economic status is generally enhanced at the time of divorce and the woman's diminished. An Urban Institute study, for example, found that the living standards for women and children fell to two-thirds of their former levels after a divorce, while the average man was slightly better off (Burkhauser & Duncan, 1988).

Although a much greater proportion of women, and particularly women who are single parents, have entered the labor force in recent years, women continue to earn lower average incomes than do men. For female heads of families who are on public assistance, the level of benefits has not kept pace with inflation. Although social security has greatly reduced the rates of poverty among the elderly, older women, and particularly minority women living alone, are much more likely to have incomes below the poverty level than are white males or those living with others (Commonwealth Fund Commission on Elderly People Living Alone, 1988; Levitan, 1990).

This review of the profile of and trends in the characteristics of the U.S. population has highlighted increasing social and economic vulnerability in general and for certain subgroups of Americans in particular.

Cross-Cutting Issues

An assessment of the impact of the availability of social status, social capital, and human capital resources on the risks of poor physical, psychological, and social health confirms that they have played an important role in exacerbating the vulnerability of many subgroups of U.S. society.

Social Status

Infants and children whose mothers are in economically impoverished circumstances are at particularly high risk of poor health (including cognitive or physical impairments, HIV/AIDS, or perinatal addiction) or being homeless. Adolescents are vulnerable because they are at a critical natural juncture in their own physical, emotional, and social development, which could be made more problematic if they are in chaotic, addictive, or abusive family situations.

The elderly often suffer a variety of losses, including economic self-sufficiency, physical or cognitive function, or the support and care of loved ones due to death or serious illness.

Both men and women are made vulnerable by gender role expectations. Single mothers are vulnerable because child care responsibilities may make it difficult for them to work full time. Even if they are working, they are likely to earn less than a male breadwinner would; the child's father may be providing little if any support; and if the mother does qualify for welfare assistance, the benefits are very limited and vary substantially across states. Drinking, smoking, and using drugs is the "macho" thing to do in many adolescent and young adult male subcultures. Family abuse and violence are directly rooted in the traditional economic and power-dependence relationships assumed between men, women, and children. Acts of violence within families often represent attempts on the part of those whom society sanctions as having power over others (husbands, parents of children, adult children of the elderly) to reinforce this position of dominance.

Elderly white males and young minority males may experience the loss of or blocked access to the job-related rewards of money, prestige, or accompanying sense of power or self-esteem. A consequence for many is a violent death—either at their own hand or as a result of violent encounters with others, often from within their own circle of acquaintances.

The origins of minorities' economic and social disadvantage lie deep in the fabric of American social and political history. Fewer than two generations of African Americans have been born since the civil rights movement of the 1960s and early 1970s that led to removing many racial barriers to jobs, schools, and housing that had evolved over years of overt racial discrimination.

Native Americans residing on reservations have been in a status of mandated dependency on federal prerogatives for generations. Many twentieth-century immigrants to the United States (a large number of whom are Hispanic or Asian) have come in search of a home, in response to the economic adversities and political conflict in their own countries.

These historical and political occurrences have had significant social, economic, physical, and psychological impacts on many foreign-born and racial and ethnic communities. U.S. policies over the past two decades have displayed vacillating levels of commitment and correspondingly mixed results in narrowing the associated racial and ethnic disparities in physical, psychological, and social health and well-being.

Social Capital

The absence of caring others in people's lives makes them especially vulnerable. Pregnant women who lack emotional or economic support from the child's father, other family members, or friends are less likely to be in a position readily to care for themselves and their child. Many chronically ill and disabled children and adults would not be able to live in their own homes without the support of family members and friends. Persons living with HIV/AIDS are particularly likely to experience the rejection or death of loved ones.

The prospect of developing mental illness, substance abuse, and violent behavior is strongly influenced by the nature and quality of connections one has with other people. Individuals who are in chaotic, addictive, or abusive family or social environments are much more likely to manifest these problems and have much less support to draw on to deal with them.

The wounds of broken relationships are particularly deep among abusing families, homeless persons, and immigrant and refugee populations. These individuals are especially likely to be bereft of a caring network of family or friends because of emotional estrangement, permanent physical separation, or death.

Human Capital

The investments that communities make in good jobs, schools, and housing and the corollary payoffs to individuals and families in terms of working, getting a good education, and having an adequate place to live directly affect vulnerability.

The diminished numbers of well-paying jobs in manufacturing and the movement of businesses and industry out of the core of major U.S. cities have resulted in a substantial loss of employment opportunities and a declining tax base for the support of public education in urban, inner-city neighborhoods. Urban regentrification and U.S. federal housing policy have sharply reduced the availability of affordable housing for low-income individuals and families in these same areas. The result of these and other changes has been the emergence of a hardcore, extremely socially and economically disadvantaged underclass, many of whom are likely to be numbered among the categories of vulnerable populations studied here: high-risk mothers and infants; people with chronic physical or mental illness or HIV/AIDS; alcohol and drug abusers; victims of suicidal, homicidal, or family violence; and homeless and immigrant populations (Braun, 1991; Jencks & Peterson, 1991; Katz, 1989; Kozol, 1991; Lynn & McGeary, 1990; Phillips, 1990, 1993; Wilson, 1980, 1989, 1990, 1996).

Population-Specific Overview

The discussion that follows reviews the effects of these social and economic changes on specific groups of the vulnerable. (See Table 4.1.)

High-Risk Mothers and Infants

The most vulnerable mothers and infants are those in a disadvantaged socioeconomic position, who experience the corollary environmental and behavioral risks associated with poverty, such as unsafe or unsupportive living situations or substance abuse.

TABLE 4.1. PRINCIPAL COMMUNITY CORRELATES OF VULNERABILITY.

Vulnerable Populations	Community Correlates		
	Social Status	Social Capital	Human Capital
High-risk mothers and infants	Minorities Adolescent and young women	Unmarried female head of family	Less than high school education Poor
Chronically ill and disabled	Minority children Elderly women	Female-headed families Living alone	Less than high school education Blue-collar job Poor Substandard housing
Persons living with HIV/AIDS	Minority men, women, children	Weak social networks	Less than high school education Unemployed Poor
Mentally ill and disabled	Minorities Adolescents Elderly	Separated, divorced, widowed	Unemployed Poor Substandard housing
Alcohol or substance abusers	Minorities Adolescent and young men	Single, separated, divorced	Less than high school education Unemployed Poor
Suicide or homicide prone	*Suicide* Adolescent and elderly white men *Homicide* Adolescent and young minority men	Single, separated, divorced, widowed Single	Unemployed Unemployed Poor
Abusing families	Infants, children, adolescents, elderly Girls and women	Weak social networks Not member of voluntary organizations	Less than high school education (especially women) Unemployed
Homeless persons	Infants, children, adolescents Women Minorities	Living alone Female-headed families Single, separated, divorced Weak social networks Not member of voluntary organizations	Unemployed Poor Substandard housing
Immigrants and refugees	Infants, children Women Minorities	Single, widowed Weak social networks Not member of voluntary organizations	Less than high school education Unemployed Poor Substandard housing

Social Status. The relative risks of inadequate prenatal care and adverse pregnancy outcomes (noted in Chapter Three) are considerably greater for African American compared to white mothers and infants. Research has examined the relative importance of social, biological, and medical factors in accounting for these differences. Substantial evidence exists that both the contemporary and historical effects of poverty and related risks (sanitation, crowding, nutrition, injury, smoking, and substance abuse) and resource disparities (income, insurance coverage) have played a major role in contributing to low birthweight and infant mortality differentials for African Americans compared to whites (Bird & Bauman, 1998; Collins & Hawkes, 1997; Hessol, Fuentes-Afflick, & Bacchetti, 1998).

The higher postneonatal mortality rates observed for Native Americans relative to whites are similarly related to the poorer socioeconomic conditions and associated problems experienced by Native American populations (unsafe environments, unemployment, family disorganization, and alcoholism) (Honigfeld & Kaplan, 1987).

The fact that Hispanics have lower rates of prenatal care utilization, in tandem with lower infant mortality rates, is hypothesized to be due to cultural factors that inhibit other risk factors associated with high-risk pregnancies, such as out-of-wedlock births, maternal smoking, and alcohol use (Scribner & Dwyer, 1989; Zaid, Fullerton, & Moore, 1996).

Social Capital. Well-developed social networks help to mediate stress and provide resources to cope with the fact of being pregnant. Such networks can, however, either encourage or discourage a woman from seeking prenatal care, depending on the particular attitudes or beliefs of network members. Inner-city African American women are more likely to be unmarried, to rely on female relatives or friends, and to feel a lack of social, emotional, and material support during their pregnancy. The presence (or absence) of strong social networks can directly affect whether they receive encouragement or support (child care, for example) to seek prenatal care (St. Clair, Smeriglio, Alexander, & Celentano, 1989; Turner, Grindstaff, & Phillips, 1990).

Human Capital. Mothers with less than a high school education are much more likely to have inadequate prenatal care and poor pregnancy outcomes (Institute of Medicine, 1985, 1988d). The impact of mother's education has been variously explained by the father's education, family income, a higher probability of being employed, a greater awareness of preventive health practices, and more coping resources (Cleland & van Ginneken, 1988). Based on analyses of data from United Nations–sponsored surveys in over thirty countries, Cleland and van Ginneken (1988) estimated that the economic advantages associated with mother's education (such as having adequate income and housing) accounted for about half of the education-related differentials observed in infant and child mortality rates.

Multilevel modeling of neighborhood risk factors, such as per capita income, unemployment, and crime rates, has documented the role of these macrolevel social factors in explaining higher rates of low birthweight among inner-city residents in the United States (O'Campo, Xue, Wang, & Caughy, 1997).

Chronically Ill and Disabled   *Men*   *Elderly women*

The availability of social, economic, and community resources directly affects the prospects for physical, psychological, and social functioning among the chronically ill and disabled of all ages.

Social Status. Chronically ill children have been characterized as children with special needs or special health care needs. These include the traditional categories of children who are physically or cognitively disabled, as well as an increasingly prevalent number of those with "new morbidities," such as developmental, learning, and behavioral problems, eating disorders, allergies, and asthma—conditions thought to have large psychosocial components attributed to the growing proportion of children who experience parental divorce, are born to single-parent families, or are raised in low-income, low-education households (Perrin, 1998; Pless, 1998; Shelton, Jeppson, & Johnson, 1989; Zill & Schoenborn, 1990).

The risks of death or disability from injury are much greater for poor and African American and Native American compared to white, economically advantaged children. The risks of having no or inadequate prenatal care, less than an optimum birthweight, or congenital or birth-associated disabilities are greater for minority and economically disadvantaged mothers and infants. Some disability (such as ventilator dependency) is, in fact, created by the high-technology interventions employed to save high-risk newborns (Office of Technology Assessment, 1987b).

The probability of being disabled increases substantially with age. However, an important emphasis in public health and health care research is on the causes and correlates of functional disability among the elderly and the interventions most likely to "compress morbidity" in terms of the number of years individuals experience illness or disability as they age (Olshansky & Ault, 1986), enhance "successful aging" (Roos & Havens, 1991), and increase "quality-adjusted life years (QALYs)" (Rothenberg & Koplan, 1990). Trend data from the U.S. Bureau of the Census Survey of Income and Program Participation (SIPP) suggest that substantial declines have occurred in the prevalence of selected functional limitations (difficulty in seeing, lifting and carrying, climbing, and walking) among the elderly since the mid-1980s (McNeil, 1997).

Nonetheless, the feminization of poverty, particularly among the elderly, as well as the growing proportion of elderly women living alone, compound the prospect of poor health and associated functional dependence for women as they age (Commonwealth Fund Commission on Elderly People Living Alone, 1987, 1988; Stone, 1989).

Social Capital. The social support provided by kinship and friendship networks plays an important role in mitigating the risks of chronic illness. Elderly married individuals, especially men, are much more likely to engage in preventive be- haviors, such as eating breakfast, participating in physical activity, and having their blood pressure checked, than their unmarried counterparts (Schone & Weinick, 1998). Controlling for race and income differentials, individuals who live in communities with high concentrations of female-headed families are more likely to die prematurely than those who do not, which may be associated with the types or magnitude of social support available to such families (LeClere, Rogers, & Peters, 1998; Mansfield, Wilson, Kobrinski, & Mitchell, 1999).

A great deal of research has focused on the impact of caregiving and social support available to the elderly from family or friends for reducing the need for institutionalized care. The physiological and psychological benefits appear to be greatest when this care maximizes the individual's own perceived goals and ca- pacity for independence (Magaziner & Cadigan, 1988; Manton, 1989).

Human Capital. Long-term economic deprivation has been found to have an important impact on health status, functioning, and mortality (Liao, McGee, Kaufman, Cao, & Cooper, 1999; Rahkonen, Lahelma, & Huuhka, 1997). The cumulative effects of residential segregation and poverty are, for example, cred- ited with higher rates of morbidity (illness) and mortality (death) due to cardio- vascular and other chronic diseases among U.S. blacks (Diez-Roux, Northridge, Morabia, Bassett, & Shea, 1999; Hart, Kunitz, Sell, & Mukamel, 1998; Kingston & Smith, 1997).

Job-related stressors, threats to employment security, and chronic unemploy- ment have been found to be associated with higher rates of morbidity and mor- tality (Blank & Diderichsen, 1996; Ferrie, Shipley, Marmot, Stansfeld, & Smith, 1998; Mansfield, Wilson, Kobrinski, & Mitchell, 1999). The jobs that working- age adults assume affect the likelihood of their being injured and subsequently unable to work. The incidence of injury tends to be highest for laborers, particu- larly those involved in the construction and mining industries (Griss, 1988; Na- tional Center for Health Statistics, 1989b). The working-age disabled are more likely to have less than a high school education, to be poor, and to have been em- ployed in blue-collar jobs than are their nondisabled counterparts (International Center for the Disabled, 1986; Office of Assistant Secretary for Planning and Evaluation, 1995).

Individuals, especially the elderly, who live in unsafe neighborhoods are less likely to engage in regular physical exercise activity (Centers for Disease Control and Prevention, 1999c; Yen & Kaplan, 1998). To maximize the ability of disabled elderly and others to live in their homes and function on their own, adaptations to their housing are often required (Manton, 1989).

Persons Living with HIV/AIDS

A complex profile of social and economic disadvantage has contributed to the spread of HIV/AIDS, particularly among minority men, women, and children.

Social Status. The disproportionate occurrence of HIV/AIDS among socially and economically disadvantaged urban inner-city populations has been referred to as a "syndemic," resulting from "the set of synergistic or intertwined and mutual enhancing health and social problems facing the urban poor" (Singer, 1994, p. 933). The impoverishment of women and those who are single parents contributes to the prospect of domination and violence by male sex partners, the corollary exposure to or use of alcohol or drugs, and, in an increasing number of cases, prostitution for sex or other drug-related economic activity. High rates of unemployment and associated drug-related activity among minority males increase their risk of contracting HIV/AIDS. The sharing of needles for illicit drug injections or even sharing sewing needles for cosmetic purposes, such as do-it-yourself tattoos or body piercing, is also more likely to occur among the poor (Chavkin, 1995; Farmer, Connors & Simmons, 1996; Zierler & Krieger, 1997). The spread of HIV/AIDS into rural areas of the United States has also disproportionately affected low-income minority populations, and particularly women (Berry, 1993; Graham, Forrester, Wysong, Rosenthal, & James, 1995).

Social Capital. The advent of HIV/AIDS has called into question the traditional concepts of family and social supports available to mediate the stress that leads to high-risk behavior, as well as to assist in caring for those with the illness. Infants and children with HIV/AIDS face the prospect of being abandoned by their families because the parents, who are themselves likely to be infected with the disease, either have died or are physically, financially, or otherwise not able to care for the infant (Chavkin, 1995; National Research Council, 1993; Ramirez-Valles, Zimmerman, & Newcomb, 1998). The emergence of a well-kept family secret from the closet when a young homosexual male contracts the disease has challenged the capacity of many families and communities to deal openly with the issue. The resulting discrimination and fear of reprisal have tended to drive many at-risk individuals underground instead of encouraging them to seek appropriate information or counsel (Levine, 1990; Macklin, 1989).

Effective social networks within the gay male community have facilitated the sharing of information requisite to reducing the prevalence of high-risk sexual practices. Identifying sociometric linkages among HIV drug users and their sexual partners assists in pinpointing likely points of educational or behavioral intervention within these high-risk populations (Auerbach, Wypijewska, & Brodie,

1994; Friedman et al., 1997; National Research Council, 1993; Normand, Vlahov, & Moses, 1995).

Human Capital. The school dropout rates for minority adolescents are higher than those of whites, so that they are less likely to have the benefit of school-based sex or HIV/AIDS education programs. Community-based educational efforts often fail to orient their messages to the unique language, literacy, or cultural aspects of high-risk racial and ethnic communities (Kirp et al., 1989).

In the early stages of the epidemic, persons living with HIV/AIDS were often dismissed from their jobs, with a resultant loss in income and insurance benefits required to obtain adequate medical care. Subsequent amendments to the civil rights bill barred dismissals from employment due to having AIDS and levied fines on companies that did so (American Public Health Association, 1989). Yelin, Greenblatt, Hollander, and McMaster (1991) found, in a study in San Francisco, that half of those with HIV-related illness were physically unable to continue working two years after the onset of symptoms. Unstable housing situations experienced by persons living with HIV/AIDS can also result in less access and continuity of care, as well as poorer functional health status (Arno et al., 1996).

Mentally Ill and Disabled

Mental illness has been attributed to both biological and environmental determinants. The dominant model in the study of the psychosocial causes of mental illness emphasizes the role that stressful life events, particularly those that require a great deal of change or adaptation (both positive events such as marriage and negative ones such as the loss of a spouse), play in producing mental illness. Both social resources (such as social support) and personal resources (such as a sense of personal control or mastery) can mediate the effects of these stresses. The stresses and the resources for dealing with them are, however, differentially distributed by age and gender, minority status, poverty level, family structure, and employment status.

Social Status. Adolescence and young adulthood are important periods for the onset of major mental illness, such as unipolar major depression, bipolar illness, phobias, and drug and alcohol abuse and dependence. The major social stressors associated with the onset of mental illness in children are poverty, minority group status, having parents who were mentally ill or alcoholic, living in divorced or single-parent families, having experienced serious abuse or neglect, or having a major chronic illness. Poor, single, female heads of households experience particularly high levels of stress and mental illness as a result of both diminished social support and the increased environmental stressors associated with poverty (Administration for Children, Youth and Families, Children's Bureau, 1999; Johnson, Cohen, Brown, Smailes, & Bernstein, 1999; Wyshak & Modest, 1996).

The effects of minority status on mental health are associated with the influence of socioeconomic disadvantage. Baker (1987) has pointed out that the mental health of African Americans at all stages of the life cycle is affected by their membership in a "victim system," which includes historical and existing barriers to equivalent educational and job opportunities. These in turn limit educational and economic attainment, which lead to poverty and exacerbate the stress on both individuals and families. Research comparing minorities (particularly African Americans and Hispanics) and whites has found that after controlling for age, gender, education, and income, differences in mental health status observed between racial or ethnic groups tend to diminish or disappear (Golding & Lipton, 1990).

The major stressors that have been found to be associated with greater mental illness among Native Americans, particularly children, are recurrent otitis media (middle ear infections) and the consequences for learning disabilities and psychosocial deficits, fetal alcohol syndrome, physical and sexual abuse and neglect, parental alcoholism, family disruption, and poor school environments (McShane, 1988; Office of Technology Assessment, 1990).

Social Capital. Family disruption (through death or divorce, for example) has been found to be associated with a greater prevalence of both adult and childhood mental disorders. Individuals who lack social support, from family or other sources, have been found to experience more stress, and hence greater mental illness, than those who did not have this stress-buffering resource available to them. This is particularly the case for individuals who lack personal coping resources as well, such as feelings of self-esteem and personal mastery (Rosenfield, 1989; Tweed, Schoenbach, George, & Blazer, 1989).

Human Capital. Two major theoretical explanations—social stress and social selection—have traditionally been used to account for the greater prevalence of mental illness among individuals with lower socioeconomic status (SES). The social stress explanation suggests that rates of some types of disorders are higher in lower-SES groups because of the greater environmental adversity they experience, such as unemployment, inadequate housing, and crime. The social selection explanation argues, particularly with respect to rates of schizophrenia, that persons with these disorders or characteristics predisposing them to these disorders drift down or fail to rise out of the lower-SES groups. The factors that predispose schizophrenia in this case may be due to genetics or intrauterine events that influence subsequent neurological development.

Dohrenwend (1990) has pointed out that psychiatric epidemiology has tended to focus on the microlevel (individual and psychological) correlates of stress rather than macrolevel (environmental and societal) correlates, such as SES. He argues, however, for a more in-depth, analytic look in understanding both the structural and psychological dynamics of socioeconomic status that could account for the persistent differences in serious mental illness by SES. For example, unemployment, particularly chronic unemployment, as well as the resulting lowered self-esteem, have been found to be associated with poorer mental health status, although the precise causal direction of the relationship between these factors is difficult to determine.

Alcohol or Substance Abusers

The origins of substance abuse have been examined from the physiological, developmental, and cultural perspectives, that is, from the point of view of the contributions of neurobiological mechanisms (effects on dopamine transmission), particular events in an individual's normal life course (such as adolescence or aging), as well as the values and norms derived from families, peers, and the larger social environment (such as drinking attitudes and practices).

Social Status. Adolescence is a period in which a high probability exists for initiating drinking, smoking, and the use of drugs. This stage of development is characterized by more risk taking in general in the context of the normal developmental task of transition to the independence of adulthood, as well as a heightened susceptibility to the influence of peers on behavior. The initiation of the use of certain substances during the teen years (such as alcohol, smokeless tobacco, or marijuana) appears to increase the propensity for, or serve as a gateway to, the use of more serious or addictive drugs (such as cigarettes or cocaine) later. Excessive use of these gateway substances and progression to more serious substance abuse or dependence are often associated with a complex of other problem behaviors, such as poor school performance, truancy, or delinquent criminal behavior (Archambault, 1989; Bailey & Hubbard, 1990; Ellickson, Collins, & Bell, 1999; Henderson & Anderson, 1989; Jones & Battjes, 1990b).

Research on the neurological mechanisms of addiction has documented that the reinforcing properties of different substances (such as nicotine and cocaine or marijuana and heroin) may map on the same underlying neurological structures, thereby supporting the idea that common substrates for these addictive substances exist. This and related genetic research may therefore help to explain clinical and epidemiological observations that the use of gateway substances may well give rise to the use of others (Koob & Le Moal, 1997; Pich et al., 1997; Tanda, Pontieri, & Di Chiara, 1997; True et al., 1999).

Adolescence is also a period of transition toward separation from family. Research suggests that at other stages of the life course, separation, loss, or isolation from family or caring others through divorce or death can give rise to the onset of serious substance abuse problems. Although the elderly have lower rates of use of alcohol, around 2 to 10 percent of the elderly are estimated to have problems with alcohol abuse or dependence. For some elderly, late-onset alcoholism may be a response to serious losses of physical, psychological, or social functioning (Lawson, 1989).

The pattern of distribution of mental health and related substance abuse disorders also varies by gender. Underlying affective disorders are more often manifested in substance abuse (alcoholism and drug abuse) among men and in clinical depression among women (Regier et al., 1990; Robins & Regier, 1991).

Cultural factors play a large role in influencing the patterns of substance use and abuse for different racial and ethnic groups. The use of certain drugs (such as peyote) has been a component of traditional religious and spiritual practices in some Hispanic and Native American subcultures. The role of alcohol in the social life of different racial and ethnic subgroups (such as the Irish, Italian, Muslim, and Jewish cultures) also influences the levels and patterns of consumption across these groups. Both advertising and cultural norms attribute desired gender role characteristics (such as the image of being "macho" for males or "liberated" for women) to smoking or the use of smokeless tobacco (Beauvais, Oetting, Wolf, & Edwards, 1989; Brown & Tooley, 1989; Collins, 1996; Eden & Aguilar, 1989; Moncher, Holden, & Trimble, 1990).

Social Capital. Families play a significant role in the development and transmission of substance use and abuse practices. Research has demonstrated a genetic link with alcohol abuse and, to some extent, drug abuse. The impact of biological vulnerability on alcohol and drug abuse is, however, intertwined with the corollary influences of the family and the larger social and cultural environment of which the individual is a part (Pickens & Svikis, 1988; Plant, Orford, & Grant, 1989; Reich, Cloninger, Van Eerdewegh, Rice, & Mullaney, 1988).

Substantial evidence exists that both the presence and quality of family ties and the attitudes and practices of families themselves are correlated with individual members' propensity to drink, smoke, or use drugs. Rates of alcoholism, smoking, and drug use are higher among adults and children in families in which the parents are divorced or separated or in which there is considerable family dysfunction or disorganization. Substance abuse may, however, be either a cause or a consequence of family dysfunction and dissolution (Chilcoat, Breslau, & Anthony, 1996; Wolfinger, 1998).

Human Capital. The patterns of substance use and abuse by income and education vary for different substances. The prevalence of smoking is less among those with higher levels of education and income, whereas the opposite is the case for the use of alcohol. Cocaine was traditionally a drug of the rich and heroin that of the poor. The availability of crack and other cheaper forms of cocaine has resulted in its wider use among low-income populations (Escobedo, Anda, Smith, Remington, & Mast, 1990).

Unemployment and underemployment are both correlates and consequences of substance (particularly alcohol and drug) abuse. Rates of substance abuse are higher among the unemployed. Lost earnings potential is also substantial for those who are unable to work regularly because of problems with alcoholism, drugs, or smoking-related illnesses. On the other hand, being employed can present a double hazard for smokers who work in occupations for which there is also a high risk of exposure to dust, fumes, or toxic chemicals (Mullahy & Sindelar, 1989; Sterling & Weinkam, 1989).

Suicide or Homicide Prone

Elderly white men [handwritten margin note]

Biological, psychological, and sociological explanations have been offered for intentional acts of violence that culminate in suicides or homicides. Biological theories focus on the correlation of genetic or biochemical indicators with violent intentions or acts. Biopsychiatric models examine the role of aggression in human development and behavior. Psychiatrically or psychologically oriented explanations of suicide and homicide explore the role of losses of or separation from significant love objects, poor self-esteem, mental illness, and substance abuse. In addition, strong support exists for sociological explanations of violence, which emphasize the impact of social status (age, gender, race), social integration (or support), and ecological (labor market) factors (Hardwick & Rowton-Lee, 1996; Lawrence, 1994; Pettit, 1997; Raine, Brennan, Mednick, & Mednick, 1996; Reiss & Roth, 1993).

Social Status. Poverty, sexism, and racism, and the resultant differentials in wealth and power, are credited with being significant predictors of violence (Gibbs, 1988; Stark, 1990).

Widow [handwritten margin note]

Stark (1990) argued that interpersonal violence is basically a "friendly affair" rooted in patterns of male-female and related power dominance and abuse. Children who are abused or grow up in environments in which they witness substantial violence are more likely to perpetuate these patterns in their own adult lives (Canetto & Sakinofsky, 1998; Durant, Pendergrast, & Cadenhead, 1994; Fitzpatrick, 1997; Osofsky, Wewers, Hann, & Fick, 1993).

Among Hispanics, suicidal and homicidal tendencies have been found to be higher among those with psychiatric diagnoses, alcohol and drug abuse, lower educational attainment, lower incomes, or who were divorced or separated (Martinez, 1996). However, cultural factors such as familism (a strong orientation toward the authority and ties of family) and fatalism (attribution of circumstances to factors that humans are powerless to change) have been credited with moderating suicide rates for Hispanics (Hoppe & Martin, 1986).

The risk factors associated with higher rates of suicide among Native Americans include a history of mental health problems, having another family member or friend who committed suicide, alcohol problems, and a history of sexual or physical abuse (Grossman, Milligan, & Deyo, 1991). The collapse of traditional Native American ways of life and religion, high unemployment, and sending children to boarding schools have been credited with exacerbating chaotic family structures and associated substance abuse that give rise to higher rates of suicide and interpersonal violence (Berlin, 1987; EchoHawk, 1997).

Social Capital. Durkheim posited the role of social integration (or ties) with others (through families, friendships, neighborhoods, work, or voluntary associations, for example) as predictors of suicidal behavior. He identified three types of suicide that could result from isolation from a human community (egoistic), total identification with such a community to the extent that one's own self-interests are denied (altruistic), or ambiguity and uncertainty regarding one's roles in or contributions to such a community as a result of major political or economic changes (anomic) (Gibbs, 1988; Kreitman, 1988; Leenaars, Yang, & Lester, 1993).

Homicide and suicide rates are higher among individuals in chaotic or abusive family environments (Rudd, 1990; Tolan, 1988). Lack of parental supervision at home and lack of family involvement in school are considered to be important factors in contributing to violent incidents in schools (Mushinski, 1994). The rates of suicidal ideation and attempts among gay, lesbian, and bisexual adolescents are much higher than among heterosexual adolescents, which has been attributed to family and societal homophobia and rejection (Fergusson, Horwood, & Beautrais, 1999; Remafedi, 1999; Safren & Heimberg, 1999). The high suicide rates among the elderly are attributed to illness, economic insecurity, and the losses and associated loneliness, isolation, and depression that result from the death of a spouse or adult children moving away during this stage of life (Achté, 1988; Grabbe, Demi, Camann, & Potter, 1997; Kposowa, Breault, & Singh, 1995).

Rates of firearm-related crime are higher in communities in which there are lower levels of social capital, reflected in group membership and social trust. These problems are exacerbated in neighborhoods that are racially segregated or for which there has been substantial economic disinvestment and decline (Fullilove et al., 1998; Kennedy, Kawachi, Prothrow-Stith, Lochner, & Gupta, 1998; Peterson & Krivo, 1993; Wilkinson, Kawachi, & Kennedy, 1998).

Human Capital. Ecological explanations have focused on the role of broad economic or demographic trends, such as the unemployment or competition resulting from downturns in the economy, growing income inequality, and a large age cohort seeking access to limited employment or educational opportunities (Dooley, Catalano, Rook, & Serxner, 1989a, 1989b; Stack, 1996–1997; Szwarcwald, Bastos, Viacava, & de Andrade, 1999). Trends related to racial or economic ghettoization; overcrowding; locally unwanted land uses; temporarily obsolete, abandoned, or derelict industrial sites; and related deterioration in area businesses and housing are correlated with high rates of violence in urban neighborhoods (Greenberg & Schneider, 1994; Morenoff & Sampson, 1997; Stack, 1996–1997; Wallace & Wallace, 1998). The availability and ownership of firearms have also been found to be highly associated with violent death rates (Cummings, Koepsell, Grossman, Savarino, & Thompson, 1997; Kaplan & Geling, 1998; Kaplan, Adamek, & Johnson, 1994).

The high rates of male (particularly young white male) suicides have been attributed to the increased ambiguity and loss of power associated with changing gender roles, as well as the increasing difficulties in general, given shifts in the U.S. economy, in finding and retaining well-paying jobs (Sanborn, 1990). Increased rates of violence turned inward (suicide) have resulted because white males tend to blame themselves for perceived personal, educational, or professional failures, since societal expectations and objective opportunities for success have traditionally been greater for them (Osgood & McIntosh, 1986).

The high rates of violence turned outward (homicide) among black males have been attributed to responses to blocked opportunities, exacerbated and sustained by racial and socioeconomic discrimination, diminished levels of investments in inner-city schools and institutions, and the growth of the drug economy in many minority neighborhoods (Fullilove et al., 1998; Kennedy, Kawachi, Prothrow-Stith, Lochner, & Gupta, 1998; Peterson & Krivo, 1993; Phillips, 1997; Wilkinson, Kawachi, & Kennedy, 1998). An estimated 8.6 percent of black non-Hispanic males twenty-five to twenty-nine years of age were in prison in 1997, compared to 2.7 percent of Hispanic males and 0.9 percent of white males in the same age group (Beck & Mumola, 1999).

Abusing Families

The principal correlates of family violence are rooted in the differential availability of personal, social, and human resources (see Figure 1.2): the social inequality associated with the statuses of age, gender, race, and income, among others, and the social isolation of families and individuals reinforced by norms of privacy and patriarchal dominance that have traditionally governed family life in our and other societies (Gelles & Cornell, 1990; Straus, 1988).

Social Status. Initially child abuse was identified and defined as a medical problem, based on the evidence gathered by physicians in the early 1960s and 1970s of childhood injuries that clearly resulted from externally imposed trauma. This early characterization led to the medical-clinical identification of the battered child syndrome and the exploration of the causes of this and other forms of violence among intimates from individually oriented psychiatric and psychopathological perspectives on the mental health of the batterer (Helfer & Kempe, 1987). With the availability of more empirical evidence on the perpetrators, as well as the victims, of intimate violence, theory development in this area has shifted from micro (individual) to more macro (societal) levels of explanations and analysis. These include perspectives that emphasize patterns of abuse or neglect as learned behaviors that lead to intergenerational cycles of violence (social learning theory); the fact that there are rewards (such as control and dominance) as well as costs (risk of arrest) associated with such behaviors (exchange theory); and that fundamental social inequalities, such as those associated with men's and women's gender roles and differential access to wealth in our society, help to empower and sanction a culture of intrafamily and interpersonal violence (social-situational or social systems theory).

Typically wide power differentials exist between the subject and object of maltreatment, linked to the social statuses they occupy respectively. Furthermore, maltreatment most often occurs at the interstices where the relative power differentials between groups tend to be the greatest (parent-to-child, husband-to-wife, and caretaker-to-dependent elderly). Patterned modes of interaction between these groups that lead to violence are clearly rooted in long-standing historical, sociocultural, and social-structural norms. Tenets such as "spare the rod, and spoil the child" and related child-rearing practices have been and continue to be endorsed in many U.S. families. The "rule of thumb" refers to eighteenth-century law that a husband had the right to chastise his wife physically, as long as the stick or strap he used was no wider than his thumb. Patriarchal systems of family organization have traditionally assumed that the male is the head of the family, that boys must be trained to be manly and dominant, and that girls learn to be feminine and submissive.

Social Capital. Social isolation is also a defining characteristic of many abusing families. The families in which child or spousal abuse occurs are much less likely to participate in organized community or religious activities or to have informal social ties with neighbors or other friendship networks. The abused elderly are particularly likely to be invisible, since they may have been relocated from their own homes to be cared for by a child or other relative and are less likely to participate in external activities, such as going to work regularly, that would carry them into contact with other people. Further, the perpetrators of maltreatment often use force or intimidation to insulate their victims from social contact and thereby avoid detection.

Human Capital. Empirical evidence regarding the perpetrators and victims of maltreatment points clearly to the socioeconomic origins of the problem. The profile of abusive families, outlined in Chapter Three, highlighted the fact that rates of abuse were highest in families in which poverty and related unemployment or underemployment and inadequate housing were problematic, and in which the male head of the household experienced considerable status insecurity or inconsistency, relative to his desired goals and expectations. The risk of intrafamilial violence is also exacerbated when the women involved have less education or occupational skills for achieving economic self-sufficiency, and thereby the means for removing themselves from the abusive situation (Hotaling, Finkelhor, Kirkpatrick, & Straus, 1988a; 1988b; Vinokur, Price, & Caplan, 1996; Wolfner & Gelles, 1993).

The dependence of elderly on others resulting from the loss of physical or cognitive functioning, and the corollary loss of power and control over personal or financial resources, have been found to be associated with caregivers' propensity to abuse or neglect their dependent charges (Quinn & Tomita, 1986; Steinmetz, 1988).

These and other reported correlates of intrafamilial abuse or neglect (such as alcoholism or the intergenerational transmission of learned behaviors) do not fully explain these outcomes. Further, a substantial proportion of families that possess many or all of the characteristics of abusive families do not evidence these behaviors.

A fundamental look at the elements of the social structure that promote and sanction the power and dominance of certain individuals over others and reinforce the isolation, rather than the ties, between people is an important place to begin to mediate the harm to some of the most vulnerable in our society: those who are dependent on their very survival on intimate others who injure or neglect them.

Homeless Persons

The major reason for the growing number of homeless men, women, and children in the past two decades is the diminished availability of affordable housing for people who are poor or at risk due to other limitations in physical, psychological, or social functioning, such as mental illness, substance abuse, or family violence.

Social Status. Social, political, and economic trends have made it increasingly difficult for low-income people to afford a roof over their heads, and a diminished stock of low-income housing has increased the price of units (Burt, 1992; Institute of Medicine, 1988c; Rossi, 1989, 1990).

Children and youth are an increasingly visible and vulnerable component of the homeless population. An estimated 68,000 to 100,000 children are thought to be homeless at any given time. Homeless children are much more likely to experience physical, mental, emotional, educational, developmental, and behavioral problems and less likely to have obtained basic preventive health care services, such as immunizations, compared to children who are not homeless (Bassuk, Weinreb, Dawson, Perloff, & Buckner, 1997; General Accounting Office, 1989b; Shulsinger, 1990; Weinreb, Goldberg, Bassuk, & Perloff, 1998; Wood, Valdez, Hayashi, & Shen, 1990; Zima, Bussing, Forness, & Benjamin, 1997).

Very young children are likely to be accompanied by their mothers. However, there are an increasing number of runaway, throwaway, or homeless youth (older children and teenagers) as well, living on their own with little or no contact with kin. Many such youth literally deem themselves homeless rather than runaway, since their families have forcibly expelled them from their homes. These families are often ones in which there were problems of physical, sexual, substance, or other abuse (General Accounting Office, 1989b; Pennbridge, Yates, David, & Mackenzie, 1990; Ringwalt, Greene, Robertson, & McPheeters, 1998).

Women and minorities are also particularly vulnerable groups of homeless. The prevalence of mental illness appears to be greater among homeless women, while alcohol and substance abuse are more prevalent among homeless men, as is the case in the general population. Homeless women are uniquely vulnerable to unwanted pregnancies, adverse birth outcomes, and sexual and physical assault. Among low-income women, being pregnant may put them at a higher risk of homelessness. The traditional social and economic inequities by race and gender, reinforced by the increasing proportion of women, children, and minorities among the poor, also contribute to their increasing number among homeless persons (Anderson, Boe, & Smith, 1988; Bassuk, 1993; Bassuk & Weinreb, 1993; Weitzman, 1989).

Social Capital. A unique and particularly important characteristic across all categories of homeless persons is their social isolation. The homeless are much less likely to have regular or strong social ties with family, friends, or other social networks, which further increases their vulnerability to other disabilities or deprivations. Rossi, Wright, Fisher, and Willis (1987, p. 1339) conclude, "The implication of widespread social isolation is that the literal homeless lack access to extended social networks and are therefore especially vulnerable to the vagaries of fortune occasioned by changes in employment, income, or physical or mental health."

Studies of the social networks for homeless families and children document that their relationships with network members are complex and may yield either negative or positive consequences for them. Such networks may offer some measure of emotional support or provide temporary housing. On the other hand, they may represent family contexts that put them at high risk of violence or abuse from which they have sought to escape, or street environments in which they have subsequently sought refuge that nonetheless put them at higher risk of drug abuse, HIV/AIDS transmission, or involvement in criminal activity. Many homeless persons also have a history of homelessness or out-of-home placement as children (Bassuk et al., 1997; Bogard, McConnell, Gerstel, & Schwartz, 1999; Ennett, Bailey, & Federman, 1999; Koegel, Melamid, & Burnam, 1995).

Human Capital. Rossi (1990), in defining the key distinction between the "old" homeless in the decades from 1950 to 1970 and the "new" homeless, concluded that most homeless persons in previous decades had some shelter (flophouses, single-room occupancy hotels, or mission shelters), although it was inadequate by any standards. Very few were literally sleeping on the streets, as do many of the contemporary homeless.

A direct relationship exists between the reduced availability of low-cost housing and the increased number of homeless. The supply of low-income housing stock has declined significantly since the 1950s, due to conversion, abandonment, fire, or demolition. The extremely low rate of replacement of low-income housing has not kept pace with this natural attrition. The reduction of low-income housing stock was accelerated in particular during the 1980s as urban renewal and associated regentrification resulted in the widespread demolition of flophouses and single-room-occupancy hotels traditionally occupied by skid row residents, and the replacement of these units with middle- and upper-class housing (such as condominiums and townhouses) and shopping or other business complexes (Burt, 1992; Institute of Medicine, 1988c; Rossi, 1989, 1990; U.S. Commission on Security and Cooperation in Europe, 1990).

A corollary policy development exacerbating the decline in affordable housing for the poor was the withdrawal of a federal role in subsidizing low-income housing alternatives. From the depression years until 1980, the federal government was the primary source of low-income housing subsidies. Since 1980, federal support has been substantially reduced, and most of the remaining subsidies represent commitments made prior to 1980. Between 1981 and 1989, the federal budget authority for subsidized housing dropped more than 80 percent (Burt, 1992; Institute of Medicine, 1988c; Levitan, 1990).

Other factors cited as major contributors to the growing number of homeless are the deinstitutionalization of the chronically mentally ill population, the expanding prevalence of substance abuse, welfare reform, and the increased social isolation resulting from marital dissolution, mobility, and family violence. Rossi (1990) pointed out, in his analysis of the old and new homeless, that in some sense, these were problems for the old as well as the new homeless. Both the former and current generations of homeless were extremely poor, had tenuous or no ties with families or friends, and suffered from disabilities associated with physical disabilities, alcohol or drug abuse, and mental illness. To the extent that these deprivations and disabilities are becoming more prevalent, particularly for certain subgroups in society, the likelihood of their being homeless will also increase. Deinstitutionalization, however, particularly exacerbated the problem of homelessness because of the failure, in implementing this policy, to develop a system of housing and other supportive services before releasing vulnerable mentally ill and disabled individuals into the community. Other causes of homelessness, especially among women and children, include welfare's not keeping up with inflation and welfare reform that has limited the time period or benefits available (Bassuk, Browne, & Buckner, 1996; Institute of Medicine, 1988c; Rossi, 1989, 1990).

Immigrants and Refugees

Refugees and undocumented persons are particularly vulnerable categories of in-migrants to the United States because of fewer economic and social resources and ties.

Social Status. Many refugees experience substantial problems in adjusting to life in the United States because of the vast cultural differences with their home countries and the traumatic and violent circumstances often associated with their exodus. For example, the Khmer refugees, many of whom were from rural areas of Cambodia, and the Hmong refugees, who were predominantly subsistence farmers from the mountains of northern Laos, experience many problems in adjusting to urban life in the United States, many in the most impoverished core of U.S. cities.

In some refugee groups, women are much less likely to have formal education; they are unable to read or write their own language, much less English. The roles traditionally assumed by such women in their own societies are often brutally disrupted by the death of a spouse or other significant family members or by the experiences of rape or sexual assault. The prevalence of depression and posttraumatic stress syndrome is great among certain refugee populations, and particularly refugee women and children, as a result (Allden et al., 1996; Caspi,

Poole, Mollica, & Frankel, 1998; Kim & Grant, 1997; McCloskey, Figueredo, & Koss, 1995; McCloskey, Southwick, Fernandez-Esquer, & Locke, 1995; Mollica et al., 1998; Quirk & Casco, 1994; Weine et al., 1995).

In some groups of immigrants, there are often groupings that clearly reflect more socially and economically advantaged versus disadvantaged statuses, based on socioeconomic level, migration cohort, or refugee status. These most disadvantaged subgroups are least likely to have had routine preventive care (such as childhood immunizations, dental and prenatal care) and to have the most and most serious health problems, such as gastrointestinal disorders, parasitic infections, respiratory disease, flu, pneumonia, tuberculosis, injuries, or, in the instance of Asian immigrants in particular, sudden unexplained death syndrome and hepatitis (Ackerman, 1997; Lin-Fu, 1988; Hargraves, 1996; Liu, Shilkret, Tranotti, Freund, & Finelli, 1998; Meropol, 1995).

A paradox that has been observed with successive cohorts of migrants to the United States, particularly among Hispanics, is that children and first-generation immigrants may in fact be healthier than those who have lived in the United States for longer periods of time. This effect has been attributed to the fact that longer-term residents are more likely to have become acculturated to U.S. society, including adopting practices such as smoking, alcohol use, and the consumption of fatty foods that put them at higher risk of developing chronic health problems (Cobas, Balcazar, Benin, Keith, & Chong, 1996; Hernandez & Charney, 1998; Popkin & Udry, 1998; Stephen, Foote, Hendershot, & Schoenborn, 1994).

Social Capital. Some subgroups have lost their families in military or guerrilla warfare in their home countries or are unable to bring family members with them because of seeking entry illegally or because of the absence of assurances of the means of supporting them once in the United States. The mental health effects of displacement are profound for many immigrant, and especially refugee, populations. U.S. immigration policy has contributed to the separation of refugee families, once in the United States, by "scattering" or making sure such populations are broadly dispersed throughout the country. As a result, they are often socially isolated, an isolation that is reinforced by language barriers and, in the instance of undocumented persons, fear of being discovered by Immigration and Naturalization Service officials (Fullilove, 1996; Westermeyer, 1987).

Immigrants who can enter the United States as refugees from those countries for which such a status is formally granted under U.S. law have greater legal access to systems of support and services than is the case for undocumented persons. As will be seen in Chapter Six, legislation such as California's Proposition 187, as well as the federal Welfare Reform Act of 1996, did, however, substantially reduce the availability of benefits for legal residents as well.

Human Capital. Many immigrant groups, such as Mexican nationals who migrate to the United States, are pulled by the lure of better jobs and higher wages, as well as the fact that other family members are likely to have migrated already.

Refugees, such as those from Cuba and Southeast Asia, are pushed out of their home countries because of domestic or foreign policies, and associated military conflicts, from which they seek to flee. Some groups of undocumented persons, such as Mexican nationals, leave their country primarily for economic reasons and others, such as Central American refugees, primarily to escape political or military conflicts. They have not sought permanent legal residence status in the United States, often because of federal immigration policies that preclude their doing so. The groups for which there has been the largest influx of immigrants and refugees during the past two decades (Cuba, Southeast Asia, and Central America) are directly related to U.S. foreign policy and military intervention in those areas (Lundgren & Lang, 1989; Massey & Espinosa, 1997; Nicaragua Health Study Collaborative at Harvard, Centro para Investigaciones y Estudios de Salud Publica & Universidad Nacional Autonoma de Nicaragua, 1989; Rumbaut, Chavez, Moser, Pickwell, & Wishik, 1988).

Immigrants with an official refugee status have been termed "overdocumented" because of the paperwork and screening required to certify their health and prospect for economic self-sufficiency; "undocumented" persons have none of these same credentials; and "documented" immigrants fall somewhere in between in terms of status and entitlements, though the benefits to documented immigrants were also diminished under the 1996 Welfare Reform Act.

Undocumented persons have the most tenuous legal and social status, networks of family or community support, and financial or other resources for sustaining themselves in U.S. society. The Immigration Reform and Control Act of 1986 attempted to reduce the flow of undocumented persons to the United States by imposing sanctions on employers who knowingly hired them (Bean, Vernez, & Keely, 1989).

An undetermined number of undocumented persons continue to work in the United States. They are likely to be employed in the least desirable, lowest-paying jobs—as agricultural day laborers, dishwashers, or janitors or in the garment industry sweatshops of big cities, for example. They generally have no job security, health benefits, or salaries that even approximate the minimum wage. They live in crowded, substandard, unsanitary housing in the impoverished areas of large cities, or in Third World–like rural poverty in the *colonias* (rural slums) along the U.S.-Mexico border (Rumbaut, Chavez, Moser, Pickwell, & Wishik, 1988).

Conclusion

There are deep roots or fundamental causes of vulnerability to poor health grounded in the social and economic circumstances at the individual, family, community, and societal levels. The analysis in this chapter focused on social status, social capital, and human capital resources as fundamental social determinants of vulnerability. This chapter does not, however, fully explore the specific risk factors and mechanisms through which these determinants may operate for the array of dimensions of poor physical, psychological, and social health examined. As documented in Chapter Ten, there is a need for cross-disciplinary analytic research to document these influences.

Chapters Five and Six describe the programs and methods of paying for services, lodged in specific assumptions regarding what investments might make a difference, that have been developed to mitigate the causes and consequences of vulnerability to poor health. Chapters Seven through Nine assess the extent to which these initiatives have succeeded in improving access, reducing costs, and enhancing the effectiveness of care provided to the most vulnerable identified in this and previous chapters.

CHAPTER FIVE

WHAT PROGRAMS
ADDRESS THEIR NEEDS?

preventive
treatment services
longterm care

This chapter identifies the major programs and services that have been developed or proposed to address the health and health care needs of vulnerable populations, in the context of an underlying continuum of care for the vulnerable. Efforts to prevent poor health are of equal importance to (or perhaps of greater importance than) those to restore maximum functioning for people who already have serious physical, psychological, and social health problems. (See Figure 5.1.)

Such a continuum would encompass programs and services designed to (1) inhibit the onset of problems initially (preventive services); (2) restore a person who is already affected to maximum functioning (treatment services); and (3) minimize the deterioration of function for people with problems that are not curable (long-term care services). The programs and services currently available to support this continuum of care for the vulnerable include, respectively, (1) primary prevention activities related to community resource development and public health programs and services; (2) treatment services delivered primarily through the medical care and related professional service delivery systems; and (3) long-term care institutional and community-based programs and services. The major assumption underlying this continuum is that people can be made less vulnerable if the objective of maximizing physical, psychological, or social capacity undergirds each stage of the caregiving process.

However, existing programs and services, particularly in the treatment and long-term care sectors, have not necessarily had this broader concept of maximizing patient functioning as either an explicit or implicit focus. Further, the organization and integration (more often lack of integration) of these programs do not typically acknowledge the emergence and evolution of vulnerability over the

FIGURE 5.1. CONTINUUM OF CARE FOR VULNERABLE POPULATIONS.

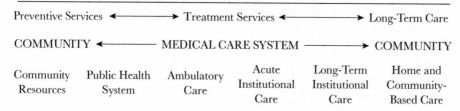

life course of individuals, as well as its essential roots in the communities from which people emerge and to which they return after being treated by the formal professional service delivery systems.

The presentation and discussion of programs in this chapter is of necessity illustrative rather than exhaustive. This overview is intended to set the stage for a more evaluative look in the chapters that follow regarding the adequacy, cost, and quality of existing programs and services for mitigating, if not eliminating, the vulnerability of those most at-risk.

Cross-Cutting Issues

The current profile of programs and services to address the health and health care needs of vulnerable populations falls far short of an integrated continuum of care.

Preventive Services

The roots of vulnerability lie deep in the sentiments and social arrangements that characterize contemporary society. The major social experiments of the 1960s, such as the War on Poverty, were relatively short-lived, and the demonstration and research projects to evaluate their impact documented a correspondingly mixed record of success. Commitments to programs that did demonstrate some effectiveness during this period, such as Head Start and Community/Migrant Health Centers, were reduced in subsequent decades.

In the 1970s and 1980s, U.S. domestic policy promulgated a diminished and decentralized federal role, along with a free market orientation, to solving domestic social and economic problems. These policies, along with major shifts in the U.S. economy during this same period (inflation, recession, loss of jobs in manufacturing and industry, and a corresponding growth in the service economy), conspired to exacerbate the socioeconomic origins of vulnerability. Although the economy and rates of unemployment improved during the 1990s, the number of part-time and low-wage positions continued to grow, and the number of income assistance supports and their level relative to inflation for persons receiving assistance diminished. The net consequence was growing income disparities between the working poor and higher-income families, as well as the reinforcement of a hard-core impoverished underclass in many U.S. cities and rural communities.

The social and economic roots of public health problems, such as those of high-risk mothers and infants, the mentally ill, and homeless persons, among others examined here, are well documented. Nonetheless, contemporary public health and medical care interventions focus primarily on the behavioral, environmental, and clinical correlates and consequences of socioeconomic disadvantage rather than on sociopolitical prescriptions to remedy it.

The Public Health Service Objectives for the Nation provide a philosophical basis as well as a concrete set of means and ends for improving the health and well-being of many of the vulnerable populations examined here. However, a major Institute of Medicine report (1988b) on public health concluded that the infrastructure for delivering public health messages and programs is poorly organized and managed and underfunded.

The lifestyle or individual-change-oriented bases of many interventions (such as how to stop smoking or drinking or say no to drugs) often fail to take into account the larger social milieu of the family or neighborhood in which the individual lives, which can have a major influence on the success of these initiatives. In addition to not being well researched in terms of their effectiveness, legally oriented interventions, such as mandatory testing for drugs or HIV antibodies, raise serious ethical questions regarding the rights of the affected individuals.

Although there is not a clear distinction in the delivery of prevention-oriented services in the public health and private medical care systems, the private medical care system has tended to focus on providing treatment services. Many front-line medical providers have not been trained and have no particular incentive (due to lack of reimbursement, for example) to include prevention-oriented procedures in their practices (such as HIV/AIDS, injury, or family abuse risk assessment). As will be discussed further in Chapter Seven, organizational or financial barriers may also preclude some particularly at-risk groups (such as high-risk mothers and children or elderly minorities) from getting even traditional prevention-oriented medical services, such as prenatal care, immunizations, or regular blood pressure screening.

Treatment Services

A complex, costly, highly technology-oriented and specialized system of medical care has evolved in this country, the primary focus of which is treating or curing disease. Many people, however, may present with problems in physical, psychological, or social functioning, which medical care providers have not necessarily been trained to identify or treat (such as mental illness, substance abuse, and child maltreatment). The complex origins of many of these problems lie outside the domain that medical providers traditionally address and are not readily fixed (or cured) by high-technology, medical silver bullets. Furthermore, the individuals may return directly to environments (such as abusing homes or living on the streets) that exacerbate their medical problems or make it harder to carry out medically prescribed follow-up care.

The acute medical care system has become a very expensive place of last resort for many of the vulnerable who have not reaped the benefits of earlier, more fundamental investments in their health and well-being through good schools, jobs, or housing or education about good health maintenance practices or access to preventive health care services. This is manifested in the expensive and technology-intensive hospital care needed by high-risk newborns that could have been avoided with adequate prenatal care or the child with cognitive impairments that could have been prevented by early case identification and treatment for lead poisoning, for example. The increasing role of managed care in providing health care presents new challenges for including those who are likely to have the most severe and correspondingly most costly health problems.

Long-Term Care

The deinstitutionalization movement (or discharge of the mentally ill from public and private hospitals) has focused on moving people out of depersonalized and bureaucratic institutional environments into less restrictive home or community settings. One of the problems with deinstitutionalization is that it encouraged or pushed individuals (particularly the mentally ill) to leave institutions without shifting resources to community-based care alternatives for those who had serious limitations in physical, psychological, or social functioning.

There is some evidence that a *re*institutionalization movement is occurring. Local jails and prisons increasingly are being filled with people who are mentally ill, homeless, drug dependent, HIV infected, or perpetrators of violence. Nursing homes house a substantial proportion of the growing number of young people with serious cognitive or mental impairments. Intensive care units of major inner-city hospitals are feeling the strain and costs of increasing numbers of HIV-positive or crack-dependent infants or ventilator-assisted children and adults, who have no home or family to go home to.

A parallel and equally important trend is the development of more community-based options as treatment and support alternatives for many categories of the vulnerable: meals on wheels to the homebound elderly, friendly visitor volunteers to persons living with HIV/AIDS, street outreach to homeless runaway youth, and alcohol or drug user peer support groups, among a multitude of others. Families continue to bear a large part of this caregiving burden for many of the vulnerable. Others have no one from a close circle of family or friends to help.

The focus of community-based, long-term care programs and services is to provide directly or support others in providing the complex array of services required to care for people who have serious, long-term limitations in physical, psychological, or social function. Because of the fragmentation and poor coordination of these services across many medical and social service sectors, case managers are often employed to create a system of care for an individual, where none exists in the community.

Population-Specific Overview

Population-specific evidence reviewed here argues for developing a more integrated, community-oriented, continuum of care for vulnerable populations.

High-Risk Mothers and Infants

Research on preventing low birthweight and reducing infant mortality has highlighted the importance of a comprehensive, coordinated system of care to serve high-risk mothers and infants (Hayes, 1987; Institute of Medicine, 1985, 1988d; National Commission to Prevent Infant Mortality, 1988a; Office of Technology Assessment, 1988; Public Health Service, 1989; Southern Regional Project on Infant Mortality, 1989). (See Table 5.1.)

Preventive Services. Public health programs provide a variety of prevention-oriented maternal and child health services. Title V of the Social Security Act authorized the establishment of the Maternal and Child Health (MCH) and Crippled Children Services (CCS) programs (now the Program for Children with Special Health Care Needs), and Title X of the Public Health Service Act provided federal funding for family planning services. The U.S. Department of Agriculture has supported the Special Supplemental Food Program for Women, Infants and Children (WIC), as well as the Food Stamp Program for welfare-eligible mothers, to enhance the availability of adequate nutrition for poor pregnant women and their children. Maternity and Infant Care Projects, Community and Migrant Health Centers, and National Health Services Corps physicians have also been major providers of care to women in many low-income neighborhoods. These programs have, however, experienced diminished levels of funding over the past two decades. This has been due to the use of block grant funding to states (that is, providing funds that specify support in particular areas, such as maternal and child health, but not the support of specific programs), as well as political pressures to reduce support for social service programs in general and family planning and abortion-related services in particular (Kotch, 1997).

Family life (sex) education and related behavioral risk education programs (relating to HIV/AIDS, smoking and substance abuse, and childhood injury) are available in some schools. Many at-risk teenagers are not reached by these programs, however (Dryfoos, 1990).

Prenatal care is the major medically oriented primary prevention intervention to enhance positive pregnancy outcomes (Institute of Medicine, 1988d; Public Health Service, 1989). Physicians are also encouraged to counsel their patients

TABLE 5.1. PRINCIPAL PROGRAMS AND SERVICES FOR HIGH-RISK MOTHERS AND INFANTS.

Preventive Services	*Treatment Services*			*Long-Term Care*	
	Ambulatory		*Institutional*		
Public Health System	**Preventive Services**	**Treatment Services**	**Acute Care**	**Long-Term Care**	**Home and Community-Based Care**
Family planning	Prenatal care	High-risk mother and infant care services	Level I or II delivery	Step-down units	Child protective services
Community outreach and case finding	Pre- and post-pregnancy counseling	Abortion services	Birth centers		Home visiting
Nutritional services	Well-baby care	Smoking and substance abuse cessation programs	Neonatal intensive care		School-based clinics
Sex education					Case management
AIDS education					
Smoking and substance abuse prevention					

regarding family planning and the risks associated with pregnancy and to encourage well-baby checkups and immunizations.

The Early and Periodic Screening, Diagnosis, and Treatment (EPSDT) program provides nutrition, vision, dental, and hearing screening; a physical history and exam; and immunizations to children who are covered by Medicaid. In 1988, only 20 to 30 percent of eligible children were estimated to have received this service. The Omnibus Budget Reconciliation Act of 1989, however, included provisions to expand the number of participating providers and allow more flexibility in scheduling screenings, to enhance Medicaid-eligible children's access to the program (Yudkowsy & Fleming, 1990). Data from evaluations of selected states tracing the impact of these provisions documented that although the proportion of children served had increased from 1989 to 1992, only around half (43 to 54 percent) of Medicaid children who were expected to have had at least one well-child visit had actually done so (Herz, Chawla, & Gavin, 1998). Medicaid managed care programs offer the possibility of increasing the provision of covered screening and preventive services to eligible child enrollees.

The Head Start Program, which began in 1965 in the Office of Economic Opportunity and is now administered by the Administration for Children and Families, provides education, social services, and health programs to disadvantaged preschoolers, most of whom are minority. This program also provides well-child screening and immunizations. Since its inception, Head Start has served more than 15 million children. In 1997 only about 40 percent of the 800,000 children eligible for the program participated (Children's Defense Fund, 1999). Infant stimulation and early childhood intervention programs help reduce the risk of cognitive and physical impairments among low birthweight, premature, or otherwise at-risk infants and children (Infant Health and Development Program, 1990).

Treatment Services. The relationship of adverse pregnancy outcomes to maternal smoking and alcohol use, as well as the increased incidence of drug-exposed infants, have resulted in an expanded interest in smoking and substance abuse cessation programs for pregnant women.

A focus of perinatal care demonstration and research projects has been the development of regionalized systems of perinatal care services, including the integration of services among hospitals having differing levels of capacity to handle high-risk newborns. Level III hospitals serve as regional centers and have the capacity for providing long-term newborn intensive care. Level II hospitals can provide short-term respiratory support, and Level I hospitals provide newborn care and have no special units for seriously ill infants.

Evaluations of regionalized perinatal network demonstration projects, such as the federally supported Maternity and Infant Care Program-Improved Pregnancy Outcome Program and the Robert Wood Johnson Foundation's Perinatal Program and Rural Infant Care Program, as well as other regionalized perinatal service systems, demonstrate that the availability of Level III hospitals, and the appropriate integration of a system of referrals among the different level institutions, results in improved perinatal outcomes, particularly the reduction of the birthweight-specific death rates for very low birthweight infants. Neonatal intensive care for high-risk newborns is expensive to provide. Furthermore, these hospital-based regionalized systems of service have not been successful in reducing the overall incidence of low birthweight infants in the populations they serve (Gortmaker, Clark, Graven, Sobol, & Geronimus, 1989; McNellis, 1988; Office of Technology Assessment, 1987a; Robert Wood Johnson Foundation, 1985, 1986).

Long-Term Care. The risks for high-risk infants and their families remain high once they leave the hospital. Programs and services to reduce child abuse and neglect, including parenting skills training, social support, and child care, may be important to ensure the infant's health and well-being after discharge (Cohn & Lee, 1988). School-based clinics and day care arrangements provide needed support for teenage mothers at risk of dropping out of school prior to graduation (Dryfoos, 1990).

Many mothers may need case management assistance to apply for and negotiate the fragmented and poorly integrated set of services for which they are potentially eligible (Issel, 1996). Home visiting of families with special needs has long been a component of public health nursing and social work practice. With the increased fragmentation of families, home visiting, with its systems of social support and care systems, offers promise as both an immediate and long-term strategy to assist high-risk mothers and their infants (General Accounting Office, 1990c; National Commission to Prevent Infant Mortality, 1989).

Chronically Ill and Disabled

Research on the prevalence of disability, the factors that lead to it, and the interventions that could be designed for the prevention, treatment, and long-term care associated with functional incapacity have led to an increasing recognition of the need for a regionalized, comprehensive, coordinated continuum of programs and services to address the needs of the chronically ill and disabled (Allen & Mor, 1998; Bonnie, Fulco, & Liverman, 1999; Institute of Medicine, 1991b; Center for Vulnerable Populations, 1992; Hinton-Walker, 1993; National Research Council, 1985, 1988). (See Table 5.2.)

Preventive Services. The Public Health Service Year 2010 Objectives for primary prevention interventions include educational programs on proper nutrition, smoking, and substance abuse and how to prevent injuries in the home and workplace, as well as encouraging increased participation in a regular program of exercise for all ages. In addition to these individual-oriented public health interventions, there are recommendations to reduce environmental risks of injury through regulations governing lead paint and product, motor vehicle, and firearms safety (U.S. Department of Health and Human Services, 1998).

Prenatal care is an important medical care–oriented intervention to detect and avert the risks of infant and early childhood disability (Institute of Medicine, 1988d). Newborn screening can help detect phenylketonuria (PKU) or congenital hypothyroidism, for example. Vision and hearing screening can help identify and lead to the correction of these impairments for both children and the elderly. Screening for lead paint poisoning, cancer, hypertension, and diabetes permits the early detection and management of these problems (Beers, Fink, & Beck, 1991; Institute of Medicine, 1991b; Needleman, 1991).

There is a growing emphasis on prevention-oriented interventions for the elderly, including the development of educational programs emphasizing home safety, nutrition, physical fitness, and medications management (Fries, 1989; Institute of Medicine, 1991b, 1991c; Office of Technology Assessment, 1989). The Centers for Disease Control and Prevention Disabilities Prevention Program is intended to build state and local capacities to prevent the primary onset and secondary consequences of developmental, as well as injury- and chronic illness-related, disability (Viano, 1990).

Treatment Services. Smoking is a significant risk factor for major chronic illnesses, such as cancer, heart disease, and chronic obstructive pulmonary disease, and alcohol is an important risk factor for cirrhosis. Programs to reduce the prevalence of these risk factors are important in enhancing both the primary and secondary prevention of serious chronic illness and associated functional limitations.

Care for long-term chronic disease often requires continuous, comprehensive, coordinated case management of clinical and social services over an extended period of time (Scott & Rantz, 1997). The onset of secondary disabilities associated with chronic illness (such as impaired vision resulting from diabetes) can be delayed or prevented if the appropriate medical regimens are introduced and the patient follows them. A particular problem in the care of chronically ill, and particularly elderly, patients is the medical management of multiple prescriptions. Many elderly experience serious physical or emotional side effects as a result of overmedication. The chronically ill and disabled may also have extensive needs for rehabilitation therapies, such as occupational, physical, and speech therapy, as well as durable medical equipment or assistive devices, such as prostheses or wheelchairs (Institute of Medicine, 1991b; Stein, 1989).

Adequate regionalized emergency medical and trauma center services are important in reducing the risk of death or long-term disability of intentional or unintentional injury. Chronically ill and disabled adults and children often face long and expensive hospital stays or long-term stays in hospital intensive care units. The expenditures for these services under Medicare are greatest during the last year of life (Bonnie, Fulco, & Liverman, 1999; Eggert & Friedman, 1988).

TABLE 5.2. PRINCIPAL PROGRAMS AND SERVICES FOR CHRONICALLY ILL AND DISABLED.

	Preventive Services	Treatment Services	Institutional		Long-Term Care	
	Ambulatory		Institutional		Long-Term Care	
Public Health System	Preventive Services	Treatment Services	Acute Care	Long-Term Care	Home and Community-Based Care	
Nutritional services	Prenatal care	Chronic disease management	Acute hospital care	Nursing homes	Home health care	

Smoking and substance abuse prevention	Screening
	  Newborn
	  Lead
	  Cancer
		Medications management	Intensive care	Hospices	Caregiver respite	

	Hypertension	Rehabilitation therapies		Social health maintenance organizations	Day care
					  Child
					  Adult	

Injury prevention programs
  Childhood
	Diabetes
	  Vision
		Durable medical equipment				

Home	Hearing	Emergency medical services			Home-delivered meals	
Work						
		Smoking and substance abuse cessation programs			Home visiting	
Exercise programs						
					Housekeeping services	
Environmental risk abatement programs						
Lead					Transportation services	
Product safety						
Motor vehicle safety					Case management	
Gun control						
					Independent living centers	
Education						
Infant stimulation					Board and care homes	
Early childhood intervention					Life care communities	

					Education
					  Special education
					  Vocational training
					  Rehabilitation	

Long-Term Care. Research on long-term care programs and services for the chronically ill and disabled has increasingly documented the importance of community-based options to institutionalized care, on forging more effective linkages between acute and long-term care services, and in developing more patient-centered models and standards of care (Allen & Mor, 1998; Bowlyow, 1990; Browne et al., 1995; Koff, 1988; Miller, 1997; Patrick & Peach, 1989; Stein, 1989; Strauss & Corbin, 1988; Weissert, Cready, & Pawelak, 1988). Comprehensive, coordinated, family-centered systems of care are particularly critical for children with special health care needs (Shelton, Jeppson, & Johnson, 1989; Stein, 1989). One of the dilemmas for children with special needs and their families is the discontinuity that results when they reach an age (such as eighteen) at which they no longer qualify for care and coverage under programs for which they were previously eligible (Sawyer, Blair, & Bowes, 1997).

The U.S. Department of Education, Office of Special Education and Rehabilitative Services, supports state efforts in providing special education and related services to disabled children from birth to age twenty-one. The Basic Vocational Rehabilitation Service Program supports the states in assisting physically and mentally disabled individuals to become gainfully employed, regardless of age (Office of Assistant Secretary for Planning and Evaluation, 1996; Seltzer, 1998; Seltzer & Essex, 1998).

Nursing homes are the primary providers of institutionalized long-term care. Projections estimate that at least 36 percent of Americans who turned forty-five in 1995 will enter a nursing home at some point in their lives (Merlis, 1999). Advanced age, physical dependency, cognitive impairment, and lack of social support are some of the major predictors of nursing home admission (Roy, Ford, & Folmar, 1990; Shapiro & Tate, 1988; Weissert & Cready, 1989b; Weissert & Harris, 1998). Hospices provide an alternative for palliative care for terminally ill patients (Torrens, 1985).

Life care communities, independent living centers, and board and care homes provide options for individuals who either elect not to or cannot continue to live in their own homes because of mental or physical limitations (General Accounting Office, 1989a; Moon, Gaberlavage, & Newman, 1989; Tell, Wallack, & Cohen, 1987). Under Title III of the Older Americans Act, Area Agencies on Aging have provided home-delivered meals, as well as a number of other support and referral services, for homebound elderly (American Association for Retired People, 1991). The Robert Wood Johnson Foundation Interfaith Volunteer Caregivers and Family Friends Projects provide examples of using volunteers to provide needed social support for the homebound elderly and disabled children and their families, respectively (Robert Wood Johnson Foundation, 1989, 1990).

The home care industry has burgeoned in an effort to respond to the growing number of adults and children who could live in the community if required medical and social support services are provided (Commonwealth Fund Commission on Elderly People Living Alone, 1989; Spohn, Bergthold, & Estes, 1988). However, the majority of the care for the community-dwelling disabled is still provided by family or friends. About 70 percent of the elderly receiving help with activities of daily living and instrumental activities of daily living reported receiving this care from unpaid caregivers. Of those receiving such care, almost 80 percent reported receiving help from relatives, the vast majority of whom were wives or daughters of the elderly person (National Center for Health Statistics, 1990c).

Programs to support the caregiver are essential if they are to continue to assume these roles. An important component of caring for the caregivers is to provide respite or homemaker services to reduce the day-to-day stress associated with taking care of a seriously ill or impaired family member (Montgomery, 1988). Social day care programs for both the elderly and disabled children provide options for more independent living, as well as respite for family caregivers (Hedrick et al., 1991; Robert Wood Johnson Foundation, 1990).

Two primary approaches have been developed for trying to integrate and coordinate services for the chronically ill and disabled: the brokered model and the consolidated delivery system model. In the brokered model, case management is typically used to coordinate services on behalf of clients, but restructuring of provider organizations is generally not required. In the consolidated models, comprehensive services are provided within a single organizational system, which assumes financial risk under a capitated contractual arrangement.

Case management has been used as a means for coordinating the complex array of medical and social services required by the elderly and disabled, although the organization and objectives (patient care, cost containment, or service coordination) of various case management models differ substantially (Capitman, 1988; Carcagno & Kemper, 1988; MacAdam et al., 1989; Shaughnessy & Kramer, 1990).

Social health maintenance organizations (S/HMOs) and the federally support Program of All-Inclusive Care for the Elderly (PACE) projects represent more consolidated models. S/HMOs are designed to cover long-term as well as acute, primary, and preventive health care on a prepaid basis. The S/HMO model emphasizes continuous case management, home care, and social services as alternatives to institutionalization (Harrington & Newcomer, 1991; Leutz, Greenlick, & Capitman, 1994; Newcomer, Harrington, & Friedlob, 1990). PACE, authorized by the Balanced Budget Act of 1997, features a comprehensive delivery system and integrated Medicare and Medicaid financing, modeled on a successful S/HMO in San Francisco: On Lok Senior Health Services (Health Care Financing Administration, 1998c). With the increasing penetration of managed care organizations among Medicare and Medicaid populations, such entities also represent important avenues for developing consolidated models of caring for the chronically ill and disabled (Allen, 1998; Estes & Close, 1998).

Persons Living with HIV/AIDS

Given that there is no known cure for HIV infection, HIV/AIDS programs have focused on the need for prevention and risk reduction through a variety of community- and individual-level interventions. The 1990 Ryan White CARE Act and the Centers for Disease Control and Prevention HIV Prevention Community Planning Initiative, as well as private foundation initiatives, such as the Robert Wood Johnson Foundation AIDS Health Services Program (AHSP), have attempted to catalyze consortia and related collaborative networks for developing comprehensive, coordinated systems of care for persons with AIDS. These initiatives have met with only limited success due to the lack of effective communication and cooperation among the diverse interests represented by HIV/AIDS populations and service providers in many communities (Coyle, Boruch, & Turner, 1991; Institute of Medicine, 1986, 1988a; McCann, Wadsworth, & Beck, 1993; Miller, Turner, & Moses, 1990; Mor, Fleishman, Allen, & Piette, 1994; Mor, Fleishman, Piette, & Allen, 1993; Osborne, 1996; Turner, Miller, & Moses, 1989). (See Table 5.3.)

Preventive Services. Prevention-oriented programs are directed to three principal audiences: the general public, target populations in particular communities, and individual clients. Mass media campaigns have been a major focus of the Public Health Service and Centers for Disease Control and Prevention initiatives to increase generalized public awareness of HIV/AIDS risks. These have included the dissemination of educational materials and videos, the preparation and airing of public service announcements, the National AIDS Hotline, the National AIDS Information Clearinghouse, outreach to the entertainment community, and public health communication assistance to state AIDS programs (Coyle, Boruch, & Turner, 1991; Davis, 1991).

Peer-led, community-based programs, particularly those that involve role modeling and participation by populations like those that are representative of the populations being targeted, have proven to be successful in ameliorating high-risk behaviors (Centers for Disease Control and Prevention, 1996; Centers for Disease Control and Prevention AIDS Community Demonstration Projects Research Group, 1999; Kegeles, Hays, & Coates, 1996; Mane et al., 1996; Rietmeijer et al., 1996). Social marketing of condoms to at-risk communities to prevent HIV/AIDS transmission represents another promising strategy for reducing the spread of the disease (Cohen et al., 1999). Health education and risk-reduction projects, such as the CDC National Partnerships Program, have also focused on involving community-based organizations, including schools, PTAs, community youth service programs, churches, and labor unions, in targeting HIV/AIDS prevention education and behavioral change interventions (O'Donnell et al., 1999; Williams, Scarlett, Jiménez, Schwartz, & Stokes-Nielson, 1991; Woods, 1998).

Street outreach programs are designed to deliver HIV/AIDS prevention messages, materials, and service referrals to high-risk persons outside traditional health care or social service delivery settings. Such strategies appear to be most effective when coupled with community change models that engender efforts to shift the behaviors and norms within the high-risk subgroups (intravenous drug users, for example) as a whole (Centers for Disease Control and Prevention, 1993a; Stimson, Eaton, Rhodes, & Power, 1994).

TABLE 5.3. PRINCIPAL PROGRAMS AND SERVICES FOR PERSONS LIVING WITH HIV/AIDS.

| | Preventive Services | Treatment Services | Institutional | Long-Term Care | Long-Term Care |
| | Ambulatory | Ambulatory | | | |
Public Health System	Preventive Services	Treatment Services	Acute Care	Long-Term Care	Home and Community-Based Care
Media campaigns	Sexual and drug history taking	Posttest counseling	Acute hospital care	Nursing homes	Home health care
AIDS education and risk-reduction projects Community based School based	Pretest counseling	HIV/AIDS treatment therapies	Intensive care	Hospices	Caregiver respite
Testing and counseling	Testing				Family/partner support or therapy
Safer-sex education	Substance abuse cessation programs				Volunteer services
Substance abuse prevention programs					Case management
Street outreach for high-risk populations					

An increasing mode of HIV/AIDS transmission, particularly among women and newborns, is through intravenous drug use (Turner et al., 1989). Syringe and needle exchange programs have been documented to be successful in reducing the frequency of needle sharing among intravenous drug users, without stimulating increased drug use. Such programs may not necessarily be successful in ultimately preventing the transmission of HIV in the drug using population (Bruneau et al., 1997; Normand, Vlahov, & Moses, 1995; Schwartz, 1993; Watters, Estilo, Clark, & Lorvick, 1994).

Enhanced prevention intervention programs that emphasize safer sex practices, condom use, and safe needle exchange, with clients being served through public health, drug treatment, or sexually transmitted disease clinics, represent individual-level avenues for reducing behaviors that are likely to put them at higher risk of contracting HIV/AIDS (Centers for Disease Control and Prevention, 1993b; McCoy, McCoy, & Lai, 1998; NIMH Multisite HIV Prevention Trial Group, 1998).

Treatment Services. Primary care physicians can play an important role in taking detailed sexual and drug use histories and in doing pretest counseling for patients who present themselves as being, or whom the provider judges to be, at risk of HIV/AIDS (McMurchie, 1993; Samet et al., 1995). Posttest counseling by medical providers is also necessary to advise patients of the outcome of the test and to advise patients regarding the importance of risk-reduction behaviors or, should the test be positive, the probable course of the disease and subsequent care needs. Since the mid-1990s, antiretroviral therapies have been successful in prolonging the lives of persons living with HIV/AIDS. The 1994 AIDS Clinical Trials Group protocol number 76 findings, which documented that the administration of zidovudine during pregnancy and childbirth could reduce the chance that the child of an HIV-positive mother would be infected by about two-thirds, led the Public Health Service to develop guidelines encouraging the counseling and testing of pregnant women for HIV infection (Renaud & Kresse, 1997; Stoto, Almario, & McCormick, 1999).

The prevalence of HIV/AIDS and drug use is high among prison populations, which compels attention to providing care for these high-risk populations while incarcerated, as well as facilitating referral or access to services once released (Dixon et al., 1993; National Research Council, 1993).

Many AIDS patients are in and out of the hospital with the immune deficiency–related morbidities associated with AIDS (such as pneumonia or neurological impairment). An important component of HIV/AIDS care is early intervention and intensive case management services in community-based health care delivery organizations for persons living with HIV/AIDS. The principal case management models for HIV/AIDS care are the broker, service management, and managed care models. In the broker model, case managers develop care plans and make referrals but have no control of funding sources. Under the service management model, case managers can authorize services and control funding, usually through funding caps. In the managed care model, providers are financially at risk for exceeding cost caps. The broker model has most often characterized HIV/AIDS case management, and HIV/AIDS care services remain fragmented and poorly coordinated in many communities (Mor, Fleishman, Allen, & Piette, 1994; Schore, Harrington, & Crystal, 1998).

Long-Term Care. Some parallels, but important differences as well, exist with respect to the long-term care needs of persons living with HIV/AIDS and the chronically ill and disabled. Both populations are heavily dependent on formal or informal systems of care over prolonged periods of time. However, with appropriate treatment, persons living with HIV/AIDS can experience intermittent, sustained periods when they are able to function normally, which may be less often the case for elderly or disabled persons with deteriorative cognitive or physical impairments (Mor, Fleishman, Allen, & Piette, 1994).

Furthermore, nursing homes are the primary institutionalized long-term care option available to the infirm elderly. Many of these institutions are not geared to serving younger populations or those with alternative (gay or drug use) lifestyles. AIDS hospices, which have sprung up in many communities, principally through volunteer efforts, provide a palliative, humane, and generally lower-cost alternative as a place to die than hospitals or nursing homes for persons with AIDS (Mechanic & Aiken, 1989).

The availability of home health care services to AIDS patients is largely a function of the extent to which they have third-party coverage. Many persons with AIDS, because of their rejection by their families as a result of their homosexuality or the absence of stable systems of family support in many cases among IV drug users, lack traditional family-based systems of care. Gay and lesbian friendship networks do, however, provide much of the informal social, emotional, and material support for persons living with AIDS and their companions or other caregivers (Macklin, 1989; National Research Council, 1993; Riley, Ory, & Zablotsky, 1989).

An array of community-based volunteer services programs has emerged to provide services to persons living with AIDS similar to that available to the elderly through the Office of Aging, such as home-delivered meals, home visiting, housekeeping, and transportation (Robert Wood Johnson Foundation, 1994; Shelp, DuBose, & Sunderland, 1990; Velentgas, Bynum, & Zierler, 1990).

Mentally Ill and Disabled

Early in the twentieth century, seriously mentally ill patients were institutionalized in state and county mental hospitals. During and after World War II, a greater awareness of the poor conditions in these institutions and a theoretical reorientation toward the role of the environment in influencing mental health led to the emergence of a community mental health movement and an impetus for the deinstitutionalization of mental patients. This new community-based care perspective received considerable support from the Kennedy administration, culminating in the Community Mental Health Center Act of 1963. This act and a series of amendments that followed encouraged the states to devote matching funds to community-based centers providing an array of mental health services. The number and growth of these centers and related community resources for caring for the mentally ill was less than anticipated due to lack of sustained political support, as well as funding, at the national and state levels.

The community mental health movement nonetheless catalyzed the large-scale deinstitutionalization of the mentally ill. Other factors, in addition to the ideological and political underpinnings, that provided an impetus for deinstitutionalization included the wider availability of psychotropic drugs that could be used to control or modify patient behavior on an outpatient basis, the belief that community care would be a less expensive alternative, and court decisions guaranteeing institutionalized patients rights to treatment that many states deemed too expensive to continue to assure (Grob, 1991; President's Commission on Mental Health, 1978a, 1978b, 1978c; U.S. Department of Health and Human Services, 1999). (See Table 5.4.)

Preventive Services. Prevention interventions in mental health may be classified as universal, selective, or indicated, based on the scope of the groups to which they are targeted. Universal preventive interventions are primary prevention strategies targeted to the general public or a whole population that has not been identified based on individual risk. Selective preventive interventions are targeted to individuals or groups whose risk of developing mental disorders is significantly higher than others, based on their biological, psychological, or social risk factors. Indicated preventive interventions are directed to high-risk individuals who have minimal, but detectable, signs or biological markers foreshadowing a serious mental disorder (Mrazek & Haggerty, 1994).

Universal and selective prevention strategies to reduce the onset of learning, developmental, behavioral, and related mental disorders in children include adequate prenatal care, newborn screening (particularly for PKU), infant stimulation, and early childhood intervention programs for high-risk children (premature infants, minority, and poor children), as well as parenting skills programs for their parents (Institute of Medicine, 1989d). Good maternal and child nutrition is also essential to ensure the developing infant and child's cognitive and physical development. Family planning, particularly for adolescent women and their sexual partners, will help to reduce the risk of pregnancy among teenage women, for whom the stresses and poor outcomes of pregnancy are likely to be the greatest.

Other important areas of universal prevention include programs to reduce unintentional injuries for children due to lead paint or other poisoning, or from motor vehicle or other accidents or injuries for adults and children that are likely to lead to serious cognitive impairment. Screening for lead paint poisoning or the psychological testing of at-risk children and adults through schools or clinic settings can also assist in the early identification of those who have or are most likely to develop cognitive or mental health impairments (Lorion & Allen, 1989).

TABLE 5.4. PRINCIPAL PROGRAMS AND SERVICES FOR MENTALLY ILL AND DISABLED.

	Ambulatory		Institutional		Long-Term Care
	Preventive Services	Treatment Services			
			Treatment Services	Long-Term Care	
Public Health System	Preventive Services	Treatment Services	Acute Care	Long-Term Care	Home and Community-Based Care
Education	Prenatal care	Outpatient mental health services	Short-term inpatient mental health services	Long-term inpatient mental health services	Family/caregiver support or therapy
Parenting skills	Screening	Crisis response services			Home visiting
Infant stimulation	Newborn				
Early childhood intervention	Lead				Child/adult protective services
	Psychological	Substance abuse cessation programs			
Nutritional services					Education
					Developmental
					Special education
Substance abuse prevention					
					Vocational
Family planning					Skills training
					Rehabilitation
Stress reduction programs					
					Community residential care
Consultation and education					Family care homes
					Halfway houses/
Environmental risk abatement programs					Psychosocial Rehabilitation
Lead					Board and care homes
Motor vehicle safety					Satellite housing
Injury prevention programs					Day treatment or partial care
Childhood					
Home					Psychiatric rehabilitation
Work					Educational
					Vocational
					Residential
					Case management
					Protection and advocacy

The relationship of substance abuse and mental impairment has also been recognized in encouraging selective prevention programs to inhibit alcohol and drug use, particularly among adolescents and pregnant women. Federal funding for substance abuse prevention and treatment has often been linked to mental health services provision through, for example, the Drug Abuse Prevention and Control Act, and the combined Alcohol, Drug Abuse, and Mental Health block grant.

Consultation and education services provided to clients seen at community mental health centers are illustrative of an indicated preventive mental health intervention. Evaluations suggest, however, that the centers often devote only a small proportion of staff time and resources to these activities. They also fail to implement a number of recommendations emanating from an American Psychiatric Association Task Force review of successful mental illness prevention programs (Dowell & Ciarlo, 1989). More research is needed to identify the most efficacious universal, selective, and targeted strategies to prevent the onset of mental disorders (General Accounting Office, 1989d; Lorion & Allen, 1989; Mrazek & Haggerty, 1994).

Treatment Services. Outpatient psychiatric services are delivered through the specialty mental health and general medical care sectors. The principal providers of outpatient specialty mental health services, in order of numbers of admissions, are multiservice mental health organizations (which provide at least two of three services: inpatient, outpatient, or partial care), freestanding outpatient clinics, nonfederal general hospitals, private psychiatric hospitals, Veterans Administration medical centers, and state and county hospitals (Witkin et al., 1998).

Depression, anxiety, and related mental disorders are estimated to be present in approximately 25 percent of the patients seen on an ambulatory basis by primary care physicians (Mechanic, 1990; Schulberg & Burns, 1988; Schurman, Kramer, & Mitchell, 1985). Emergency and crisis response services, as well as substance abuse cessation programs, are also components of treatment-oriented outpatient mental health services.

Managed care has assumed an increasing role in the delivery and financing of public and private mental health care services. Managed behavioral health care provides mental health and related behavioral substance abuse services through either health maintenance organization or related preferred provider arrangements. Services are financed through the capitation of enrollees or negotiated carve-outs to permit the separate pricing of such services (Center for Mental Health Services, Substance Abuse and Mental Health Services Administration, 1998; McFarland, 1994; Mechanic, 1998).

Long-Term Care. Prior to the community mental health movement, state and county mental hospitals were the major providers of long-term institutional care. With the deinstitutionalizaton movement, the numbers of the mentally ill in such institutions dropped sharply. There has, however, been a substantial growth in the number of private psychiatric hospitals, nonfederal general hospitals with psychiatric services, and residential treatment centers for emotionally disturbed children (Witkin et al., 1998).

Many mentally retarded and mentally ill children and adults are still being cared for by their families. The provision of family and caregiver respite and therapy services is important for continuing to support and strengthen their ability to sustain their caregiving role. Home visiting and child and elder abuse and neglect services also serve to monitor and enhance the capacities of at-risk families to provide for a disabled family member (Office of Technology Assessment, 1986).

Although the community mental health movement is fragmented and poorly developed in many communities, it has given rise to a number of home- and community-based long-term care options (Craig, 1988a). Support for educational services to mentally retarded and mentally ill adults and children is provided through the developmental disabilities, special education, and vocational rehabilitation and training programs (Seltzer, 1998; Seltzer & Essex, 1998). Partial care services provide an option to traditional inpatient and outpatient mental health services. With these arrangements patients can be admitted to day treatment programs or stay overnight, but be free to go to a job or other community activities during the day (Witkin et al., 1998).

Housing has been one of the most pressing community care needs for persons with cognitive or mental impairments since the advent of deinstitutionalization. Major options are family care arrangements (including foster family care); psychosocial rehabilitation facilities, such as halfway houses or other transitional care facilities; board and care homes; and satellite housing dispersed throughout the community (Rosenfeld et al., 1997; Segal & Kotler, 1989). With the limited availability of these specific housing options and the diminished availability of low-income housing in general, the number of mentally ill who are homeless has increased as well. As high as 50 percent of the homeless population has been estimated to have serious mental illness. Nursing homes, jails, and prisons also represent important de facto institutional providers of long-term care for the seriously mentally ill (Goldstrom, Henderson, Male, & Manderscheid, 1998; Kessler et al., 1998).

A variety of public and foundation-sponsored programs have supported the development of community housing, social service, educational, and related service capacity for serving the chronically mentally ill and homeless. The National Institute of Mental Health Community Support Program for the chronically mentally ill, the comparable Child and Adolescent Service System Program, and the Program of Assertive Community Treatment, as well as the Robert Wood Johnson Foundation Mental Health Services Development Program and the Mental Health Services Program for Youth, among others, were intended to facilitate the availability of a comprehensive, coordinated system of care for these populations (Beachler, 1990; Jaskulski & Robinson, 1990).

The psychiatric rehabilitation model emphasizes the importance of the individual's own needs assessment and decision-making processes for maximizing functioning in "working, living, and learning" in the community (Farkas & Anthony, 1989). The Fairweather Lodge Experiment, for example, created a community-based residential facility to train discharged hospital patients to live together in a supportive, family-like environment and to seek jobs in the community. The rates of rehospitalization were lower and sustained employment higher for patients who participated in these arrangements compared to those who were trained in the hospital and then simply discharged to the community (Segal & Kotler, 1989).

A range of case management models has been developed to serve the serious and persistent mentally ill. These vary in their relative emphasis on program personnel's versus the client's assessment of needs, and linking the client to services versus trying to enhance the client's own strengths and capacities for obtaining what he or she needs (Damron-Rodriguez, 1993; Robinson & Toff-Bergman, 1990).

State mental health protection and advocacy programs oversee placement decisions made by agents acting on behalf of the mentally ill and disabled through guardianship, protective order, or community commitment procedures (Scallet, Marvelle, & Davidson, 1990).

Alcohol or Substance Abusers

Alcohol, drug, and other substance abuse are typically long-term problems associated with an array of physical, psychological, and social correlates and consequences. A broad-based, multifaceted approach to prevention, treatment, and long-term care is required to address the onset and progression of these problems through the complex and interactive stages of use, abuse, dependence, abstinence, recovery, and relapse (Gerstein & Harwood, 1990; Haack, 1997; Institute of Medicine, 1987, 1989c, 1990). (See Table 5.5.)

Preventive Services. Considerable debate surrounds whether prevention efforts should focus more on restrictive legal means for limiting the supply or availability of alcohol, drugs, or other addictive substances versus community- or individual-oriented educational programs to diminish individuals' interest in or susceptibility to initiating the use of these substances. The supply-oriented approach is grounded in a moral model (drug use is morally wrong and deserving of punishment), while the use-reduction framework assumes a disease model (addiction is a biological or genetic disease that requires treatment and rehabilitation) (Jarvik, 1990; Marlatt, 1996, 1998; Reuter, 1991).

A variety of legal means have been used to restrict the availability and use of drugs, alcohol, and tobacco. State and federal laws impose criminal penalties on those who have been found to be supplying or using certain substances (such as

TABLE 5.5. PRINCIPAL PROGRAMS AND SERVICES FOR ALCOHOL OR SUBSTANCE ABUSERS.

Preventive Services	Treatment Services				Long-Term Care	
	Ambulatory		*Institutional*		*Long-Term Care*	
Public Health System	**Preventive Services**	**Treatment Services**	**Acute Care**	**Long-Term Care**	**Long-Term Care**	**Home and Community-Based Care**
Legal deterrence Criminalization Interdiction Restricted access	Counseling Individual Family	Pharmacological Agonist Antagonist Symptomatic	Hospital-based treatment programs	Therapeutic communities Rehabilitation units		Skills development Social Vocational Stress management
Screening		Behavioral Verbal therapy Contingency management Conditioning therapy				Peer support self-help Alcoholics Anonymous Narcotics Anonymous
Media campaigns						Halfway houses
						Aftercare programs
Substance abuse prevention programs Affective education Social influence Social skills training						Worksite/employee assistance programs
						Correctional facilities

cocaine or heroin). Federal law enforcement agencies (such as the Federal Bureau of Investigation, Central Intelligence Agency, and Border Patrol) have assumed major roles in halting (interdicting) shipments of designated substances to the United States.

State and local laws impose restrictions on where and to whom alcoholic beverages or cigarettes are to be sold. State dram shop laws assign liability to servers and owners of establishments that sell alcoholic beverages to obviously intoxicated customers, and drunk driving laws impose fines or penalties on individuals who are deemed to be legally intoxicated in efforts to both deter and punish such behaviors (Graitcer, 1989; Worden, Flynn, Merrill, Waller, & Haugh, 1989). Economic controls imposed at the governmental level, by increasing the price of substances such as alcohol and cigarettes through high rates of taxation or for illegal drugs through increased penalties for selling or possessing them, can reduce the incidence and quantity of use (Bach & Lantos, 1999; Becker, Grossman, & Murphy, 1994; Chaloupka & Wechsler, 1997; Chaloupka, Grossman, & Saffer, 1998; Grossman & Chaloupka, 1998).

Mandatory, as well as voluntary, testing or screening (particularly for drugs) is a controversial intervention that employers, insurers, the military, and criminal justice officials have used to deter potential users or detect, punish, or refer those who are found to be using or abusing such substances (Gust & Walsh, 1989). Private physicians and therapists are often in a position to counsel high-risk patients or families about the prevention or treatment of substance abuse. Screening programs to identify alcohol and drug problems among health and social service agency clients provide useful opportunities for the development of interventions or systems of referral for these populations (Weisner & Schmidt, 1993).

Community-based programs for the prevention of alcohol, tobacco, and other drug use are grounded in public health approaches that focus on multiple systems and providers within the community, community empowerment, and development and are designed to influence the host, agent, or environment within high-risk communities. Major public and private mass media campaigns about the dangers of drug, alcohol, tobacco, and other substance abuse represent one such type of intervention. These social marketing campaigns are intended to provide antidotes to the massive advertising conducted by the alcohol and tobacco industries to sell their products, which are often directed to particular market segments, such as women, adolescents, or minorities. Other programs include community-based skills training through a variety of community institutions (schools, police, local government) and the involvement and empowerment of local community organizations and neighborhoods (Aguirre-Molina & Gorman, 1996; Anderson, 1994; Fisher et al., 1998).

A number of states have coalitions for the prevention and control of tobacco use, which engage in a variety of public education, lobbying, and research and development efforts to diminish the use of tobacco products (Centers for Disease Control and Prevention, 1990b). A variety of private advocacy groups as well, such as Mothers Against Drunk Driving and Students Against Drunk Driving, have launched major media and public education campaigns to encourage safer practices (including the use of designated drivers) or the development or enforcement of stricter anti–substance abuse legislation.

Primary prevention-oriented programs, rooted in psychosocial theories of the etiologies of drug and related substance abuse, have been developed to target particularly at-risk groups such as adolescents (Bell & Battjes, 1990; Jones & Battjes, 1990a). These initiatives may be broadly classified as traditional versus psychosocial prevention methods.

The traditional approaches are mainly informational or affective. Informational methods emphasize potential dangers and efforts to arouse fears as a deterrent to use. Affective or humanistic education methods were designed to enhance overall self-esteem and encourage responsible decision making. Research on these approaches has shown little demonstrable impact on reducing the use of drugs or other addictive substances.

The two major psychosocial approaches—social influence and personal and social skills training—are rooted in somewhat different theories of causality. The social influence approach recognizes the role that the social influence of family and peers has on adolescents in particular in engaging in high-risk behaviors. Programs based on this approach have attempted to make participants aware of these influences, teach specific coping skills ("Just Say No"), and correct misperceptions of social norms regarding those behaviors (such as acquainting students with the fact that most people do not smoke).

Personal and social skills training builds on the social influence approach but emphasizes that these behaviors are basically learned through modeling and reinforcement. Programs based on these assumptions focus on learning skills such as self-control, assertiveness, or tension reduction that may be useful in resisting the temptation or invitation to engage in these behaviors. Evaluations of programs based on these models have demonstrated greater success in preventing the onset of adolescent smoking and drug use (Bangert-Drowns, 1988; Ellickson & Bell, 1990a, 1990b; Gerstein & Green, 1993; Graham, Johnson, Hansen, Flay, & Gee, 1990; Noland et al., 1998; RAND, 1998a; Tobler, 1986).

Treatment Services. The treatment of substance abuse disorders is multifaceted and involves an array of providers and interventions, often based on competing theoretical conceptions of underlying causes. Most long-term treatment programs for substance abusers are guided by one of three perspectives: (1) the physiological or biological perspective, underlying the medical model; (2) the psychological perspective, which informs psychotherapy and behavior therapy; and (3) the sociocultural perspective, which informs the social model (Barrows, 1998). Treatment has been variously characterized according to the mode of intervention used (pharmacological, psychological, or social), as well as the location at which services are provided (outpatient, inpatient, residential, or community based) (Gerstein & Harwood, 1990; Institute of Medicine, 1990).

There are three major pharmacological interventions involving the use of prescribed medications:

- The substitution of a medication that has actions that are similar to the abused drug but are much less physically or psychologically harmful, such as methadone treatment for heroin addiction or the use of nicotine chewing gum by smokers, on a long-term or short-term basis to suppress withdrawal symptoms during detoxification
- Treatment with a medication that blocks the effects of the abused drug, such as naltrexone treatment for heroin addiction
- Treatment with medications to relieve some of the symptoms associated with using the addictive drug, such as the insomnia and anxiety associated with opiod withdrawal

Psychologically and socially oriented therapies include the following:

- Individual, family, or group counseling and psychotherapy (verbal therapy)
- Systematic scheduling of positive or negative consequences as incentives for behavioral change, based on Skinner's principles of operant conditioning (contingency management)
- Systematic exposure to drug-related stimuli in the absence of abuse behavior to reduce or eliminate feelings of drug craving, based on Pavlov's principles of classical conditioning (conditioning therapy)
- Long-term treatment in a closed residential setting, emphasizing abstinence and learning new attitudes and behaviors (therapeutic community)
- Teaching skills in areas (such as the social or vocational) where deficits are thought to contribute to abuse (skills development)
- Groups such as Alcoholics or Narcotics Anonymous in which recovering abusers share their experiences and support one another in remaining free of the substance (peer support self-help groups) (National Institute on Drug Abuse, 1991)

The vast majority of federal dollars in the United States have been allocated to law enforcement and incarceration to reduce the supply of drugs, although treatment has been demonstrated to be more effective in reducing long-term drug use (Amaro, 1999). Both supply- and use-reduction policies have been criticized as giving insufficient attention to the changing epidemiology of drug use (the declining prevalence in the general population and increased volume of use among hard-core users) and attendant harm to addicts, others, and society. Harm-reduction policies, which have their origins in the Netherlands and other European countries, shift the focus from reducing the supply or use of drugs to the harmful consequences or effects of addictive behavior and ways to reduce these effects. Examples include drug legalization and syringe and needle exchange and bleach provision programs, condom distribution, and the creation of safe and healthy working conditions for addicted prostitutes (Broer & Garretsen, 1995; Caulkins & Reuter, 1997; Marlatt, 1996, 1998; Reuter & Caulkins, 1995; Roche, Evans, & Stanton, 1997).

Long-Term Care. The regimens and facilities in which alcohol- and substance abuse–related services are rendered reflect a varied mix of both treatment and long-term-care-oriented services. There are five major types of care provided:

- Detoxification (medical)—use of medication under treatment of medical personnel to reduce or eliminate the effect of the drug in a hospital or other twenty-four-hour care facility
- Detoxification (social)—systematic reduction or elimination of the effects of the drug in a specialized nonmedical facility by trained personnel with a physician on call
- Rehabilitation/recovery—planned program of professionally directed evaluation, care, and treatment for the restoration of functioning
- Custodial or domiciliary—provision of food, shelter, and assistance on a long-term basis
- Outpatient or nonresidential—treatment, recovery, aftercare, or rehabilitation services in a unit in which the person does not reside, with or without medication, but including counseling and supportive services (Institute of Medicine, 1990)

Sustained abstinence or the long-term maintenance of other desired treatment outcomes is difficult for individuals who are attempting to recover from prolonged substance abuse. Relapse to these behaviors, on either an intermittent or irreversible basis, is frequently an outcome for many in recovery. Aftercare or continuing-care programs are intended to facilitate the development or maintenance of the requisite skills, as well as to effect changes in their family, work, or social environments, to facilitate the long-term maintenance of positive treatment outcomes (Tims & Leukefeld, 1988).

A variety of custodial and community-based self-help options are components of this continuing care process. Employee assistance programs (EAP) are major work site–based initiatives that have been employed in facilitating the diagnosis and treatment, as well as the continuing care, of substance-abusing employees (Brody, 1988; Gust & Walsh, 1989). Furthermore, a plethora of self-help groups based on the twelve-step recovery model (such as Alcoholics Anonymous and Narcotics Anonymous, among a multitude of others) are available to those who are in long-term recovery from chemical dependency. Results from the National Institute on Drug Abuse Collaborative Cocaine Treatment (Project Match) Study demonstrated that individual drug counseling based on the twelve-step model plus group drug counseling was more successful in reducing cocaine use among cocaine-dependent patients than group counseling alone or individual psychotherapy (Crits-Christoph et al., 1999).

Suicide or Homicide Prone

The root causes of violence often lie deep in the basic social or economic structure of human communities and families, areas that have traditionally been outside the domain of medical and public health practice. There is an increasing acknowledgment, however, of the salience of violence as a public health concern and the importance of interdisciplinary cooperation in designing programs and research to address the interrelated problems of suicide, homicide, and family abuse (Alcohol, Drug Abuse, and Mental Health Administration, 1989a, 1989b, 1989c, 1989d; Blumstein, Cohen, Roth, & Visher, 1986a, 1986b; Committee on Law and Justice, National Research Council & JFK School of Government, Harvard University, 1994; Reiss & Roth, 1993). (See Table 5.6.)

Preventive Services. Persistent poverty that results from lack of opportunities for entering the economic mainstream of society has historically been highly associated with rates of violence and homicide. Violent crime rates were high for many new groups of immigrants until opportunities opened for them to enter the industrial workforce (Gurr, 1989). In the postindustrial U.S. society, the loss of relatively well-paying jobs for semiskilled laborers in manufacturing, the corollary movement of industry out of the heart of many U.S. cities, and the resultant disinvestments in inner-city schools and neighborhoods have exacerbated the problems of many minority youth in finding meaningful and well-paying employment. The poverty, sense of relative deprivation, and resulting resentment are cited as major contributors to the epidemic of violent behavior among these subgroups. Major interventions to prevent violence, however, have not tended to focus on these fundamental social and economic underpinnings and the structural and societal changes required to address them.

As in the area of substance abuse, philosophies regarding the prevention or reduction of homicides have tended to diverge in terms of means that emphasize more punitive, legal deterrence versus educational, skills-building or risk-reduction strategies. Incarceration and capital punishment, for example, have been promulgated as means either to deter or incapacitate those who are likely to engage in violent interpersonal behavior.

Research investigating the impact of legal deterrence has not demonstrated strong and consistent support for their success in reducing homicide rates (Blumstein, Cohen, Roth, & Visher, 1986a, 1986b; O'Carroll et al., 1991; Smith, 1997). These strategies are nonetheless the major devices available to the criminal justice system, which bears the major responsibility for addressing the consequences of individual and interpersonal violence.

Studies of the causes of suicide and homicide have identified a number of factors that have become the focus of public health–oriented prevention programs.

TABLE 5.6. PRINCIPAL PROGRAMS AND SERVICES FOR SUICIDE OR HOMICIDE PRONE.

| | *Preventive Services* | *Treatment Services* | | *Long-Term Care* | |
| | *Ambulatory* | | *Institutional* | | |
Public Health System	**Preventive Services**	**Treatment Services**	**Acute Care**	**Long-Term Care**	**Home and Community-Based Care**
Legal deterrence	Case identification screening	Outpatient mental health services	Acute hospital care	Long-term inpatient mental health services	Child/adult protective services
Gun control					
Capital punishment	Psychological evaluation	Crisis intervention centers	Short-term inpatient mental health services	Residential treatment centers	Battered women's shelters
Family planning					
Parenting skills education		Substance abuse cessation programs			Peer support self-help Save Our Sons and Daughters
Substance abuse prevention					Correctional facilities
Stress reduction programs					Police and court systems
Violence prevention education					
Suicide prevention centers					

Family planning and family life education programs have been encouraged to reduce unwanted pregnancies and teach parenting and problem resolution skills as alternatives to aggressive or injury-producing acts of physical violence. Alcohol and substance abuse prevention and stress reduction programs also have the secondary benefit of reducing or eliminating risk factors that are highly correlated with individual and interpersonal acts of harm.

Curricula have been developed to teach junior and senior high school students how to alter their behaviors when cast in the role of aggressor, victim, or bystander in an effort to avert or diminish the lethality of incipient acts of interpersonal violence. Formal suicide prevention programs, available through a variety of public and private auspices (schools, community mental health centers, and private psychiatric hospitals, among others), are intended to assist in identifying individuals most at risk and to provide the individuals, families, and helping professionals information or resources to reduce the probability of suicide (Alcohol, Drug Abuse, and Mental Health Administration, 1989a, 1989b, 1989c, 1989d; Friday, 1995; Metha, Weber, & Webb, 1998; Pfeffer, 1989).

The development of valid screening tools and training health care professionals, teachers, nursing home administrators, and protective service workers in how to use them can facilitate the design of prevention-oriented interventions with those individuals most likely to inflict harm on themselves or others (Clark-Jones, 1997; Slap, Vorters, Chaudhuri, & Centor, 1989).

As with the legal-oriented approaches to deterring or averting violent behavior, more research is needed on what public health-oriented interventions are most likely to identify and reduce the potential for violence.

Treatment Services. Most treatment for suicide-related risks and behaviors has resided in the mental health services sector. "Treatment" for violence-prone behavior leading to homicide has largely been provided through the criminal justice system. Suicide crisis intervention programs and hot lines, sponsored by a variety of public and private sources, provide a resource for at-risk families or individuals. Mental illness and substance abuse are important correlates of suicidal and homicidal behavior. Programs and services to address these risk factors are also part of the continuum of care for victims of intentional harm.

Long-Term Care. The principal philosophical focus of the criminal justice system in dealing with individuals who have committed homicide or related acts of intentional interpersonal injury is incapacitation, that is, imprisonment. No particularly successful programs have been identified or implemented to intercept or modify the careers of individuals who may be on their way to a life of crime (Blumstein, Cohen, Roth, & Visher, 1986a, 1986b).

Research and support for drug and vocational rehabilitation or other programs that are likely to reduce rates of recidivism and postrelease criminal violence are very limited in poorly funded and overcrowded correctional systems in many states. Residential treatment centers, many of which are components of the criminal justice system, are an important source of treatment for emotionally disturbed, violent, or suicidal youths, although the availability and quality of the treatment in these programs are quite uneven (Flanagan & Maguire, 1990).

Important components of community-based systems of support to avert violent intentional injury include child, elder, spouse, or other family member abuse services. Suicide, homicide, and family abuse and neglect appear to be closely interrelated forms of individual and interpersonal violence. Volunteer groups, such as S.O.S.A.D. (Save Our Sons and Daughters) in Detroit, provide social and emotional support for surviving family members who have been victims of violent death. Such support groups are also important components of the aftercare process, to assist family members of suicide victims to deal with the socioemotional impact of the event (Osgood & McIntosh, 1986; Prothrow-Stith, 1995).

Abusing Families

The issues of child, spousal, elder, and other abuse among intimates have come into political and social salience during the past three decades. A variety of state and federal legislation has been enacted to try to address these problems. Nonetheless, discrete, nonoverlapping, and often poorly coordinated programs and services exist for different victims (for example, women, children, and the elderly) and perpetrators (for example, male partners, parents of young children, children of older parents) of abuse (Chalk & King, 1998; Crowell & Burgess, 1996; National Research Council Panel on Research on Child Abuse and Neglect, 1993). (See Table 5.7.)

Preventive Services. The propensity to abuse innocents and intimates lies deep in the structure of human society. Correspondingly, the interventions recommended for altering the likelihood of these behaviors lie outside the domains traditionally encompassed by public health, and certainly medical care, practice. Such proposals include:

- Altering the social and familial norms that legitimize and glorify violence, such as the acceptability of corporal punishment, media violence, and the ready availability of hand guns
- Reducing violence- and stress-provoking social and economic inequalities resulting from differential educational or employment opportunities
- Mediating the sexist character of family and society, manifest in the definition of rigid gender role expectations and differential social status and rates of pay for "women's work" (such as child care, teaching, social work, or nursing) relative to "men's work" (administration, management, accounting, or medical practice)

TABLE 5.7. PRINCIPAL PROGRAMS AND SERVICES FOR ABUSING FAMILIES.

Public Health System	Preventive Services	Treatment Services		Long-Term Care	
	Ambulatory		Institutional		Long-Term Care
	Preventive Services	Treatment Services	Acute Care	Long-Term Care	Home and Community-Based Care
Legal deterrence Mandatory reporting Presumptive arrests Restraining orders Gun control	Screening and risk assessment	Emergency medical services	Acute hospital care	Long-term inpatient mental health services	Child/adult protective services
Media campaigns	Counseling Individual Family Group	Crisis response services	Short-term inpatient mental health services		Battered women's shelters
Family planning	Substance abuse cessation programs	Outpatient medical care services			Peer support self-help Parents Anonymous Men's groups
Sex education		Outpatient mental health services			Foster care
Parenting skills education					Home visiting
Substance abuse prevention					Caregiver respite
Stress reduction programs					Day care Child Adult
Violence prevention education					Housekeeping services Transportation services Housing alternatives Legal assistance Job placement Police and court systems Welfare services Case management

- Facilitating the linkage of isolated individuals and families (such as single-parent heads of households or the elderly living alone) with networks of community-based social support services (Gelles & Cornell, 1990)

The fundamental changes entailed in this series of recommendations require a social consciousness and political commitment not yet manifest in policy-making in this and related areas affecting the health and health care of vulnerable populations.

Nonetheless, programs have been developed or suggested to intervene categorically to prevent or treat the effects of intimate violence. Interventions that have emanated from the legal versus the public health or social service sectors tend to follow conflicting philosophies, grounded in the contrasting values of "control" versus "compassion" toward abusers.

Methods of legal deterrence, such as mandatory reporting laws, presumptive (meaning mandatory) arrests when actual abuse is suspected, the imposition of civil protection (restraining) orders or peace bonds on those actually convicted (in which a defendant who violates the court's ruling restricting his contact with the persons he abused previously is obligated to pay a bond set by the court), and the support of gun control legislation represent efforts forcibly (or legally) to control or inhibit the likelihood of the occurrence of violent behaviors.

Community media campaigns and associated hot lines have been used as means to both enhance the public's knowledge and awareness of the family violence problem, as well as to encourage the reporting of suspected or actual incidents of abuse to the police or other proper authorities (Gelles & Cornell, 1990).

Public health and social service interventions, such as family planning, sex and sex abuse education, parenting skills education, substance abuse prevention, stress reduction, and violence prevention programs attempt to reduce the risks associated with unwanted or unplanned pregnancies or other interpersonal or behavioral stressors within the family. Home visitation by nurses or other social service professionals has also been demonstrated to be an effective means for reducing the likelihood of child abuse and neglect in high-risk families. These and related service-oriented programs attend to the more "compassionate" orientation that abusers may themselves be victims of their environments and that it is important to reduce the risks and increase the coping resources they need to avert the prospect of intentional or unintentional injury to an intimate in their care (Daro, 1988; Elliott, 1993; Epstein, 1990; General Accounting Office, 1990c; Loring & Smith, 1994; Neergaard, 1990; Upsal, 1990).

There has been an emphasis on encouraging a greater role on the part of public health and health care professionals in identifying and treating, or appropriately referring, cases of intrafamily violence and abuse (Bekemeier, 1995; Comerci, 1996). Family and individual counseling or substance abuse cessation programs are also often directly or indirectly intended to avert the risk of potential violence, in addition to addressing mental health or addiction problems within multiproblem families.

Such interventions may, for example, view the stress associated with social or economic factors (such as unemployment or cultural norms toward violence) as independent variables and personal and psychological variables (tendency to see violence as a problem-solving strategy, poor interpersonal or coping skills) as intervening variables that are most likely to predict which families or individuals will react to these stresses with acts of violence toward other family members (Justice & Justice, 1990).

Treatment Services. Cases of child, spousal, elder, or other intrafamilial abuse often land in outpatient medical care facilities, particularly big-city emergency rooms. For example, estimates are that approximately 22 to 35 percent of women who visit emergency departments are there because of an injury or manifestation of living in an abusive relationship. Especially severe cases may require inpatient admissions for the treatment of injuries incurred during the abusive incidents (Ernst, Nick, Weiss, Houry, & Mills, 1997; Kyriacou, McCabe, Anglin, Lapesarde, & Winer, 1998; Randall, 1990). Although poorly developed or nonexistent in most U.S. communities, hot lines or crisis response programs provide another avenue for dealing with the family or medical emergencies precipitated by incidents of abuse.

Approaches to treating child sexual and other types of abuse include a lay or paraprofessional approach using peer counseling and support, the group approach emphasizing group therapy and education, and social work that relies on individual counseling. New emphases in trying to address the multicausal and multiproblem maltreatment in many families include multidisciplinary teams of medical care and social service professionals and interagency cooperation to develop networks of case identification, treatment, and referral for at-risk families and individuals (Borduin et al., 1995; Carney, 1989; Justice & Justice, 1990).

Long-Term Care. Child and adult protective and welfare agencies are the major social service–oriented governmental institutions charged with identifying and intervening with abusing families and individuals. The level of funding and staffing for these agencies is uneven and generally inadequate across states, and the resultant caseloads often are too large for agency caseworkers to attend closely to the families most at risk.

Shelters or safe houses are one of the key sources of community-based, private sector support for battered women and their children. These agencies are largely supported by private donations and volunteer efforts and have slim operating budgets (Gelles & Cornell, 1990; Public Health Service, 1990).

Protective service, welfare, and voluntary community groups concerned with abusing families attempt to identify and provide an array of support services either to mediate the stresses on families that appear to be productive of violence or to permit the victims of abuse to gain sufficient independence to extricate themselves from the abusive environment. These services include foster care, caregiver respite, day care, housekeeping, alternative housing, transportation, and legal or job placement services.

Peer support self-help groups, such as Parents Anonymous or men's groups formed to provide peer counseling for abusers, are also important components of the treatment and long-term service continuum for this population. Sometimes convicted offenders' participation in such groups is mandated by the courts. The dropout rates for both voluntary and nonvoluntary participants are nonetheless quite high in these groups.

The police and courts remain the front lines of intervention for many incidents of domestic violence, particularly spousal abuse. Domestic disturbances have come to be diagnosed as the "common cold" of police work. Mandatory (or presumptive) arrests for suspected intrafamilial abuse are permitted in some municipalities, although how local police departments choose to handle these cases remains quite variable. To attempt to deter convicted offenders from committing acts of violence once released from custody, the courts may issue restraining orders or peace bonds (Finn & Colson, 1990; Gelles & Cornell, 1990; Thyen, Thiessen, & Heinsohn-Krug, 1995; Wells & Tracy, 1996).

Homeless Persons

The "new" homeless began to become more and more visible in U.S. cities during the early 1980s. In the absence of significant public and private initiatives at the national level, the burden of caring for homeless persons fell to local voluntary organizations, such as rescue missions or sectarian or nonsectarian charitable organizations, and municipalities. Programs serving homeless persons still rely to a large extent on these local, largely privately funded, and in many cases, volunteer-based initiatives. Over time, however, private foundations, as well as the federal government, have assumed more of a role nationally in funding programs in general and for certain categories of homeless persons (such as the chronically mentally ill). Both private and federal initiatives have sought to develop a continuum of care for providing housing and related services to homeless persons. Nonetheless, programs for homeless persons still fall far short of "curing" the problem of homelessness, as well as addressing the needs of those for whom it is already a fact of life (Burt et al., 1999; Institute of Medicine, 1988c; Rochefort, 1997; Rosenheck, Gallup, Leda, Gorchov, & Errera, 1990; Rosenheck, Frisman, & Kasprow, 1999; Stephens, Dennis, Toomer, & Holloway, 1991; U.S. Conference of Mayors, 1999; U.S. Commission on Security and Cooperation in Europe, 1990). (See Table 5.8.)

Preventive Services. As with other vulnerable populations, preventing homelessness requires societal and political investments that lie outside the domain of traditional public health and medical care practice.

Three major types of housing can be effective in preventing homelessness: low-income, supportive, and emergency housing. Federal policy has manifested a decade-long retreat from ensuring decent housing for low-income

TABLE 5.8. PRINCIPAL PROGRAMS AND SERVICES FOR HOMELESS PERSONS.

Public Health System	Preventive Services	Treatment Services		Long-Term Care	
	Ambulatory	Treatment Services	Institutional	Long-Term Care	Home and Community-Based Care
	Preventive Services	Treatment Services	Acute Care	Long-Term Care	Home and Community-Based Care
Housing Low income Supportive Emergency	Prenatal care	High-risk mother and infant care services	Acute hospital care	Long-term inpatient mental health services	Homeless shelters
Street and community outreach	Immunizations	Chronic disease management	Short-term inpatient mental health services	Residential placement	Housing alternatives
Family planning	Health screening Infectious disease Chronic disease	HIV/AIDS treatment therapies			Food assistance
Parenting skills education	Psychological evaluation	Outpatient mental health services			Education School-based programs Vocational
Nutritional services		Substance abuse cessation programs			Battered women's shelters
AIDS education		Emergency medical services			Child/adult protective services
Substance abuse prevention		Outpatient medical care services Dental care services Tuberculosis treatment services			Welfare services Case management

Americans. There is also a paucity of specialized or supportive housing for vulnerable subgroups of the homeless that other systems of caring have failed, such as the physically disabled, mentally ill, abused women and children, and alcohol and drug users. Emergency housing is particularly important for the new homeless (many of whom are mothers and children) who find themselves suddenly without a roof over their heads because of a family crisis (such as domestic violence) or an economic crisis (such as a job layoff) (Institute of Medicine, 1988c; Shinn et al., 1998).

In addition, a variety of other outreach and prevention-oriented services are needed to prevent or ameliorate the complex, and often serious, health problems that homeless persons experience. Street and community outreach, particularly for mentally ill adults and runaway or homeless youth, is useful in identifying those individuals who may be most at risk of harm from living on the streets (victims of robbery, violence, or sexual exploitation, for example).

Homeless women and adolescent female runaways are much less likely to afford or use birth control than are other women. Correspondingly, they are more likely to have higher rates of pregnancy than housed women. They are also quite likely in many cases to be escaping abusive family environments. The provision of family planning and associated parenting skills education is then increasingly important for the growing number of women of childbearing ages among homeless persons.

Homeless persons, and particularly homeless women and youth, are more likely to be at risk of substance addiction and HIV/AIDS. Behaviorally oriented interventions, such as providing free condoms or sterile needles, are likely to be more effective than traditional educational or attitude change approaches for altering high-risk behaviors among these subgroups (Nyamathi, Stein, & Brecht, 1995).

Many homeless persons not only do not have a roof over their heads, but also do not know the source of their next meal. Soup kitchens, pantries, and shelters have been mainstays in providing food for homeless persons, as well as other groups of the poor (Bowering, Clancy, & Poppendieck, 1991; Clancy, Bowering, & Poppendieck, 1991; Rauschenbach, Frongillo, Thompson, Anderson, & Spicer, 1990). A number of the health problems of homeless persons, particularly among homeless children (under- or malnutrition, anemia, skin disorders, developmental delays, elevated cholesterol), are associated with poor or inadequate nutrition. Poor nutrition also puts pregnant, homeless women at risk of having low birth-weight babies or other adverse birth outcomes. Expanding and targeting federal food programs for the poor, such as WIC and food stamps, as well as increasing the amounts of fruit, vegetables, and lower-fat foods in homeless shelters and meal programs, represent avenues for ameliorating the health effects of poor nutrition among homeless persons (Gelberg, Stein, & Neumann, 1995; Wood, Valdez, Hayashi, & Shen, 1990).

A related and important component of medical care for vulnerable homeless persons is prenatal care and well-child care for homeless pregnant women and children. Homeless children are much less likely to have received routine immunizations. Respiratory ailments, tuberculosis, skin conditions, and venereal and other infectious diseases are more prevalent among homeless adults, relative to the general population, as are dental and mental health problems. Mobile vans, shelter-based, and freestanding clinics have been used in a number of communities to provide screening and referral services for homeless persons (Brickner, Scharer, Conanan, & Scanlan, 1990; Gelberg, Panarites et al., 1997; McAdam, Brickner, Scharer, Crocco, & Duff, 1990; Zolopa et al., 1994).

Treatment Services. A number of unique characteristics of homelessness exacerbate the effective delivery of medical care and other services to this population (Institute of Medicine, 1988c). These include the circumstances of living on the street, which make it difficult to implement a successful treatment plan (keeping a supply of medication or resulting side effects, such as drowsiness, that might make them more vulnerable to exposure or violence); the multiplicity and diversity of their health, social, and economic needs (including mental, physical, and substance abuse problems; inadequate incomes; and lack of housing and a stable food supply); their isolation resulting from the lack of supportive family or friends; and their distrust of traditional health and mental health care or other professionals because of bad experiences while under care previously (Gallagher, Andersen, Koegel, & Gelberg, 1997; Gelberg, Gallagher, Andersen, & Koegel, 1997).

The Robert Wood Johnson Foundation Health Care for the Homeless (RWJF-HCH) project attempted to incorporate principles in the design of health care programs for homeless persons that would better match their serious and multifaceted needs. The nineteen projects differed considerably in design, evolving primarily according to the model deemed most appropriate by the local broad-based community coalitions responsible for the programs. The RWJF-HCH programs did tend to share the following elements in common, however: a holistic treatment approach, which took into account the social and economic, as well as medical care, needs of homeless persons (such as where they slept, got food, and the benefits to which they were entitled); street and community outreach to establish a conduit for service or benefit provision; a well-trained and empathetic staff and continuity in the personnel seen; a multidisciplinary team approach and range of services to address their diverse medical, mental, social, and economic needs; and case management and coordination to facilitate continuity and follow-up. The Health Resources and Services Administration Health Care for the Homeless (HRSA-HCH) program took over the RWJF-HCH program and expanded the number of cities where it operated (Stephens, Dennis, Toomer, & Holloway, 1991).

Other major federally funded programs to serve homeless persons, such as the Veterans Administration Homeless Chronically Mentally Ill and Health Care for Homeless Veterans programs (Rosenheck, Gallup, Leda, Gorchov, & Errera, 1990; Rosenheck, Frisman, & Kasprow, 1999), the National Institute of Mental Health Community Mental Health Services Demonstration Program (Sargent,

1989), and the Access to Community Care and Effective Services program of the Substance Abuse and Mental Health Services Administration (Rosenheck et al., 1998), among others, have also incorporated many of the key components of the RWJF-HCH projects.

Hospital emergency rooms remain the major source of care for homeless persons on an urgent or episodic basis in many U.S. cities or localities. Many homeless persons have not applied for or have failed to retain eligibility for benefits, such as Temporary Assistance for Needy Families, Social Security Disability Insurance, or Supplemental Security Income (because of the lack of a permanent address or the red tape required), that might entitle them to coverage for health care services through Medicaid or Medicare. Having such coverage may be particularly important when acute medical or mental health care is needed. Otherwise homeless persons are likely to be inadequately served or go unserved ("dumped") by institutions unwilling or unable to assume a larger financial burden for patients who cannot afford to pay for their care (Institute of Medicine, 1988c; U.S. Commission on Security and Cooperation in Europe, 1990).

Long-Term Care. Particular problems that homeless persons with complex, chronic mental or physical problems experience are that they have neither a home nor supportive caregivers to provide them home care. Nursing homes may refuse to take them because they have no means of paying for their care or the institution may be unwilling to take on what they perceive to be problem patients. Homeless persons themselves are often unwilling to consider being cared for in traditional institutional settings because of prior negative experiences or a preference for a more independent life on the streets (even though middle-class health care providers view this as an extremely tenuous or threatening way of life).

Through volunteer or local municipal efforts, converted apartment buildings and shelters have been used to establish convalescent or respite units linked to, but separate from, health care institutions, to provide a place for homeless seriously ill persons to go after discharge. A residential placement program of the Veterans Administration secures supervised housing alternatives in the community—in private residences or personal board and care homes—for patients who are to be discharged from VA facilities. Creative and resourceful discharge planning is a particularly important need for homeless persons (Institute of Medicine, 1988c).

Shelters have provided the backbone of community-based service provision for homeless persons in many U.S. cities. Soup kitchens, food pantries, and other emergency food assistance programs are also important initiatives for addressing the paired problems of hunger and homelessness. The Stewart B. McKinney Homeless Assistance Act and associated Federal Emergency Management Agency, locally generated revenues, state grants, and Community Development and Community Services Block Grants are important sources of support for these programs (U.S. Conference of Mayors, 1999).

Protective service agencies and battered women's shelters, as well as school-based programs and vocational educational or job placement programs, could be links in the chain of service provision for homeless persons, particularly homeless women and children, although in most cities communication and coordination among agencies serving these populations are either poorly developed or nonexistent (Anderson, Bee, & Smith, 1988; Chenoweth & Free, 1990).

Outreach and case management are key components of the major public and private programs described earlier for serving homeless persons. Case management for homeless persons has been variously viewed as a critical means to identify and coordinate a diverse and fragmented array of services on their behalf, as well as a poor and unsatisfying substitute for the failure to undertake fundamental reforms of the systems (actually nonsystems) of care for homeless persons, as well as the array of other vulnerable populations numbered among them (the physically and mentally ill, persons living with AIDS, alcohol and substance abusers, victims of family abuse or neglect, among others) (Institute of Medicine, 1988c).

Immigrants and Refugees

Most immigrants, documented or otherwise, confront cultural, social, and economic barriers in adjusting to life in the United States. The programs and activities developed to serve immigrants depend to a large extent on the values and political objectives underlying U.S. foreign and immigration policies.

One set of opinions, for example, is guided by the strongly held values and attitudes of nativism, racism, protectionism, and xenophobia, which attempt to exclude or limit the influx of the foreign born to the United States, as well as the assumption of any collective or societal responsibility for their welfare. An opposite perspective calls for a more open policy, principally due to the fact that many of those who were forced or sought to leave their homeland did so as a direct or indirect consequence of U.S. foreign political, military, or economic policy. This point of view argues that since those seeking refuge were made vulnerable by U.S. foreign policies, there is a corollary collective (or societal) responsibility to attempt to address and provide for their needs. Still another opinion is that certain categories of immigrants, such as foreign workers, should be encouraged to come to the United States, because they bring a specialized set of skills or are willing to work for lower wages than U.S. citizens, and thereby enhance the competitive position of U.S. industry and agriculture. In this case, they are assumed to be entitled to those benefits they earn through participation in the labor market and the corollary social class of which they become a member.

These and other values have variously guided the formulation of U.S. immigration policies at different times, as well as the programs and services to which immigrants and refugees are entitled (Bean, Vernez, & Keely, 1989; Rumbaut, Chavez, Moser, Pickwell, & Wishik, 1988; Simon, 1991; Smith & Edmonston, 1997). (See Table 5.9.)

TABLE 5.9. PRINCIPAL PROGRAMS AND SERVICES FOR IMMIGRANTS AND REFUGEES.

| *Preventive Services* | *Treatment Services* | | | *Long-Term Care* | |
| | *Ambulatory* | | *Institutional* | | |
Public Health System	**Preventive Services**	**Treatment Services**	**Acute Care**	**Long-Term Care**	**Home and Community-Based Care**
Family planning	Prenatal care	Emergency medical services	Acute hospital care	Long-term inpatient mental health services	Education Literacy/language Training
Nutritional services	Immunizations	Outpatient medical care services	Short-term inpatient mental health services		Housing alternatives
Health education	Health screening Infectious disease Chronic disease	Outpatient mental health services			Transportation services
Infectious disease control	Psychological evaluation	Dental care services			Legal assistance
Environmental risk abatement programs Housing Sanitation					Job placement
					Voluntary agency (Volag) refugee assistance Child/adult protective services Welfare services Case management

Preventive Services. Many immigrant and refugee populations are exposed to substantial health risks as a function of inadequate public health or preventive-oriented care, as well as the hazardous, overcrowded, and unsanitary living and working conditions that characterized their lives prior or subsequent to arrival in the United States (Loue, 1998; Toole & Waldman, 1990).

The most socially and economically disadvantaged immigrants and refugees in particular may benefit from basic, traditional public health services. This includes the maintenance of community standards and services regarding housing, sewage, and garbage pickup in areas in which large immigrant or refugee populations reside. Although many cultural factors come into play in designing and delivering such services, basic health education and nutritional services may help to prevent the onset or spread of preventable diseases.

Refugees are required to undergo health screening and to demonstrate a level of physical and mental health and associated support requisite to ensuring their ultimate economic self-sufficiency, once they are permanent residents of the United States. Undocumented persons are very unlikely to have any screening of this kind (such as for tuberculosis or hepatitis). Substantial proportions of subgroups of migrant and refugee children are also not likely to have had routine immunizations, which greatly increases their risk of contracting preventable childhood diseases.

The fertility rates of certain refugee and immigrant women are quite high. Yet substantial educational and cultural barriers may exist to providing family planning and prenatal care services to such populations (Kulig, 1990; Rumbaut, Chavez, Moser, Pickwell, & Wishik, 1988).

Treatment Services. Access to medical care services through private or institutional providers is limited by the same financial and organizational barriers that exist for other groups with a similar profile of socioeconomic status and associated entitlements such as Medicaid. In addition, cultural or language factors may dictate where immigrants and refugees can or choose to go for care, such as community or neighborhood health centers, rather than hospital outpatient departments, or to private providers of the same race or cultural background, rather than to "foreign" (U.S.) physicians.

Both legal and illegal refugee groups have often experienced serious psychological, in addition to physical, trauma resulting from themselves' or family members' being tortured or from witnessing loved ones killed. U.S. immigration policies have also contributed to the stresses that refugees experience by scattering family members or providing very time-limited support for resettlement, for example. Policies and programs to treat as well as prevent posttraumatic stress syndrome and the associated psychological manifestations resulting from extremely stressful premigration and resettlement experiences are needed for many subgroups of refugees (Westermeyer, 1987; Westermeyer, Callies, & Neider, 1990).

The dental health needs of immigrants and refugees, particularly children, have been found to be substantial, due to inadequate nutrition or preventive or treatment-oriented dental care services (Hernandez & Charney, 1998).

Long-Term Care. One of the major problems that many immigrants and refugees experience is that they are unable to speak, read, or write English or in some cases are illiterate in the language spoken in their country of origin. English-language and literacy classes are an important component of community support for these new arrivals. Other important support services and resources for refugees and immigrants are job placement, housing, transportation, or welfare or in some cases legal assistance in these or related areas (Broughton, 1989; Rumbaut, Chavez, Moser, Pickwell, & Wishik, 1988).

Voluntary refugee assistance agencies (Volags), sponsored by religious, cultural, or human rights groups, among others, play a large role in obtaining the necessary sponsorship and support (for housing and employment, for example) needed by groups and individuals seeking admission to the United States under an official refugee status. Groups of volunteers also serve as a kind of underground railroad for "refugees" who are fleeing their homeland but are not eligible for official refugee status under existing U.S. immigration policy.

Child or adult protective services agencies may be drawn into dealing with cases of apparent abuse or neglect on the part of immigrant or refugee families, reported by health care or other professionals. These cases may, however, be surrounded with ambiguity and misunderstanding, due to language barriers, differing child-rearing norms, or folk or indigenous medical care practices that may not be fully understood by the accusing professional. Formal or informal case management services are provided refugee populations through public (child protective services, welfare) or voluntary (Volag) refugee assistance agencies.

Conclusion

There is a need for a comprehensive, coordinated continuum of care for vulnerable populations, encompassing an array of prevention, treatment, and long-term care services, as well as the de facto absence of such a continuum in caring for the vulnerable at present. The next chapter examines who pays for the current complex and diverse array of programs and services to care for the vulnerable.

CHAPTER SIX

WHO PAYS FOR THEIR CARE?

Major legacies from the proliferation of health and social legislation in the mid- to late 1960s are the Medicare and Medicaid programs. Medicare is a federal social insurance program that provides essentially universal entitlement to selected health care benefits for persons sixty-five years and older and to disabled workers under age sixty-five. Medicaid is a means-tested (or income eligibility–based) program for categories of individuals eligible for benefits through state public assistance programs or the federal Supplemental Security Income (SSI) program for the aged, blind, and disabled. Medicare provides uniform benefits across states, while Medicaid, a combined state-federal program, is characterized by wide variability in the services covered in different states.

Medicare and Medicaid are the principal payers for health care services for the vulnerable who qualify for these programs. Private health insurance benefits are principally available to people who are working full time and their dependents, although the majority of the uninsured are in households with either full- or part-time workers. The number of Americans with no private or public health insurance has increased dramatically in the past decade due to cutbacks in health benefits in both the governmental and industrial sectors, in response to the accelerating costs of medical care.

This chapter profiles the patchwork of public and private sources of payment for the care of the vulnerable, as well as which groups are likely not to have any safety net of coverage.

Cross-Cutting Issues

The profile that emerges for many vulnerable Americans is that of a sieve, rather than a safety net, of coverage for care delivered through a financially constrained, publicly supported tier of institutions and providers.

Public Payers

Medicaid is a major source of coverage for many of the vulnerable, particularly high-risk mothers and infants, the chronically ill and disabled, persons living with HIV/AIDS, and those with official refugee status. Federal and state legislation has attempted to expand coverage to low-income women and children. The aged, blind, and disabled in financial need who qualify for SSI are automatically eligible for Medicaid. About half of those receiving SSI are eligible because of mental disorders or retardation. The actual benefits provided by Medicaid are, however, quite variable across states and have become more restrictive in some states because of a diminished federal role in financing that program.

Medicare covers physician and hospital services for the elderly but provides very limited support for long-term care services for this or other categories of eligibles. People under age sixty-five who qualify for Social Security Disability Income (SSDI) are eligible for Medicare, but only after a two-year waiting period.

State governments assume a large role in financing mental health services and patient care services for persons living with HIV/AIDS, particularly those with no public or private insurance coverage.

Managed care is assuming an increasingly important role in both the public and private financing of medical care. The challenge is how to balance the need to contain costs within capitated methods of financing with the inclusion of particularly high-risk populations in such plans.

Private Payers

Private insurance is available primarily to people who work and their dependents. Many of the vulnerable are not employed because physical, psychological, or social limitations in functioning preclude their doing so, or they have lost their jobs as a result of associated illnesses or injuries. Certain groups that are working (such as undocumented immigrants or refugees) are nonetheless quite likely to be employed in jobs that do not offer health benefits. The private health insurance benefits for certain categories of problems (such as mental illness or substance abuse) have traditionally been more limited and have become even more so. Private insurers have also developed a variety of devices for ensuring that high-risk groups (such as persons who are HIV positive or technology-assisted children) are either excluded from coverage or have constrained benefit ceilings or high cost-sharing provisions. A related issue is that an increasing number of the low-income working population are likely to decline the health insurance coverage offered through their work because of the high premiums or cost-sharing provisions.

The Uninsured

An estimated 44.3 million (16.3 percent of) Americans are without public or private insurance of any kind (U.S. Bureau of the Census, 1999a). Individuals and families may also rotate in and out of being insured as a consequence of changes in employment, earnings, or family structure. Certain categories of the vulnerable (such as homeless persons, undocumented persons, and young minority victims of violence) are very likely to be uninsured. Others may lack adequate coverage for covering their complex or costly health care needs (such as children with special health care needs). Clearly distinct tiers of service are available for the poor or medically indigent versus those with insurance who have mental health or substance abuse problems. This is also increasingly the case in the medical care system, as publicly supported hospitals and clinics face increased demands in providing care for the array of vulnerable groups who have neither the financial resources nor coverage to pay for it.

The final chapter presents recommendations for knitting together a more effective safety net of coverage out of the current patchwork of public and private financing. (See Table 6.1.)

Population-Specific Overview

The insurance coverage status of the array of vulnerable populations examined here will be reviewed in the discussion that follows.

High-Risk Mothers and Infants

Medicaid is the primary source of payment for poor, pregnant women. Nonetheless, over one in four women of reproductive age have no coverage for maternity-related care.

Public and Private Payers. Changes in the Medicaid program related to restrictions or expansions in eligibility, welfare reform, the growth in Medicaid managed care, and the Child Health Insurance Program (CHIP) have had major impacts on the care and coverage of high-risk mothers and infants. The Omnibus Budget Reconciliation Act of 1981 eliminated many of the working poor and their dependents from eligibility by limiting deductions for work-related expenses, child care, and earned income, and by tightening the Aid to Families with Dependent Children (AFDC) resource requirements. Since that time, in the context of worsening trends in child and infant health indicators, a series of

TABLE 6.1. PRINCIPAL PAYERS FOR VULNERABLE POPULATIONS.

Vulnerable Populations	Public Payers	Private Payers	The Uninsured
High-risk mothers and infants	Medicaid is primary payer for low-income pregnant women.	Private insurers provide limited coverage for maternity care.	Around one in four women are uninsured at the beginning of their pregnancy.
Chronically ill and disabled	Medicare is primary payer for 65+ and for disabled under 65 through SSDI. Medicaid is primary payer for nursing homes for 65+ and disabled poor through SSI, medical indigence.	Private insurers provide very limited or no coverage for long-term care.	Around one in six working-age adults with serious functional limitations are uninsured.
Persons living with HIV/AIDS	Medicaid is primary payer for persons living with HIV/AIDS through TANF or SSI.	Private insurers largely refuse to insure persons with AIDS and those who are HIV positive.	From 20 to 29 percent of persons living with HIV/AIDS are uninsured.
Mentally ill and disabled	State governments are primary payers for specialty mental health services.	Private insurers tend to provide more limited coverage for mental than for physical health care benefits.	Vast majority of clients in public tier are uninsured. Around 10 percent in private tier may be uninsured.
Alcohol or substance abusers	Federal, state, and local governments are primary payers for public tier of services.	Private insurers are primary payers for private tier of services.	Vast majority of clients in public tier are uninsured. Around 11 to 13 percent in private tier may be uninsured.
Suicide or homicide prone	Criminal justice system is primary payer for costs of homicide-related deaths. Medicare may be payer for most elderly suicides.	Private insurers are payers for subset of suicide-related deaths.	Majority of homicide victims are likely to be uninsured.
Abusing families	Criminal justice and social service systems are primary payers for costs of family abuse. Medicaid may be major payer for abused children and Medicare for the elderly.	Private insurers are payers for subset of abuse victims.	Many of the victims of abuse in two-parent families with an unemployed wage earner may be uninsured.
Homeless persons	Public entitlement and insurance programs cover very small number of the homeless.	Private insurers have little or no role in providing coverage for the homeless.	Vast majority of homeless have no insurance.
Immigrants and refugees	Medicaid provides time-limited coverage for those with official refugee status.	Private insurers cover only immigrants and refugees in jobs with benefits.	Vast majority of undocumented immigrants and many employed legal immigrants are uninsured.

expansions have been directed at increasing the proportion of low-income women and children eligible under Medicaid.

The primary thrust of subsequent legislation was to decouple Medicaid from eligibility for the AFDC program, through permitting states to extend Medicaid coverage to pregnant women whose family incomes reached 185 percent of the poverty level and, in 1990 by mandating coverage for those with incomes up to 133 percent of the poverty level. States were also permitted to expedite the eligibility determination process through dropping the assets test for eligibility; using a shortened application form; introducing presumptive, expedited, or continuous eligibility procedures; and stationing Medicaid eligibility workers outside welfare offices. Subsequent legislation gave the states the option of providing Medicaid coverage for enhanced services dealing primarily with behavioral, attitudinal, and nutritional factors.

The Personal Responsibility and Work Opportunity Reconciliation Act (the Welfare Reform Act) of 1996 has also had major impacts on the eligibility of pregnant women and their infants for Medicaid. The Temporary Assistance for Needy Families (TANF) created by that act essentially broke the link between welfare and Medicaid, in that Medicaid was not an automatic benefit to those qualifying under TANF, as it had been to individuals and families who received AFDC benefits. Eligibility for Medicaid was, however, still tied to AFDC-related income guidelines. TANF mandated that any woman who is capable of working should do so in order to continue to receive benefits. By taking away Medicaid benefits at the relatively low AFDC income eligibility threshold, a level at which few workers can either obtain or afford private coverage, the TANF rules in effect penalize low-income mothers for working. A consequence was that a large proportion of women lost Medicaid benefits without corollary access to private coverage (Heymann & Earle, 1999; Short & Freedman, 1998).

By and large, these laws did not directly address issues related to the accessibility and quality of care provided to Medicaid-eligible women. The types of benefits covered vary greatly by state, eligibility determination and application procedures remain complex and cumbersome, the rate of reimbursement to providers is lower than their average fees, and an estimated 29 percent of doctors providing obstetric services refuse to accept Medicaid patients. Many poor women do not have Medicaid coverage because of program access barriers or the fact that their income falls above restrictive state income eligibility guidelines (Barber-Madden & Kotch, 1990; Cunningham & Monheit, 1990; Dubay, Kenney, Norton, & Cohen, 1995; Ellwood & Kenney, 1995; Hill, 1990; Mitchell, 1991; Perloff, Kletke, Fossett, & Banks, 1997; Sardell, 1990; Schlesinger & Kronebusch, 1990).

An important policy trend is the increased efforts by states to enroll Medicaid beneficiaries in managed care. The percentage of the Medicaid population enrolled in managed care increased from 14.4 percent in 1993 to 53.6 percent in 1998 (Health Care Financing Administration, 1998b). These initiatives were intended both to improve access and contain the costs of care to pregnant women and children under Medicaid. However, evaluation studies of the effect of both Medicaid expansions and Medicaid managed care have shown mixed results with respect to increasing access to prenatal care services and improving birth outcomes. Although women may obtain care earlier in the pregnancy, birth outcomes are not necessarily enhanced. The most successful initiatives appear to be ones that provide targeted and expanded services to particularly at-risk women (Baldwin et al., 1998; Griffin, Hogan, Buechner, & Leddy, 1999; Levinson & Ullman, 1998; Piper, Mitchel, & Ray, 1994; Ray, Mitchel, & Piper, 1997).

The availability of private health insurance coverage has been documented to exert a strong, positive influence on women's decision to work and a strong negative impact on continued welfare participation (Moffitt & Wolfe, 1993). Nonetheless, private sector coverage has diminished for low-income workers and their dependents. National survey data on trends in insurance coverage from 1977 through 1996 documented that children in poor and low-income working families experienced the greatest estimated decline in private coverage (Weinick & Monheit, 1999). One in five children in single-parent families was uninsured in 1996, which is one-third more than in 1977. The percentage of children in two-parent families with public coverage doubled between 1987 and 1996, from 6 percent to nearly 13 percent. This increase occurred primarily among poor families and those with only one working parent, which was consistent with expansions in the Medicaid program during this period. The diminished availability of private coverage for children with working parents was attributed to the decline in real earnings for full-time workers and the loss of jobs in the industrial sector to the service sector, where employers were less likely to offer health insurance.

CHIP, enacted in 1997, was intended to expand coverage for families and children though Medicaid or other state-initiated programs. The trend toward the diminished availability of private coverage, particularly for low-income workers and their dependents, continues unabated. There is some concern that the availability of expanded public coverage through either Medicaid or CHIP will, in effect, further crowd out the provision of private coverage through work for these groups (Selden, Banthin, & Cohen, 1999).

The Uninsured. Around 40 million Americans are estimated to be uninsured, with women in the childbearing years being disproportionately represented. Only around two-thirds (64 percent) of pregnant women in the United States are estimated to have private coverage that covers all or part of their care related to childbirth. Approximately 26 percent of women have no insurance at the beginning of their pregnancy, and 15 percent have none by the time of delivery (York, Grant, Gibeau, Beecham, & Kessler, 1996). Those without coverage are disproportionately young, unmarried, minority, and poor. Title V of the Social Security Act, which authorized the establishment of the Maternal and Child Health and Crippled Children Services programs (now the Program for Children with Special Health Care Needs), provides support for safety net providers of care for uninsured, as well as insured, high-risk mothers and infants.

Chronically Ill and Disabled

Three principal types of programs provide direct or indirect financial support for the chronically ill and disabled: (1) income assistance programs, such as SSDI, SSI, Veterans Administration (VA), civil service, and black lung disability programs, and worker's compensation; (2) health insurance programs, including Medicare, Medicaid, as well as VA and Civilian Health and Medical Program of the Uniformed Services (CHAMPUS)/TRICARE (coverage for dependents of U.S. military personnel); and (3) supportive service programs, funded through social services, mental health, and maternal and child health block grants, child welfare services, the Administration on Developmental Disabilities, and the Department of Education (Office of Assistant Secretary for Planning and Evaluation, 1996).

Public and Private Payers. SSDI benefits are available to disabled persons under age sixty-five who have previously been employed and their dependents. The definition of disability for SSDI eligibility is "the inability to do any substantial gainful activity . . . by reason of any medically determinable physical or mental impairment which can be expected to result in death or has lasted or can be expected to last for a continuous period of not less than 12 months" (Office of Assistant Secretary for Planning and Evaluation, 1996, p. 4).

Only persons who are totally disabled and whose disability is expected to be long term can qualify. According to the 1990 Survey of Income and Program Participation (SIPP), about 13 percent of the working-age population received SSDI. Significantly higher proportions of SSDI beneficiaries were found among persons with spinal cord injury (36.2 percent), mental illness (33.6 percent), mental retardation or developmental disabilities (32.7 percent), heart disease (27.2 percent), and respiratory conditions (22.6 percent) (Office of Assistant Secretary for Planning and Evaluation, 1995). SSDI beneficiaries are eligible for coverage under Medicare. However, there is a twenty-four-month waiting period, after qualifying for SSDI, to become eligible for this benefit.

The SSI program provides monthly cash benefits to aged, blind, and disabled workers who are in financial need. Unlike SSDI beneficiaries, SSI recipients do not have to have a work history. The SSDI definition of disability also applies in determining SSI eligibility. Financial need is based on countable income (including both income and assets). States, at their option, can provide supplementary payments to federal SSI. The amount of these subsidies varies considerably across states. SSI recipients were more likely to have a primary disabling condition related to their mental, rather than physical, functioning, reflected in the fact that the two groups significantly more likely to receive SSI among the disabled population were the mentally ill (25.6 percent) and those with mental retardation or developmental disabilities (43.2 percent) (Office of Assistant Secretary for Planning and Evaluation, 1995).

SSI recipients are automatically eligible for Medicaid upon receipt of SSI benefits. Unlike the link between SSDI and Medicare, there is no waiting period to establish Medicaid eligibility.

Medicaid is the largest third-party payer for institutionalized long-term care, accounting for 45 percent of the expenditures for nursing home care (Kaiser Family Foundation, 1997). Of the approximately 35.2 million persons who received services funded by Medicaid in 1995, 16.6 percent (5.8 million) were eligible because of their disability or blindness (Kaiser Family Foundation, 1997). The role of Medicaid in financing nursing home care came about largely due to the failure of Medicare or private insurance to cover these services for the chronically ill and disabled, although substantial gaps and variability in eligibility exist in the coverage provided for individuals in nursing homes and other long-term care institutions (Carpenter, 1988).

Medicaid home- and community-based service waivers, authorized under section 1915 (c) of the Social Security Act, afford states the flexibility to develop and implement alternatives to placing Medicaid-eligible individuals in institutions, such as nursing homes. The Medicaid Home and Community-Based (2176) Waiver Program (enacted in 1981) and the Tax Equity and Fiscal Responsibility Act (TEFRA) Section 134 Option for Disabled Children ("Katie Beckett" waiver enacted in 1982, named for a ventilator-assisted child whose family wished for her to be cared for at home rather than in a nursing home) provide more flexibility for providing long-term care services at home rather than in institutional settings. The 2176 waiver permits certain home care services to be covered if they are budget neutral (do not cost more than institutional care). The Katie Beckett waiver permits family income eligibility criteria to be waived in covering home care services for categories of individuals (such as ventilator-assisted children). The Omnibus Budget Reconciliation Act of 1990 provided an alternative to the 2176 waiver in financing home and community-based care under Medicaid by incorporating them as optional services for individuals with severe physical or cognitive impairments who were eligible for Medicaid (Health Care Financing Administration, 1999; Laudicina & Burwell, 1988).

Of the 39 million people covered under Medicare in 1996, around 13 percent (5 million) were disabled people under age sixty-five. The vast majority was also covered for physicians' services under Part B (Kaiser Family Foundation, 1999). Medicare is a major payer for hospital and physician services, but has a more limited role in financing long-term institutional care for the chronically ill and disabled. The expansion of home health care benefits under Medicare since 1974 has resulted in substantial increases in expenditures for that benefit under Medicare, however.

Approximately 25 to 30 percent of all disabled Medicare enrollees under age sixty-five are covered by Medicaid. Disabled Medicare enrollees with incomes below the poverty level are also entitled to have Medicare Part B premiums, coinsurance, and deductibles covered through Medicaid in many states (Kaiser Family Foundation, 1999).

Programs funded under maternal and child health block grants, particularly Programs for Children with Special Health Care Needs, play a significant role in the care of chronically ill children. Services vary across states, but most fund screening and treatment of disabling conditions, case management, and counseling. Compared to funding for health and health-related services, financial support for community-based support services for families of children with impaired mobility (such as respite care, after-school care, homemaker services, and summer camp) is largely lacking. The range of services for chronically ill children covered by firms offering health insurance to employees and their dependents is often limited, and the deductible and coinsurance are rates high, thereby forcing families to bear a large share of the costs of their child's care (Fox & Newacheck, 1990).

An increasing number of chronically ill children and the elderly are being enrolled in managed care plans due to state-mandated enrollment of Medicaid-eligible individuals in such plans, as well as federal initiatives to encourage the wider availability of managed care alternatives for Medicare recipients (Fama, Fox, & White, 1995).

The Uninsured. Children and working-age adults with substantial limitations in functioning are much less likely to be covered under private insurance compared to their nondisabled counterparts. According to the 1994–1995 SIPP, 22.7 percent of persons twenty-two to sixty-four years old with disabilities had no public or private coverage, compared to 17.1 percent of people in this age group who were not disabled. Around one in six (16.7 percent) working-age adults with serious functional limitations lacked either public or private coverage (McNeil, 1997).

A study conducted by ICF, Inc. and the Brookings Institute on alternatives for financing long-term care endorsed the growth of public and private risk-sharing options. That study called for a universal, social insurance–based long-term care program to be added to Medicare, rather than one linked to the more categorical, welfare-based Medicaid program, which is de facto currently the system of financing long-term care (Rivlin, Wiener, Hanley, & Spence, 1988; Wiener & Rubin, 1989). The issue of long-term care insurance and medical savings accounts as means for financing the costs of extended illness has remained a salient one in federal health care reform debates (Pepper Commission, 1990; Wiener & Hanley, 1990).

Persons Living with HIV/AIDS

Public insurers, most notably Medicaid, and to an increasing extent Medicare, are the major payers for persons living with HIV/AIDS.

Public and Private Payers. National estimates of the percentage of persons living with HIV/AIDS covered by Medicaid have ranged from 29 percent to 50 percent. Up to 90 percent of all children with AIDS have been estimated to be covered by Medicaid (Diaz et al., 1994; Fleishman & Mor, 1993; Health Care Financing Administration, 1998a; RAND, 1999). The proportion of persons living with HIV/AIDS with Medicaid varies considerably by state because of differing eligibility requirements and covered benefits. Persons living with HIV/AIDS may become eligible for Medicaid through state categorically needy programs—generally through TANF for women and children and the SSI disability program for adult males—or, when available, a state's program for the medically needy (Buchanan, 1996).

Data from the 1996 HIV Cost and Services Utilization Study estimated that 19 percent of persons living with HIV/AIDS were covered by Medicare (RAND, 1999). Medicare is available to individuals receiving social security benefits, including the elderly, the disabled who qualify under SSDI, as well as enrollees in the End-Stage Renal Disease Program. The vast majority of persons living with HIV/AIDS receiving Medicare benefits have qualified under the SSDI program. To become eligible for SSDI and attendant Medicare benefits, persons living with HIV/AIDS must meet SSDI requirements for both prior work history and disability. Disabled persons can begin to collect cash social security benefits five months after the onset of their disability, but must wait an additional twenty-four months (for a total of twenty-nine months) before they become eligible for Medicare coverage (Fasciano, Cherlow, Turner, & Thornton, 1998; Schietinger & Schechter, 1998).

The Health Care Financing Administration estimated that in fiscal year 1998, the federal share of Medicaid and Medicare spending was 22 percent and 16 percent of total federal HIV/AIDS spending, respectively. In addition, the state portion of Medicaid spending for HIV/AIDS was estimated to be 46 percent of combined state and federal spending (Pine, 1998).

State budgets are also a substantial source of funds for other HIV/AIDS-related programs, such as surveillance, testing, and counseling programs; patient care; support services; and administrative activities (Rowe & Keintz, 1989).

With the development of antiretroviral therapies in the mid-1990s, the time period for persons with HIV infection progressing to full-blown AIDS has been greatly extended. The categorical disability-related eligibility requirements for Medicaid and Medicare coverage do not, however, adequately provide for the care and coverage of persons with asymptomatic HIV, who may benefit from such therapies. Medicare does not provide prescription drug benefits. State Medicaid programs also limit the price or type of HIV-related drugs included in their program formularies (Buchanan & Smith, 1994a, 1994b). Title II of the 1990 Ryan White Comprehensive AIDS Resource Emergency Act permits states to allocate funds to cover home-based health services, provide medication and other treatments, continue private health insurance coverage, or fund HIV care consortia. AIDS Drug Assistance Programs funded under this act have been used to extend and supplement drug coverage for persons living with HIV/AIDS in many states (Buchanan & Smith, 1998).

The proportion of persons living with HIV/AIDS covered by private insurance has been estimated to range from 20 to 32 percent (Diaz et al., 1994; Fleishman & Mor, 1993; RAND, 1999). Private insurers employ a variety of devices to exclude or limit coverage for persons living with HIV/AIDS, including preexisting condition screening, coverage limitations, and high premiums (Levi, Sogocio, Gambrell, & Jones, 1999). The increasing penetration of managed care in both the public and private sectors also presents challenges in setting adequate capitation rates and avoiding adverse selection or exclusion of persons living with HIV/AIDS from these arrangements (Conviser, Gamliel, & Honberg, 1998).

The Uninsured. The proportion of persons living with HIV/AIDS who have no insurance, because of the restrictive eligibility criteria imposed by both public and private insurers, has been estimated to range from 20 to 29 percent (Diaz et al., 1994; Fleishman & Mor, 1993; RAND, 1999). These include individuals who have become unemployed and lose private insurance benefits through work or who start receiving SSDI benefits that exceed income eligibility criteria for Medicaid through SSI or medically needy programs (Fleishman, 1998). Policy recommendations to reduce the number of uninsured with HIV/AIDS include private insurance market reforms, such as guaranteed issue, rating restrictions, eliminating or minimizing preexisting exclusions, and state risk pools; extending presumptive disability to persons with HIV infection under state Medicaid medically needy programs; and payment for supplemental insurance and drug coverage for Medicare-eligible individuals (Buchanan, 1996; Levi, Sogocio, Gambrell, & Jones, 1999; Schietinger & Schechter, 1998).

Mentally Ill and Disabled

State budgets are the largest sources of funding for mental health care services, although Medicaid and Medicare have assumed a larger role in paying for such services over the past decade. Managed behavioral health care is being increasingly used in the provision of both public and private mental health care services.

Public and Private Payers. The principal payers for mental health services in 1994 were as follows: state mental health agencies (24.5 percent) or other state (5.5 percent) or local government sources (8.1 percent); Medicaid (19.7 percent), Medicare (14.0 percent), or other federal sources, such as CHAMPUS or the VA (5.3 percent); client fees (17.7 percent); contract funds (1.4 percent); and all other sources (3.8 percent) (Witkin et al., 1998).

The benefit design of Medicaid and Medicare and the deficit financing role of state mental health authorities (meaning they are the payer of last resort for patients not covered from other sources) have resulted in the respective payers' mainly covering certain types of services. State psychiatric hospitals are principally funded by state mental health authorities. Those funded by a mix of state mental health authorities and local governments primarily include psychiatric outpatient clinics, psychiatric day/night facilities, multiservice mental health organizations, state and local government-operated general hospital psychiatric units; and other residential treatment centers. Residential treatment centers for emotionally disturbed children tend to be supported by state and local sources of funds for education or criminal justice rather than mental health. Private psychiatric hospitals and general hospital psychiatric units are mainly supported through private insurance and patient fees (Witkin et al., 1998).

Federal income support programs, such as SSDI, SSI, TANF, and food stamps, assist mentally ill individuals in obtaining nonmedical support services. The Alcohol, Drug Abuse and Mental Health, Community Development, and Social Services block grants are the largest federal block grant funding sources for services and resources for the mentally ill and disabled (Craig, 1988b).

Most mentally ill Medicaid beneficiaries qualify through being eligible for SSI benefits because of their disability and income levels. Mandatory services provided under Medicaid cover the basic mental health care needs of acutely ill patients in hospitals and nursing homes. Considerable variability exists across states in the optional services covered to facilitate the care of the mentally ill in the community (such as reimbursement for freestanding outpatient clinic services, prescription drugs, case management, rehabilitation, and home health care). Small residential facilities, such as halfway houses, adult foster homes, crisis centers, or institutions for mental disease, do not qualify for Medicaid (Taube, Goldman, & Salkever, 1990). The burgeoning costs of care for mental health care services within state Medicaid programs have led to the increasing use of waivers to permit Medicaid-eligible individuals to be enrolled in managed behavioral health care arrangements (Busch, 1997; Feldman, Baler, & Penner, 1997; Frank, McGuire, Notman, & Woodward, 1996; Kastner, Walsh, & Criscione, 1997).

Medicare coverage for mental health services is limited, although it has expanded since the early 1990s. Mentally disabled individuals become eligible for Medicare principally through their enrollment in the SSDI program. Medicare does not, however, cover many of the social support and other long-term care services needed by the chronically ill in general or mentally ill individuals in particular.

Part A of Medicare imposes a lifetime limit of 190 days of care in freestanding psychiatric hospitals and 90 days in a general hospital within a benefit period (uninterrupted hospital stay). Medicare Part B coverage for physician services in inpatient settings is the same for mental and physical treatment. Coverage in outpatient settings differs, however. Part B pays 80 percent of approved charges after a deductible is met for treatment of physical disorders, but only 50 percent of treatment for mental disorders (with the exception of patients with Alzheimer's disease, to which the 80 percent coverage rule applies) (Bartels & Colenda, 1998; Cano, Hennessy, Warren, & Lubitz, 1997; Rosenbach & Ammering, 1997; Sherman, 1996).

The vast majority of large employers cover inpatient and outpatient mental health care and related substance abuse services, and the majority cover intensive nonresidential treatment, such as partial hospitalization. The proportion covering nonhospital and intensive nonresidential treatment—respectively, 52 percent and 64 percent in 1997 among the most prevalent plans—has increased but nonetheless remains lower than for other services. Based on 1997 data, around three out of four employer-sponsored plans placed greater restrictions on behavioral health care than on general medical coverage (Buck, Teich, Umland, & Stein, 1999; Buck & Umland, 1997).

Managed behavioral health care programs are becoming a dominant means of financing mental health and substance abuse services in both the public and private sectors. Payment for services is generally in one of two forms: a monthly flat fee per enrollee paid in advance (generally referred to as an administrative services only payment) or a monthly per capita payment under which the managed behavioral health care organization (MBHCO) is at risk for the cost of all the administrative and clinical service costs. A network of providers is under contract to provide the agreed-on behavioral health care services. These benefits are usually negotiated as carve-outs, meaning they are priced and provided separately from general medical care or other services. The challenge in setting the per capita rates for such services is how to minimize moral hazard (incentives to increase the unnecessary use of covered services) and adverse selection (MBHCOs' tendencies to exclude high-risk cases from coverage) (Dial, Kantor, Buck, & Chalk, 1996; Feldman, 1998; Frank, McGuire, & Newhouse, 1995; Manderscheid & Henderson, 1996; Mechanic, 1996c; Shore, 1996).

The Uninsured. Data from the National Center for Health Statistics and National Institute of Mental Health (NIMH) showed that a larger portion of psychiatric patients are uninsured compared to medical-surgical patients. Based on the 1986 National Hospital Discharge Survey, 9.5 percent had no insurance, compared to 7.6 percent of all patients. According to 1981 NIMH data on the mental health services sector, 10.4 percent of discharges from general psychiatric units, 5.0 percent from psychiatric hospitals, and 62.0 percent from public mental hospitals were not insured (Frank, 1989). Problems of the absence or inadequacy of coverage are greatest for the long-term chronically mentally ill, who require a comprehensive array of inpatient and outpatient mental health as well as related social services (Frisman & McGuire, 1989; Grazier, 1989; Robinson, Meisel, & Guthierrez, 1990).

Alcohol or Substance Abusers

Although the proportion of alcohol and substance abuse services covered by private third-party insurance has increased substantially in recent years, the largest overall source of support continues to be federal, state, or local funds. However, distinct types and tiers of services have emerged in response to the evolution of private versus public sources of funding.

Public and Private Payers. Federal funding for drug abuse grew substantially from 1969 to 1974, stabilized, and then declined before beginning to grow again in 1986. From 1969 to 1975, the federal government put the majority of its anti–drug abuse resources into treatment and prevention rather than criminal justice. In the mid-1970s the trend was reversed, and in 1989 the lion's share (69 percent) of federal anti–drug abuse expenditures was in the criminal justice area.

In 1976 the federal government paid for 42.5 percent of drug treatment, and state and local governments paid for 48.2 percent. The balance came from private sources (5.0 percent) or other donations (4.3 percent). In 1989, the federal share was down to 17.4 percent, which included Medicaid, Medicare, or other public insurance (10.6 percent), welfare and social service payments (3.7 percent), and federal categorical grants (3.1 percent). The state and local share declined to 34.8 percent, while the share covered by private sources increased considerably to 42.5 percent: 29.3 percent by private third-party payers, 11.2 percent by client out-of-pocket payments, and 1.9 percent private donations. The balance (5.4 percent) was from other sources (Gerstein & Harwood, 1990; National Institute on Drug Abuse, 1990).

Two distinct tiers of drug abuse treatment have emerged, linked directly to the means of paying for care. The public tier programs are either publicly owned or private, not-for-profit programs that obtain their revenues mainly from local, state, or federal agencies. This public tier is composed mainly of large, multisite residential and methadone programs and outpatient clinics. They principally serve clients who are indigent or uninsured, and are largely an adjunct to the criminal justice system.

The private tier largely contains private providers who serve patients with private insurance or sufficient resources to pay for treatment themselves. This tier evolved primarily from hospital inpatient units that focused on alcohol treatment, but now includes a substantial outpatient and aftercare focus. In 1989 the private tier treated 22 percent of all reported admissions and received 41 percent of system revenues. It averaged $2,450 in revenues per admission, compared to public system revenues of $1,240 per admission (Gerstein & Harwood, 1990).

The funding of alcohol treatment has followed trends similar to that of drug abuse treatment in terms of diminished federal support relative to increased private support over time. In 1982, the percentage distributions of funding sources, compared to 1989, were as follows: federal programs (16.8 versus 4.8 percent), state or local (34.7 versus 35.3 percent), public welfare (1.6 versus 1.5 percent), public insurance (6.9 versus 8.5 percent), private insurance (26.4 versus 31.9 percent), client fees (9.8 versus 13.2 percent), and other (3.7 versus 4.7 percent) (Institute of Medicine, 1990; National Institute on Drug Abuse, 1990).

Separate public and private service systems also exist for the treatment of alcohol problems. The vast majority of funding for programs receiving government support from state alcoholism agencies comes from state, local, or federal sources, and the opposite is the case with private sector specialty programs in which the vast majority of admissions are covered by private insurance or patient fees (Institute of Medicine, 1990).

Medicare and Medicaid pay a relatively small percentage of alcohol and drug abuse treatment costs overall. Neither Medicare nor Medicaid has specific benefits for the treatment of alcohol or drug abuse. Both programs tend to categorize treatment of these problems under mental disorders, with attendant limitations in coverage and benefits under Medicare and wide variability in optional services covered under Medicaid. Neither provides coverage for the educational, vocational, and psychosocial services that are generally considered to be an important component of rehabilitation and maintenance for substance abuse (relapse prevention) (Institute of Medicine, 1990; Rogowski, 1993).

A 1997 survey of companies with ten or more employees showed that the majority provided substance abuse treatment coverage. The percentages of plans covering specific substance abuse treatment among the plans with the largest enrollments were as follows: inpatient detoxification (87 percent), outpatient counseling (84 percent), outpatient detoxification (76 percent), intensive nonresidential (59 percent), nonhospital residential (50 percent), case management or referral (49 percent), and methadone maintenance (18 percent). Most plans imposed substantial limitations on benefits. The most frequently imposed limits were the amount payable per year or the number of inpatient days or outpatient visits per year (Buck, Teich, Umland, & Stein, 1999).

The Uninsured. Anywhere from 31 million to 92 million Americans have been estimated to have no or inadequate drug abuse treatment coverage. This assumes that 31 million people have no health insurance at all, and around 48 million people with private insurance and 13 million people on Medicaid have no or very limited benefits (Gerstein & Harwood, 1990). The vast majority of clients seen in the public drug and alcohol abuse treatment sectors have no insurance. Around 11 to 13 percent of the treatment costs for those seen in the private sector in 1986 were paid directly by the clients themselves (Institute of Medicine, 1990).

Suicide or Homicide Prone

The agencies and institutions that bear the costs associated with attempted or completed suicides and homicides reside in a variety of sectors. A number of the correlates and predictors of violent deaths, such as depression, suicidal ideation or attempts, aggressive behavior, and family discord or abuse, tend to be treated within the mental health care sector. Alcohol and substance abuse is treated within both the general mental health and alcohol and drug abuse treatment sectors. The extent of coverage for mental health and substance abuse services, as well as the direct medical care costs for individual victims of suicide and homicide, is a function of the type of plan and benefits for which they might be insured.

Public and Private Payers. Those individuals most likely to be suicide victims (white males) are likely to have private insurance coverage or Medicare.

Other sectors, such as the criminal justice and social service systems, absorb a great deal of the costs of dealing with the consequences of violent death due to homicide and suicide. Violent (and particularly drug-related) crime is an important component of expenditures within the criminal justice system.

Major social services activities administered by the U.S. Department of Health and Human Services that also provide direct or indirect support for programs to prevent suicide and related violent or abusive behaviors include the Social Services, Community Services and Alcohol, Drug Abuse, and Mental Health Block Grants, Head Start, Child Welfare Services, Foster Care, Child Abuse and Neglect Program, the Older Americans Act, the Runaway Youth Act, and the Adolescent Family Life Program (Silverman, 1989).

The Uninsured. Those most likely to be both the perpetrators and victims of homicide (black and Hispanic males) are least likely to have insurance. In some cases, they may qualify for publicly subsidized coverage (through the VA or possibly Medicaid, for example). The coverage provided for these services under both public and private plans remains limited. Gunshot injuries have been estimated to cost around $2.5 billion in lifetime medical costs, a large proportion of which is not covered by insurance, since victims of firearm-related violence are more likely to be uninsured or are eligible for medical care assistance under government programs that do not fully reimburse trauma costs (Cook, Lawrence, Ludwig, & Miller, 1999; General Accounting Office, 1991).

Abusing Families

The principal payers for the costs associated with maltreatment are the agencies and institutions that address the short- and long-term needs of abusing families: child protective services and welfare systems, foster care, regular and special education, police departments, juvenile and adult court and detention facilities, substance abuse treatment programs, and public health departments, in addition to medical care and rehabilitation services providers (Daro, 1988).

Public and Private Payers. The medical care costs of the injuries resulting from abuse, many of which are treated in hospital emergency rooms, are covered by the family's or individual's insurance. Daro (1988) projected the hospitalization costs for all those children reported to have suffered serious physical injury from maltreatment ($n = 23,648$). The resulting impairments included brain damage, skull fractures, bone fractures, internal injuries, poisoning, and burns. Assuming that only half of the children required hospitalization for an estimated 5.2 days (the average length of stay for children with bone fractures), Daro estimated that the inpatient costs of treatment would exceed $20 million. The vast majority would be paid by Medicaid, since many of the children on which the estimates were based received public assistance.

Medicare is the principal payer for the medical care costs associated with injuries or illness experienced by noninstitutionalized abused dependent elderly (Filinson & Ingman, 1989; Steinmetz, 1988).

The Uninsured. Estimates of the number of uninsured among victims of intimate abuse are not available. Unemployment, underemployment, and associated economic stresses often characterize such families. The rates of uninsurance are likely to be highest among families that do not qualify for benefits through TANF/AFDC, but in which the main wage earner is either out of work or employed in a low-paying or part-time job with no benefits.

Homeless Persons

The vast majority of homeless persons have no means of paying for care. Most are uninsured. A very small number have some form of public or private insurance coverage.

Public and Private Payers. Data on homeless clients in the 1996 National Survey of Homeless Assistance Providers and Clients documented that 40 percent had some means-tested benefit, including AFDC (10 percent), General Assistance (9 percent), SSI (11 percent), food stamps (37 percent), and Medicaid (30 percent). In addition to the 30 percent who said they had coverage for medical expenses through Medicaid, 7 percent reported coverage through the Department of Veterans Affairs, 4 percent through private insurance, and 10 percent through other types of insurance. The percentages receiving these benefits tended to be higher among clients in homeless families and lower among single homeless clients (Burt et al., 1999).

The Homeless Eligibility Clarification Act, which was part of the Anti-Drug Abuse Act of 1986, provided that people without a fixed home or mailing address could not be denied eligibility for Medicaid, food stamps, AFDC, SSI, veterans' benefits, job training. or other programs. A focus of the Health Resources and Services Administration Health Care for the Homeless and Department of Veterans Affairs–Health Care for Homeless Veterans (VA-HCHV), as well as other programs serving homeless persons, is to assist those who are eligible in obtaining benefits (Rosenheck, Frisman, & Kasprow, 1999; U.S. Commission on Security and Cooperation in Europe, 1990).

The Uninsured. The prevalence of physical disabilities, mental health, and drug and alcohol disorders qualifies a large proportion of homeless persons for SSI/SSDI benefits. Recipients of SSI and TANF/AFDC are generally eligible for Medicaid coverage. SSDI beneficiaries are eligible to receive Medicare after a two-year waiting period. Health insurance coverage is low among the homeless population due in large part to their low rates of participation in such programs. The Welfare Reform Act of 1996 removed many previously eligible individuals from receiving benefits, which exacerbated the lack of coverage among multi-problem homeless persons (those with substance abuse or mental health problems, for example). Fifty-five percent of the clients in the 1996 Urban Institute survey of homeless assistance providers and clients reported they had no medical insurance of any kind (Bassuk, Browne, & Buckner, 1996; Burt et al., 1999; Kreider & Nicholson, 1997).

The vast majority of homeless persons continue to slip through the cracks of the fragmented and inadequate safety net of support of health and social services that do exist for the poorest of the poor in our society, among whom the homeless are clearly numbered.

Immigrants and Refugees

"Overdocumented" immigrants (those with official refugee status) have the most formalized guarantees of support and coverage (for a period at least), and the "undocumented" (those who have entered the country illegally) the least.

Public and Private Payers. Foreign-born residents are less likely to have private insurance, Medicare, and Medicaid than those who are native born (Thamer, Richard, Casebeer, & Ray, 1997; Thamer & Rinehart, 1998).

Restrictive state laws, such as Proposition 187 enacted in 1994 in California, as well as the federal Welfare Reform Act passed in 1996, have had a profound impact on further limiting eligibility for insurance and social service benefits for foreign-born residents of the United States. Proposition 187 barred undocumented immigrant children from attending public schools and withheld all non-emergency medical care, including prenatal care and inoculations. Most of the provisions of Proposition 187 subsequently have been declared unconstitutional. Its approval did, however, serve to foster an anti-immigrant sentiment, increase the propensity on the part of providers to require documentation of legal status from foreign-born residents, and thereby inhibit potentially eligible individuals from applying for benefits (Calavita, 1996; Turshen, 1996).

The federal Welfare Reform Act reduced the benefits available to both documented and undocumented foreign-born residents. Except for selected categories of refugees and veterans, noncitizens were no longer eligible for SSI and food stamp benefits. Immigrants receiving SSI, many of whom were elderly or disabled, would also lose accompanying Medicaid benefits. Immigrants who arrived after August 22, 1996, were barred from any federal means-tested benefits for five years. After the five-year ban, new immigrants must include their sponsor's income when applying for any federal means-tested benefits. States were also given wider discretion for determining immigrants' eligibility for benefits. Undocumented immigrants were deemed to be ineligible for federal, state, or local public benefits.

To try to minimize the impact of the law on the loss of Medicaid coverage by women, children, and families receiving AFDC benefits, the Welfare Reform Act required that states continue to use their old AFDC rules that were in effect in July 1996 before the enactment of the TANF program created by the act. Welfare caseloads have diminished substantially in many states, and preliminary data suggests that there has been an accompanying, though not as a dramatic, decline in Medicaid caseloads. The federal CHIP, which provides support to states to expand coverage to uninsured children and their families, offers the prospect of providing insurance safety nets to such families. Eligibility for noncitizens may, however, continued to be restricted by federal and state statutes (Ellwood & Ku, 1998; Halfon, Wood, Valdez, Pereyra, & Duan, 1997; Norton, Kenney, & Ellwood, 1996).

Public policy regarding the health care of refugees was detailed in the Refugee Act of 1980 (Public Law 96–212). Title III of the act authorized the Office of Refugee Resettlement within the Department of Health and Human Services to (1) monitor health screening and immunization activities in overseas centers before the refugee enters the United States; (2) inspect the refugee's health documents at the port of entry; (3) notify local health departments of refugees resettling in their communities; (4) provide health assessments after relocation; and (5) facilitate the refugee's access to timely treatment through appropriate health and mental health services.

Many immigrants, as well as refugees and undocumented immigrants, are working. Those who are paid through regular payrolls have social security and state and local income taxes withheld. Immigrants pay sales taxes on their regular purchases; excise taxes on gas, cigarettes, and liquor; and property taxes on property they rent or own. Overall legal and illegal immigrants and refugees, particularly working-age adults, may well contribute more to the public coffers through these means than they take through various entitlement or income transfer programs (Calavita, 1996; Smith & Edmonston, 1997; Turshen, 1996).

The Uninsured. Immigrants are often employed in jobs or industries that pay low wages and have few or no health and other fringe benefits. Substantial proportions have no private insurance through their place of employment and do not qualify for coverage for Medicaid or other welfare benefits because what they do earn is too high or they do not fit the categoric (TANF, SSI) criteria for eligibility (Rumbaut, Chavez, Moser, Pickwell, & Wishik, 1988; Thamer, Richard, Casebeer, & Ray, 1997; Thamer & Rinehart, 1998). This dilemma is reflected particularly in the high rates of Hispanics nationally (35.3 percent) without health insurance for the entire year (in 1998) compared to other racial and ethnic groups: non-Hispanic whites (11.9 percent), blacks (22.2 percent), Asian and Pacific Islander (21.1 percent) (U.S. Bureau of the Census, 1999a).

Conclusion

There are distinct public and private tiers of paying for services for vulnerable populations, as well as some troubling trends regarding cutbacks on the part of private payers in providing coverage for the most vulnerable; growing gaps in the safety net of coverage for those served in the public sphere; as well as a large number of individuals experiencing poor health who may be without coverage of any kind for all or part of the year. The absence of resources for purchasing needed services, as well as the fragmentation of the system for providing these services, documented in the previous chapter, have major access implications for vulnerable populations. The next chapter examines the impact of these organizational and financial barriers on access to needed services for the vulnerable populations that are the focus of these analyses.

CHAPTER SEVEN

HOW GOOD IS THEIR ACCESS TO CARE?

Access implies that people have a place to go and the financial and other means to obtain care. The way services are organized and the methods that exist to pay for them may not always facilitate either entry or continuity, however.

Chapters Five and Six described the programs and payers that exist to provide a continuum of care for the vulnerable. This chapter reviews the evidence of organizational and financial barriers to access in the context of evaluating how well they have succeeded.

Cross-Cutting Issues

In general, the results confirmed that institutional doors are closed to many of the vulnerable; for those who do gain entry, people with few resources are likely to enter through one door and those with more resources through another; and the process of providing and paying for services itself does not always recognize the nonclinical causes or consequences of the problems that prompted the clients to seek care initially.

The distribution of providers and, more important, the effect of service availability on whether care is sought have been and continue to be central access concerns. A number of trends nationally point to the exacerbation of these issues for many of the most vulnerable: the buyout and conversion of nonprofit community hospitals by for-profit health care corporations; an increase in the rates of closure of rural hospitals and financially stressed safety net providers serving poor, inner-city populations; primary care provider flight from or reluctance to locate in these same areas; an unwillingness to serve individuals on Medicaid or who are uninsured; and the lack of cultural sensitivity of providers and the institutions in which they practice.

Many doors are closed to the vulnerable because of fear, including providers' fears of medical malpractice lawsuits from high-risk mothers or of contracting HIV infection or losing patients due to treating persons with AIDS; a community's fears of having a halfway house for the mentally ill or a shelter for battered women or homeless persons in their neighborhood; undocumented persons' fears of being detected; or refugees' fears of being referred to protective service authorities because they used folk remedies to treat a sick child.

Higher-income people and those with private insurance and their families who have mental health or substance abuse problems are likely to be seen in private psychiatric hospitals or residential substance abuse treatment centers. The poor and uninsured, on the other hand, are more likely to receive care in overcrowded and underfunded state-supported facilities, to be reinstitutionalized in local jails or prisons, or to join the ranks of the homeless population.

Systems of caring for the vulnerable are more aptly described as nonsystems, primarily because there is little integration or coordination of services across the variety of health and social service sectors required to address their needs. This is true for essentially all the categories of the vulnerable examined here.

Case managers are being used to create systems of care for individuals where none exists in the community. Consortia of institutions and agencies represent alternatives at the community level to build comprehensive, coordinated systems of care for vulnerable populations (such as those supported by the Ryan White legislation to improve services to persons living with HIV/AIDS, the Robert Wood Johnson Foundation and Health Resources and Services Administration Health Care Programs for the Homeless, as well as proposals for implementing the Public Health Service Objectives for the Nation, among others). Categorically oriented state and federal funding have historically provided incentives favoring fragmented, rather than integrated, program development. The persistence of these fiscal disincentives, as well as traditional interagency rivalries and competition, make building such consortia problematic, if not impossible, in many localities.

Financial Barriers

Some providers' doors are closed to people who cannot afford to pay the usual and customary fee for services. Almost three out of ten obstetrics providers refuse to see women on Medicaid. Diagnosis-related group (DRG)-based reimbursement under Medicare, which provides a fixed amount for the hospital services provided a patient with a given diagnosis, has encouraged some providers to discharge chronically ill elderly patients in an unstable condition. Private insurers increasingly have sought to exclude certain high-risk groups, such as persons living with HIV/AIDS, from coverage or to limit the benefits of others (with mental health or substance abuse problems, for example).

The system of financing services can be characterized as having neither parity nor equity. Parity means that levels of third-party coverage and benefits are comparable for different types of services (such as acute medical care, mental health, substance abuse, or long-term care), and equity means they are comparable for different groups of people (based on race, employment status, or public versus private sources of coverage, for example).

The physically disabled and other categories of the vulnerable that qualify for Medicare through Social Security Disability Insurance (SSDI), such as persons living with HIV/AIDS, could go without having any coverage for needed care or fail to survive the two-year waiting period. People covered by Medicaid, which provides very low rates of reimbursement in many states, or those who work in jobs that provide no coverage (as do many undocumented persons) are much more likely to confront substantial financial barriers to access than those with generous job-related benefits.

The incentives provided by both public and private insurers have discouraged the growth of integrated systems of caring for the vulnerable. Most plans cover medically related hospital and physician expenses. Only limited benefits are provided for prevention-related services or long-term home and community-based care.

Overall, a number of significant barriers exist to providing and paying for care for vulnerable populations. (See Table 7.1.)

Population-Specific Overview

The major organizational and financial barriers to access for vulnerable populations are examined in the discussion that follows.

High-Risk Mothers and Infants

High-risk mothers face a number of barriers to obtaining adequate and appropriate pre- and postconception care, including the lack of financial resources; an inadequate number and distribution of providers; a fragmented, uncoordinated, and inconvenient delivery system; and cultural and personal factors that inhibit their seeking formal medical care services (Institute of Medicine, 1985, 1988d; National Commission to Prevent Infant Mortality, 1988a; Public Health Service, 1989; York, Grant, Gibeau, Beecham, & Kessler, 1996).

Organizational Barriers. The Institute of Medicine report, *Prenatal Care: Reaching Mothers, Reaching Infants* (1988d), concluded that reducing financial access barriers through expanded public or private coverage or even increasing the numbers of providers willing to offer maternal and child health services still would not address the fact that the U.S. maternity care system ("the complicated

TABLE 7.1. PRINCIPAL ACCESS BARRIERS FOR VULNERABLE POPULATIONS.

Vulnerable Populations	Organizational	Financial
High-risk mothers and infants	The U.S. maternity care system is "fundamentally flawed, fragmented, and overly complex" (IOM, 1988d, p. 12).	Women who have no insurance or are on Medicaid face substantial financial and institutional barriers to access to maternal and child health services.
Chronically ill and disabled	The programs and services needed for caring for the chronically ill or disabled are either not available or not well coordinated in most communities.	Restrictive eligibility and coverage provisions on the part of public and private payers limit financial access for the chronically ill and disabled.
Persons living with HIV/AIDS	The main organizational barriers to care for persons living with HIV/AIDS in many cities are substantial service gaps, strained capacity, providers' fears of treating persons with HIV/AIDS, and at-risk groups' lack of information.	Private insurers overtly exclude persons living with AIDS and HIV-positive individuals from coverage, and public insurers severely restrict eligibility or covered services for persons with HIV/AIDS.
Mentally ill and disabled	The deinstitutionalization of the mentally ill without adequate community-based support services has resulted in a high risk of reinstitutionalization and homelessness.	The current system of financing mental health services lacks both parity and equity—that is, coverage comparable to medical care services and across groups, respectively.
Alcohol or substance abusers	Alcohol and substance abuse services are often poorly matched to needs due to the chronic relapsing nature of the problem, the lack of or fragmentation of services, or the unavailability of culturally sensitive treatment.	The private system sees fewer clients but receives more revenues, while the public system sees more, and more serious, cases of alcohol or substance abuse but receives fewer revenues.
Suicide or homicide prone	Both suicidal and homicidal behavior are dealt with in a fragmented and uncoordinated fashion across an array of discrete service delivery sectors in most communities.	Primary prevention programs for suicide and homicide are generally nonexistent, and the burden of caring for victims of violence tends to fall disproportionately on the public sector in most communities.
Abusing families	Programs for different categories of victims of intimate violence are poorly developed, fragmented, and uncoordinated.	Both public and private programs in family abuse tend to have limited funding, inadequate staffing, and poorly developed or supported systems of referral or placement.
Homeless persons	The organizational barriers to care for the homeless are exacerbated by their extreme poverty, unstable and unhealthy living conditions, and multidimensional health care needs.	Public support of programs and services for the homeless is limited and has failed to focus on the larger socioeconomic origins of the problem.
Immigrants and refugees	The main organizational barrier to care for immigrant and refugee populations is the unavailability of accessible and culturally sensitive providers and services.	Many immigrants and refugees experience substantial financial barriers to care due to low incomes; lack or loss of eligibility for public coverage; or the unavailability of private coverage through their work.

network of publicly and privately financed services through which women obtain prenatal, labor and delivery, and postpartum care") was "fundamentally flawed, fragmented, and overly complex" (p. 12). This system was characterized by poor service coordination, including the absence of a systematic system of referrals between maternal and child health or health department clinics and inpatient delivery sites, as well as relevant human service systems, such as welfare, housing, or schools; lack of information about where to go for care; service hours that do not accommodate women's work schedules; long waits for appointments or to be seen once at the site; language and cultural barriers; lack of alternatives for child care; and transportation problems.

This report, as well as other studies, document that many women who delay seeking prenatal care have unplanned or unwanted pregnancies. They may think that care is not important or that it is needed only if a woman becomes ill. Many poor, inner-city women, including the growing number of homeless women, are socially isolated and have no network of family or friends to support them emotionally or materially during their pregnancy. Women who abuse alcohol and drugs, or undocumented immigrants and refugees, may also fear exposure to social or legal sanctions if they seek care. The availability of a full range of maternal and child health and family planning services has also been limited by varying levels of funding under Title V of the Social Security Act and Title X of the Public Health Service Act (Perloff, Kletke, Fossett, & Banks, 1997; Moore & Hepworth, 1994; Rosenbaum, Hughes, & Johnson, 1988).

The number of physicians willing to provide obstetrician-gynecologist services, particularly to low-income, uninsured, or Medicaid-eligible women and those residing in inner-city or rural areas, has been a significant problem in many communities. Physicians' reluctance has been attributed to the low rates of reimbursement and the cumbersomeness of the payment process for Medicaid-eligible women, as well as the greatly increased risk and premiums associated with malpractice suits (Perloff, Kletke, Fossett, & Banks, 1997; Institute of Medicine, 1989a, 1989b; National Commission to Prevent Infant Mortality, 1988b). State initiatives in mandating Medicaid-eligible individuals' enrollment in managed care plans represent an effort to address the availability and willingness of providers to serve this population.

Financial Barriers. Over a fourth of women in the reproductive years have no coverage for maternity-related care. Women with private insurance are much more likely to seek prenatal care than are women who have no insurance or are on Medicaid (Braveman, Bennett, Lewis, Egerter, & Showstack, 1993; General Accounting Office, 1987; Institute of Medicine, 1988d; Oberg, Lia-Hoagberg, Hodkinson, Skovholt, & Vanman, 1990; York, Grant, Gibeau, Beecham, & Kessler, 1996). The constriction of eligibility or coverage for high-risk women under public and private systems of financing also threatens to undermine access to more costly regionalized neonatal intensive care services (McCormick & Richardson, 1995).

The Medicaid enrollment process in many states is complex and cumbersome, and many low-income women may be well into their pregnancy before they can establish eligibility. In addition to efforts to reduce the administrative barriers to obtaining Medicaid by streamlining eligibility determination procedures, many states have initiated programs to extend outreach to Medicaid-eligible women, recruit obstetrical providers into participating in the program, and add enriched nonmedical prenatal benefits (Hill, 1990). The direction of these reforms acknowledges that simply establishing high-risk women and children's eligibility for Medicaid will not be sufficient for enhancing their access to adequate perinatal care services. The availability, accessibility, and acceptability of these services must also be substantially improved (Institute of Medicine, 1988d; Lia-Hoagberg et al., 1990; Piper, Ray, & Griffin, 1990; Sable, Stockbauer, Schramm, & Land, 1990; St. Clair, Smeriglio, Alexander, Connell, & Niebyl, 1990).

Chronically Ill and Disabled

The chronically ill and disabled face a number of service availability and organizational, as well as financial barriers, in obtaining needed medical and social support services, particularly for long-term or community-based care.

Organizational Barriers. The programs and services for the chronically ill and disabled, listed in Table 5.2, are either not available in many communities or serve only limited subsets of those eligible for these services. This is particularly the case for the community-based primary and tertiary prevention-oriented programs, such as risk-reduction education or intervention programs, day care, home-delivered meals, home visiting, transportation services, and caregiver respite services. Even when they are available, there is often poor communication about or inadequate coordination among services (such as transportation and day care) to ensure that those in need are aware of and able to obtain access to them (Densen, 1991; Jones, Densen, & Brown, 1989; Nyman, Cyphert, Russell, & Wallace, 1989; Scanlon, 1988; Wallace, 1990). Case management services are often devices for insurers to contain the costs of care rather than for clients to have expanded access to needed services (Capitman, 1988). The Americans with Disabilities Act (ADA) enacted in 1990 was intended to reduce overt discrimination against the disabled primarily in the areas of employment, housing, and public accommodations (West, 1991).

The shorter lengths of stay and earlier condition-specific rates of discharge subsequent to the introduction of DRGs have highlighted the inadequate institutional and human services system capacity in many communities in providing adequate nursing home, as well as community-based, care (Scanlon, 1988). Surveys of the elderly and disabled children have documented that large proportions (half to two-thirds) have substantial unmet needs for both medical and related social support services (General Accounting Office, 1988b, 1989c; Short & Leon, 1990). Particularly pressing needs for many chronically ill disabled and their families are caregiver respite, housekeeping, or home visiting services to relieve the stress of caregiving for the large number of family members who care for their functionally restricted parent or child at home (Kosberg, Cairl, & Keller, 1990; Oktay & Volland, 1990; Stone & Short, 1990).

Rates of preventable hospitalizations for chronic illness are higher in communities in which there is poor access to primary care services (Bindman et al., 1995). Poor and minority children with chronic illness are more likely to be uninsured and to make less use of ambulatory care services, but they have more hospitalizations than their nonpoor, white counterparts (Newacheck, 1994; Newacheck, Stoddard, & McManus, 1993). Chronically ill African Americans have also been found to be less likely to have selected surgical procedures (for stage I non-small cell lung cancer and coronary artery bypass graft, for example) than whites (Greenwald, Polissar, Borgatta, McCorkle, & Goodman, 1998; Hannan et al., 1999).

Financial Barriers. Around one in six adults and children with serious functional limitations have no public or private insurance coverage. Both public and private insurers limit financial access for this population through restrictive eligibility criteria, limitations of benefits, or the cost-sharing provisions or level of reimbursement provided for covered services (Feder, 1990; Griss, 1988, 1989).

The two-year waiting period for Medicare eligibility for the SSDI population represents a significant barrier during a period in which their expenses are likely to be the greatest. Medicare is also oriented toward paying for acute medical care, particularly physician and hospital services. It does not therefore adequately cover many of the services required to prevent the onset of primary or secondary disabilities, such as preventive or wellness care or custodial or personal assistance services. It also provides very limited coverage for other services more likely to be needed by this population, such as outpatient mental health services, prescription drugs, and disposable and durable medical equipment.

Medicare pays for home health care and rehabilitation services, if these services are deemed "medically necessary" or permit "restoration of function," respectively. However, neither of these criteria might be met by individuals who have long-term, irreversible loss in physical and social functioning. Furthermore, because of the prospective payment provisions enacted under Medicare, many elderly and disabled individuals are being discharged into the community in unstable condition, without adequate posthospitalization care provisions.

Increased cost-sharing provisions associated with Medicare through co-insurance, deductibles and the Part B premium have increased the financial burden on many elderly and disabled beneficiaries as well. The typical elderly person spent about 19 percent of his or her income on health care in 1997. The low-income elderly spend an even greater share of income (35 percent) on health care (O'Brien, Rowland, & Keenan, 1999).

Medicaid (not Medicare) provides coverage for one of the most expensive components of care for the elderly and disabled: long-term nursing home care. However, its means-tested provisions have often increased, rather than diminished, the financial or cost-sharing burden on families. Families must "spend down" to the poverty level to qualify for Medicaid coverage for nursing home care, although the Medicare Catastrophic Coverage Act of 1988 did increase the allowed amount of the nondisabled spouse's monthly income and the couple's assets that could be retained. The Katie Beckett waiver allowed states the option of not counting the parents' income in determining Medicaid eligibility for services to be provided at home that were formerly covered only if the child was institutionalized.

One of the most significant equity issues with respect to the Medicaid program is the wide variability across states in optional benefits, such as physical therapy, occupational therapy, personal care, and rehabilitative services, which may not be "optional" for the long-term chronically ill or disabled (Ellwood & Burwell, 1990; Griss, 1988, 1989).

Persons deemed ineligible under public programs may still be unable to obtain or afford private insurance. Private insurers increasingly are using preexisting condition exclusion criteria, medical testing, and restrictive underwriting policies to exclude or drop categories of the disabled or seriously ill. As with the public insurers, many private policies also fail to cover the major services required to prevent primary or secondary disability, such as wellness and preventive care and long-term health and social support services (Griss, 1988, 1989; Kinney & Steinmetz, 1994).

Chronically ill individuals and their families face additional restrictions in the managed care–dominated marketplace. Health maintenance organizations tend to offer better protection against out-of-pocket expenses and generally are more likely than conventional plans to cover certain services (such as ancillary therapies, home care, and outpatient mental health care). However, they also place limits on these and other services required by chronically ill children and adults and, in particular, restrictions on access to specialty physician services. The challenge to both public and private funders of managed care services for the chronically ill and disabled is how best to ensure the affordability and accessibility of such services (Fox, Etheredge, & Jones, 1998; Fox, Wicks, & Newacheck, 1993; Neff & Anderson, 1995; Wholey, Burns, & Lavizzo-Mourey, 1998).

Persons Living with HIV/AIDS

Persons living with HIV/AIDS face an array of overt and purposeful organizational and financial barriers to needed services.

Organizational Barriers. Considerable variability exists across states and communities in the resources available to care for HIV/AIDS patients. Problems encountered in many communities include limited hospital inpatient capacity for caring for persons with AIDS; long waiting lists for outpatient clinic services; insufficient bed capacity, trained staff, or rates of Medicaid reimbursement to ensure access to nursing home care; and inadequate long-term home and community-based care, including home nursing, attendant care, case management, mental health services, substance abuse treatment, dental care, and housing for persons living with HIV/AIDS. The 1990 Ryan White Comprehensive AIDS Resource Emergency and AIDS Prevention Acts were passed to enhance resources and services to cities, states, and facilities that were particularly burdened by the epidemic (Lehrman, Gentry & Fogarty, 1998; Piette, Fleishman, Stein, Mor, & Mayer, 1993).

An important additional barrier to medical care for persons with AIDS is the fear that health care providers have themselves of contracting the disease (Daniels, 1991; Gerbert, Macguire, & Coates, 1990; Rizzo, Marder, & Willke, 1990; Sadowsky & Kunzel, 1996). Fear of AIDS has also had an impact on the willingness of medical students and residents to treat AIDS patients or to enter specialties or establish practices with high concentrations of persons with AIDS (Cooke & Sande, 1989; National Research Council, 1993). Furthermore, there is evidence that many primary care physicians, who are in a unique position to contribute to the prevention of HIV transmission by counseling high-risk patients, fail to do so (Centers for Disease Control and Prevention, 1994a).

National and local surveys have documented that large numbers of persons living with HIV/AIDS do not have a regular care provider. Substantial inequities exist by gender, race, HIV risk group, and insurance status. Whites, men, and nonintravenous drug users are more likely to obtain care through private physicians or outpatient clinics, while nonwhites, women, and intravenous drug users are more likely to use hospital emergency rooms. Fewer blacks, women, and uninsured and Medicaid-insured individuals take antiretroviral medication, which since the mid-1990s has been the recommended standard of care for persons living with HIV/AIDS. HIV-infected drug abusers are likely to have low levels of access to basic needs such as long-term shelter and food, vocational retraining, and long-term drug treatment (Bozzette et al., 1998; Fleishman, Hsia, & Hellinger, 1994; Huba & Melchior, 1994; Montoya, Richard, Bell, & Atkinson, 1997; Mor, Fleishman, Dresser, & Piette, 1992; Shapiro et al., 1999). Women living with HIV/AIDS, the majority of whom are minority and low income, appear to experience significant barriers to HIV/AIDS care in general, and dental, drug treatment, and prenatal care services in particular (Davidson et al., 1998; Hellinger, 1993b; Shiboski, Palacio, Neuhaus, & Greenblatt, 1999; Weissman et al., 1995). Many providers neglect opportunities to counsel high-risk pregnant women or fail to do an effective job in providing them relevant information or testing (Healton et al., 1996; Limata, Schoen, Cohen, Black, & Quesenberry, 1997; Phillips, Morrison, Sonnad, & Bleecker, 1997).

The rates of HIV/AIDS infection are high among prison populations, yet prisoners are less likely to have access to experimental therapies while incarcerated, and they encounter significant difficulties in obtaining needed medical and social services after release from prison (Collins, Baumgartner, & Henry, 1995; Warren, Bellin, Zoloth, & Safyer, 1994).

Studies have documented that those who may be most at risk of AIDS also know the least about it. The level of knowledge on the part of subgroups of adolescents who are likely to be most at risk (such as minorities or those who are in adolescent detention facilities) have been found to be less than those at lower risk

(DiClemente, Lanier, Horan, & Lodico, 1991; Goodman & Cohall, 1989; Hardy, 1990). These studies highlight the need for targeted and culturally sensitive educational and behavioral risk interventions to those who may be most at risk but least informed about modes of HIV transmission (Aruffo, Coverdale, & Vallbona, 1991; Eskander, Jahan, & Carter, 1990).

Financial Barriers. The federal government and the public health and health care infrastructure were slow to react to the onset of the AIDS epidemic (Bayer, 1991; Epstein, 1996; Presidential Commission on the Human Immunodeficiency Virus Epidemic, 1988; Winkenwerder, Kessler, & Stolec, 1989). Subsequently, there was a backlash in response to increased levels of AIDS funding by opponents who argued that "too much" was being spent on that illness, at a time when the death rates for other diseases, such as heart disease and cancer, were even higher (Casarett & Lantos, 1998; Murphy, 1991).

Several trends contribute to new and expanded burdens for the provision and financing of care for persons living with HIV/AIDS. Among them are new standards of care encompassing drug-based antiretroviral therapy that include protease inhibitors, which prevent the reproduction of the HIV/AIDS virus within human cells; the increasing incidence of HIV infection related to substance abuse; and declines in AIDS-related mortality due to the new therapies and enhanced treatment services, which result in extended periods of lifetime treatment for persons living with HIV/AIDS (Levi, 1998).

Substantial financial barriers exist to the receipt of care for AIDS. Some states have no explicit constraints imposed by insurance commissions prohibiting private insurers from discriminating based on sexual orientation, asking about or performing HIV antibody testing, or excluding AIDS as a covered condition. The Medicaid and Medicare programs also limit the coverage of HIV-related drugs and other services required by persons living with HIV/AIDS.

Daniels (1990) and others (Oppenheimer & Padgug, 1986) point out that the concept of "actuarial fairness" that underlies the justification for these practices directly conflicts with the requirements of "social fairness" (or justice). Considerations of fairness from an actuarial point of view argue for the exclusion, and from a social justice point of view for the inclusion, of those most at risk, from a common insurance pool.

Mentally Ill and Disabled

Major access and service availability problems for the mentally ill and disabled have resulted from shifting philosophical, political, and programmatic priorities regarding the types of facilities and services most appropriate for meeting their needs.

Organizational Barriers. The deinstitutionalization of mentally ill individuals without sufficient development of alternative community-based systems of care led early on to a revolving door of readmissions and more recently to concerns about the "transinstitutionalization" or "reinstitutionalization" of the mentally ill to an array of institutions, such as board and care homes, nursing homes, residential treatment centers, or jails, as well as being at a higher risk of having no home at all.

The 1999 surgeon general's report on mental health pointed out that one of the fundamental barriers to adequate service provision for this population was the victim-blaming stigma associated with being mentally ill and its resultant impact on public and political support for programs and services to address their needs (U.S. Department of Health and Human Services, 1999).

The elimination of categorical support for community mental health clinics with their inclusion in block grants to states in the early part of the 1980s resulted in a number of centers closing or greatly reducing the scope of services they provided (Dowell & Ciarlo, 1989). There is a shortage of community-based services, as well as case management and coordination across service systems, especially for children, the elderly, and the seriously mentally ill or retarded (Crocker, 1990; Grob, 1991; Ivey, Scheffler, & Zazzali, 1998). Rural communities in particular often lack adequate mental health care services (Fox, Merwin, & Blank, 1995; Kane & Ennis, 1996; Lambert & Agger, 1995; Rost, Zhang, Fortney, Smith, & Smith, 1998).

A pressing need for the chronically mentally ill is community-based housing. Obstacles to developing an adequate continuum of alternatives include the absence of legislation to facilitate access to such housing, poor interagency cooperation, inadequate funding, a diminished supply of public and private low-income housing stock, and community resistance to having mentally ill individuals living in the neighborhood (Levine & Haggard, 1989).

The magnitude of unmet need for mental health services is estimated to be high in many communities. Based on the Epidemiological Catchment Area study, around 30 percent of individuals with a diagnosable mental disorder go untreated, while 56 to 59 percent receive care in the general medical care sector, and only 8 to 12 percent in the specialty mental health sector (Hough et al., 1987, p. 709). Rates of untreated disorders have been estimated to be higher for women, children, elderly, blacks, and Hispanics, particularly among Hispanics who are migrant agricultural workers, are less acculturated, or lack insurance coverage (Curbow, Khoury, & Weisman, 1998; Nadelson, 1998; Office of Technology Assessment, 1986; Padgett, Patrick, Burns, & Schlesinger, 1994; Ruiz, 1993).

Financial Barriers. Although changes have been made, the system for financing mental health services still lacks parity and equity. Parity means that mental health services are as accessible and available as are general health care services to those who need them. Equity refers to coverage being equally available to all groups, based on need, rather than factors such as their income, occupational status, race, or where they live (Ridgely & Goldman, 1989).

The extent of coverage and rates of reimbursement for providers under both public and private systems of financing programs have typically been less for mental health than for general medical care services. The Domenici-Wellstone amendment in 1996 (attached to an appropriations bill), which prohibited different treatment of mental health care in terms of lifetime caps and annual reimbursement ceilings, was an effort to establish greater parity in mental health coverage. The legislation did, however, permit health plans to continue to place annual day and visit limitations on covered services and to use higher levels of cost sharing for mental health care than for other services (Frank, Koyanagi, & McGuire, 1997). In Medicaid, the rate paid for specialty psychiatric services, when provided by physicians, is lower than that paid for general medical services delivered by the same providers (Taube, Goldman, & Salkever, 1990). For Medicare patients seen on an outpatient basis, those being treated for physical illnesses have to pay 20 percent of the charges for the visits themselves, while beneficiaries being treated for mental illness have to pay half (with the exception of recent exemptions for the medical management of prescription drugs, and treatment for Alzheimer's patients) (Lave & Goldman, 1990).

People's willingness to purchase mental health care is even more sensitive to how much it costs them out of pocket than is the case for general medical care services, regardless of the nature of the problem. There is then a greater likelihood that the more they have to pay themselves, the less likely people who need mental health care services are to obtain them.

Both public and private third-party coverage have tended to provide inadequate or nonexistent attention to the comprehensive, longer-term social and health care service needs of the mentally ill and disabled. Deinstitutionalization and public financing through Medicaid have encouraged the use of nursing homes as a long-term institutional alternative for the seriously mentally ill (Glied, Hoven, Moore, Garrett, & Regier, 1997; Morrissey, 1989; Scallet, 1990).

The increasing penetration of managed behavioral health care into both the private and public sectors has illuminated access problems resulting from adverse selection, the lack of integration of clinical and community services, and the conflicting values of market- versus community-oriented providers (Surles & Shore, 1996; Tommasini, 1994).

Alcohol or Substance Abusers

The delivery system for alcohol and substance abuse services is fragmented, poorly integrated, and variably funded and developed across states. Furthermore, the unique characteristics of substance abuse addiction compound the problems in adequately addressing the needs of people with these disorders.

Organizational Barriers. Substance abuse is a chronic relapsing disorder, with identifiable stages of development (use, abuse, dependence, recovery and relapse), that has an array of physical, psychological, and social correlates and consequences. Furthermore, treatment for those affected may be mandated rather than voluntary. As a result, a variety of interventions and treatment modalities with different objectives, and focusing on different stages of the problem, have emerged to address the needs of individuals who use or abuse alcohol and drugs. These services are often poorly integrated and coordinated, particularly for those dually diagnosed with substance abuse and mental health problems (Brach et al., 1995; McCaughrin & Howard, 1996). Estimates of the proportion of persons not receiving needed treatment among those with severe drug dependence have ranged from 54 to 68 percent, based on the National Household Survey on Drug Abuse (Epstein & Gfroerer, 1998).

Jails, prisons, and the criminal justice system represent important sources of referral and treatment for the drug-abusing population. The overcrowding in many state prison systems, often due to an increase in convictions for drug-related or drug-involved crimes, has created additional strains on an already overburdened system of corrections. There is often a paucity of drug treatment programs in prisons, especially in local jails, as well as linkages with community services for drug users postrelease to reduce rearrest and recidivism rates (Freudenberg, Wilets, Greene, & Richie, 1998; Gerstein & Harwood, 1990; Leukefeld & Tims, 1993).

In addition to wide variations in the availability and adequacy of treatment for substance abuse disorders, an additional challenge is providing culturally sensitive treatment to groups most at risk, such as racial and ethnic minorities. Programs may fail to incorporate adaptations to those groups' culture or values that could facilitate the treatment process—for example, hiring bilingual staff, grounding the treatment in the client's own spiritual belief system or family context, or locating or designing the facility itself in a manner compatible with cultural tastes and preferences (Trepper, Nelson, McCollum, & McAvoy, 1997). Access to appropriate services for pregnant women who also have significant substance abuse or mental health problems is particularly problematic due to the fragmentation and lack of coordination among the prenatal care, substance abuse, and mental health care systems in many communities (Grella, 1997; Haack, 1997; Lewis, Haller, Branch, & Ingersoll, 1996; Stratton, Howe, & Battaglia, 1996).

Financial Barriers. The resources, services, and clients in the two (public versus private) tiers of care in the drug abuse treatment system differ significantly. The private system sees fewer clients but receives a larger share of treatment dollars than does the public. The revenues for inpatient and residential treatment per client in the private system are approximately three to four times those in the public system, although average outpatient revenues are similar. Compared to the private sector, public sector clients are much more likely to be long-term, serious, multiproblem cases, compounded by a recurrent history of drug abuse or dependence, unemployment, a poor education, poor health, from broken or disorganized families, and with criminal records.

The private sector has a much higher rate of unused (or excess) capacity (34 percent) than does the public sector (16 percent). The excess capacity in public

methadone maintenance programs is, on average, much smaller, however (5 percent), and the capacity across states and localities varies substantially. Waiting
times for treatment are longer for public pay patients and in settings in which
providers have higher caseloads (Gerstein & Harwood, 1990; McCaughrin &
Howard, 1996).

Wide variability exists across states in the availability and funding of alcohol
treatment services that is not necessarily correlated with variations in the need for
these services. Programs serving clients with alcohol problems are also seg-
mented based on social factors, paralleling the public and private tiers of drug
abuse treatment; for example, clients seen in hospital-based aversion-conditioning
treatment programs are likely to have much higher levels of social functioning
ing (have jobs, are in intact families, and do not have criminal records) than
those served in county police–sponsored rehabilitation centers (Institute of Medicine, 1990).

Both public and private insurance provide limited coverage of alcohol and
drug abuse treatment services. Health insurance is also oriented toward covering
medically oriented (particularly inpatient) services, which is only one part of
the complex array of social and community-based services that substance abuse
clients need. Substantial variability also exists in the types of substance abuse
providers and services that are eligible for reimbursement by private and public
insurers (particularly Medicaid), which results in a crazy quilt of coverage across
states and subgroups. Welfare reform has led to the denial of benefits to recipients with drug felony convictions and the corollary reduction of drug treatment
programs in many states, which has particularly affected access for drug-using
pregnant women (Chavkin, Breitbart, Elman, & Wise, 1998; Chavkin, Wise, &
Elman, 1998; Schmidt, Weisner, & Wiley, 1998). Managed behavioral health care
offers the possibility for better coordination and management of medical care and
related substance abuse services, but it may also significantly limit the coverage
of benefits needed to treat multiproblem enrollees (Fuller, 1994; Kunnes et al.,
1993; Wilson, 1993).

Suicide or Homicide Prone

Major impediments to the development of accessible and effective programs to
reduce the likelihood of suicide or homicide include the lack of a clear consensus,
based on well-developed theories, empirical research, demonstrations, and program evaluations, regarding how best to address what are purported to be multifactorial biological, psychological, and social origins of violent behavior.

Organizational Barriers. The problems of suicidal and homicidal behavior
are dealt with in a fragmented and uncoordinated fashion across an array of discrete service delivery sectors: the public health, medical care, mental health care,
substance abuse treatment, criminal justice, social service, and educational systems. The Public Health Objectives for the Nation call for better coordination

and integration of services across these sectors to address the Year 2010 goals to reduce violent and abusive behavior (U.S. Department of Health and Human Services, 1998). It is possible that more indirect interventions (such as economic development programs in inner-city neighborhoods or mental health or substance abuse services) may be even more effective than direct interventions (such as suicide prevention or crisis intervention centers) in affecting such behaviors. Nonetheless, direct suicide and homicide prevention programs are not well developed in many states (Rosenberg et al., 1987).

Prison overcrowding has become a major problem in many states and localities due to an increased focus on incapacitation as a means of dealing with offenders. The number of inmates occupying state correctional facilities in the United States exceeded the number that planners or architects intended for the facilities by 33 percent on average in 1995, reflecting an increase from 22 percent in 1990 (U.S. Department of Justice, 1998).

Physicians, teachers, social workers, pastors, mental health and substance abuse counselors, and other professionals need to be better trained to identify those who may be most at risk of violent behavior. Such individuals could serve as gatekeepers to identify and channel high-risk individuals and their families to appropriate prevention- or treatment-oriented services (Public Health Service, 1990). A 1994 nationwide survey of crisis intervention centers in the United States and Canada to assess the extent to which they were prepared to prevent suicide among the elderly, who have the highest overall rates of suicide, revealed insufficient training, a lack of familiarity with recent suicide trends, and limited outreach to older adults (Adamek & Kaplan, 1996).

Suicidal youth and victims of aggravated assault and family abuse are much more likely to be seen in hospital emergency rooms. Emergency room personnel could be trained in the use of protocols for identifying high-risk cases, and provided information regarding available channels and sources of referrals to assist them (Alcohol, Drug Abuse, and Mental Health Administration, 1989b; Slap, Vorters, Chaudhuri, & Centor, 1989). There is evidence that racial differences in access to emergency transportation and subsequent medical care of victims of violent assault increase the chances that African American assailants will be charged with homicide more often than white assailants would (Hanke & Gundlach, 1995).

Financial Barriers. The public and private treatment tiers in the mental health and substance abuse treatment sectors clearly serve different socioeconomic classes. The population housed in correctional facilities is increasingly minority.

Targeted primary prevention and broader social, economic, and educational programs, which could perhaps serve as a deterrent or alternative to criminal or violent behavior leading to incarceration, are either nonexistent or poorly developed in most high-risk minority and disadvantaged neighborhoods. Furthermore, many interventions may not be sensitive to the cultural differences and norms that affect who is most vulnerable to different forms of violence within a community (Alcohol, Drug Abuse, and Mental Health Administration, 1989c; Canetto & Lester, 1995; Gurr, 1989).

A number of trauma centers have closed, many as a result of the financial burden of the costs of uncompensated care for individuals with violence-related trauma. These closings have placed additional burdens on other public and private community providers for the delivery of trauma care (General Accounting Office, 1991).

Abusing Families

The major issues in caring for victims of intimate violence are inadequate services and programs, the fragmentation and lack of integration resulting from different programs focusing on discrete categories of victims of violence (children, wives, elderly, and so on), and the poor coordination across the array of sectors (medical care, public health, welfare, protective services, mental health, and criminal justice, among others) involved in service provision in general and for each group.

Organizational Barriers. Different paradigmatic approaches exist in the medical care, human services, and legal systems regarding how best to handle cases of intimate abuse. This greatly inhibits the prospect for communication and coordination of a multifaceted, interagency approach to addressing the needs of both victims and perpetrators (Knudsen, 1988).

Within child and adult protective services agencies, the values of compassion and control are often in tension or conflict. Program administrators have to weigh their agency's legalistic mandates to detect and investigate incidents of abuse and arrange for the forcible removable of the victim or restraint of the offender, against the humanistic considerations of the impact of removing the individuals from situations, which though by some "objective" standards are abusive, are nonetheless ones in which the "victims" declare they wish to stay (Carney, 1989; Fritz, 1989; Knudsen, 1988).

Similar tensions exist in considering the design of community prevention and treatment initiatives in this area. In most states and localities, the agencies and constituencies concerned with different victims of intimate abuse may rarely coordinate services and programs. For example, one agency (say, a battered women's shelter) may deal principally with addressing the needs of one affected family member (the mother), while another (the child protective services agency) deals principally with others (the children), and still another (the police) with the perpetrator of the violence (the father). Such a system exacerbates the fragmentation, confusion, and lack of integration that already plagues many abusing families.

The laws governing elder abuse are variably implemented and understood by agency officials in many states. Furthermore, virtually no laws exist to protect certain categories of victims of hidden violence, such as siblings, adolescents, or noneldery parents. Local police are often reluctant to intervene in domestic disturbances because of the issue of family privacy and the fact that many victims often drop charges against the perpetrator prior to prosecution. Adult protective services are more likely to focus on the elderly rather than cases of spousal or nonelderly adult abuse.

Although physicians may be the front-line sentinels for identifying at-risk or actual victims of abuse, many providers are not adequately trained or provided with the resources to diagnose or refer abuse victims to appropriate nonmedical networks of treatment or support (Jellinek, Murphy, Bishop, Poitrast, & Quinn, 1990; Krueger & Patterson, 1997; Randall, 1990). School-based sex abuse education and related prevention-oriented efforts are also variably available in most communities (Wurtele, 1987).

The prevalence of physical, emotional, or sexual abuse, as well as the barriers to seeking appropriate services, are often greater among low-income, minority, homeless women, and those who have been diagnosed with HIV/AIDS. Laws that encourage or mandate notification of a partner of an individual with HIV/AIDS can, for example, lead to affected women experiencing negative consequences from their partners, including rejection, abandonment, verbal abuse, or physical assault (Bassuk, Melnick, & Browne, 1998; Frye & D'Avanzo, 1994; Gielen, O'Campo, Faden, & Eke, 1997; Rothenberg & Paskey, 1995).

Financial Barriers. Governmental and private volunteer efforts in this area tend to have limited funding, inadequate staffing, and poorly developed systems of referral, placement, or social and human service resources to provide for victims of intimate violence. Furthermore, women and their children who are in domestic violence situations may be dependent on an abusive family member or partner for essential financial support, housing, transportation, and insurance, which may preclude their ability to extricate themselves from the abuse situation (Bassuk, Melnick, & Browne, 1998).

Managed care offers opportunities to network medical and community providers and services to identify and treat victims of domestic violence more efficiently and effectively. Selected plans, such as HealthPartners in Minnesota and Group Health Cooperative of Puget Sound, have undertaken initiatives to reduce the rates of domestic violence among plan members. Most managed care plans have not, however, and are unlikely to do so unless direct incentives are provided by public or private managed care contractors (Mitchell, 1997).

Homeless Persons

Access problems previously detailed for other vulnerable groups are multiplied for homeless persons. Extreme poverty; inadequate, unstable, or unhealthy living conditions; poor nutrition; the greater prevalence of mental illness; substance abuse; and sexual or physical exploitation and injury all contribute to homeless persons' being in poorer health than the U.S. population in general and the housed poor in many cities.

Organizational Barriers. Homeless persons are much less likely to have a regular source of care or transportation, and more likely to have long waits, experience hostile attitudes, or be told to go elsewhere when they do seek care. Substantial competing subsistence needs and related financial barriers also preclude their obtaining routine preventive or primary care services. Many homeless persons who experience serious acute or emergent conditions seek care in hospital emergency rooms (Gallagher, Andersen, Koegel, & Gelberg, 1997; Gelberg, Doblin, & Leake, 1996; Gelberg, Gallagher, Andersen, & Koegel, 1997; Padgett, Struening, Andrews, & Pittman, 1995; Wenzel et al., 1995).

The social stigma related to homelessness and the other problems likely to be experienced by homeless persons (HIV/AIDS, substance abuse, or mental illness) create additional impediments to the development of facilities and services in many communities (Brickner et al., 1993; Rosenheck & Lam, 1997; Takahashi, 1997). Homeless and runaway children, especially those who have lived on the streets for extended periods, are much less likely to have received adequate well-child care and more likely to have engaged in high-risk sexual or drug activity than housed youth or than other homeless youth who have been in foster or other institutional care arrangements (Ensign & Santelli, 1997; 1998; Riemer, Van Cleve, & Galbraith, 1995; Weinreb, Goldberg, Bassuk, & Perloff, 1998; Zlotnick, Kronstadt, & Klee, 1998). The needs, as well as the barriers to care, are exacerbated for pregnant homeless women and those with substance abuse or serious mental health problems (Wagner, Menke, & Ciccone, 1994; Wenzel, Koegel, & Gelberg, 1996).

The lack of integration of the public health, medical care, mental health care, substance abuse treatment, social service, and other sectors caring for discrete categories of vulnerable populations makes designing an accessible, integrated, and effective system of care for the multiproblem homeless even more difficult. Outreach and case management services have been effective in getting eligible homeless persons in for care and encouraging return visits when needed (Brickner, Scharer, Conanan, & Scanlan, 1990; Lam & Rosenheck, 1999; McMurray-Avila, 1997; Rosenheck et al., 1998; Stephens, Dennis, Toomer, & Holloway, 1991). The lack of a place to go after discharge is a major problem for many chronically mentally or physically ill homeless persons. The Veterans Administration Homeless Chronically Mentally Ill program has facilitated the development of residential treatment alternatives for homeless veterans (Rosenheck, Gallup, Leda, Gorchov, & Errera, 1990).

The demand on major sources of support for homeless persons in many cities, such as emergency food and shelter programs, in many cases exceeds the capacity of the system to meet it. The 1999 U.S. Conference of Mayors Survey of Hunger and Homeless in America's Cities found that the demand for emergency food assistance had increased 18 percent on average over the previous year. In 54 percent of the cities, emergency food assistance facilities had to turn away people in need because of lack of resources. On average across the cities, 21 percent of the requests for emergency food assistance went unmet. The requests for emergency shelter (or housing) by homeless families increased an average of 12 percent over the same period. Shelters had to turn away homeless families or individuals in 73 percent of the cities because of lack of resources. An average of 25 percent of the requests for emergency shelter were estimated to have gone unmet (U.S. Conference of Mayors, 1999).

Financial Barriers. Many homeless persons lack any type of private or public insurance coverage, which creates substantial financial barriers to care seeking.

Private advocacy groups for homeless persons and others sharply criticized the federal government for its slowness in developing program and policy initiatives for the homeless population (General Accounting Office, 1985; National Alliance to End Homelessness, 1988; Partnership for the Homeless, 1987, 1989). With the enactment of the Stewart B. McKinney Homeless Assistance Act of 1987, Congress recognized the need to supplement mainstream federally funded housing and human services programs with funding specifically targeted to assist homeless people. The agencies charged with the implementation and oversight of the McKinney Act have also been subject to severe criticism for the restrictions (relating to the complex application process, matching funds requirements, and funding stream, among others) that made it difficult for grantees to get programs in place in a timely fashion; the lack of responsiveness of the programs to local needs and priorities; as well as the foot dragging and delays on the part of agencies charged with both the expenditure and oversight of program funds (General Accounting Office, 1990b, 1999; U.S. Commission on Security and Cooperation in Europe, 1990).

Twenty-four percent of the homeless clients in the 1996 Urban Institute survey of homeless assistance providers and clients reported that they needed medical attention in the past year but were not able to get it. Almost half (46 percent) indicated that they did not go to a dentist when one was needed. These high levels of unmet need are exacerbated by the low rates of public or private insurance coverage among the homeless (Burt et al., 1999).

As with other vulnerable populations, the root causes of homelessness lie deep in the social, economic, and political structure. *Homelessness in the United States*, a report by the U.S. Commission on Security and Cooperation in Europe (1990, p. 68), concluded:

> The Executive Branch and Congress should act to address growing poverty and larger socio-economic issues such as unemployment, an insufficient minimum wage, the lack of affordable housing and health care, and education deficiencies. The federal government should provide, in addition to funding, moral leadership and a comprehensive strategy designed to address larger socio-economic problems, of which homelessness is just a symptom.

Immigrants and Refugees

The type and magnitude of access problems differ for documented legal immigrants, overdocumented refugee populations, and undocumented persons. However, the common factors affecting access for all of these groups are the availability and affordability of services and their acceptability and adequacy for those in need of care.

Organizational Barriers. Availability refers principally to the types of providers that are present in areas where immigrants and refugees tend to live and whether the providers' doors are open to them. Some providers require that patients present proof of citizenship or permanent residence status to be eligible for services. Undocumented immigrants, who fear detection and subsequent deportation, will be reluctant to seek care. Furthermore, some facilities may make little or no accommodation to serving immigrant and refugee populations by failing to have bilingual providers or translators to facilitate patient-provider communication.

Community outreach and follow-up, through identifying people at risk and facilitating their access to needed medical care, are important components in extending service availability. Mobile vans and storefront clinics have been used to provide health screening, immunizations, and referrals of at-risk immigrant and refugee populations in urban neighborhoods, as well as isolated rural communities along the U.S.-Mexico border.

As Rumbaut, Chavez, Moser, Pickwell, and Wishik (1988, p. 177) point out, "The delivery of health care to immigrants and refugees is, of course, not merely a technical-medical orientation or a bureaucratic-financial transaction, but also a social relation in a culturally defined situation." The acceptability and adequacy of services being proffered to these populations are substantially affected by "social and cultural problems of miscommunication, misinformation, misunderstanding and mistrust in the relationship between provider and patient" (p. 170). The principal factors that generate or exacerbate these problems are language barriers and cultural beliefs and practices that differ between the providers and the populations being served. These difficulties can give rise to a reluctance to seek care initially, a failure to follow prescribed medical regimens, a fear and distrust that inhibits the pursuit of subsequent follow-up care, and poor treatment outcomes (Loue, 1998; Rumbaut, Chavez, Moser, Pickwell, & Wishik, 1988; Siddharthan, 1990).

Financial Barriers. The affordability of services is principally a function of whether people have insurance or other personal resources to pay for care.

State and federal laws, such as Proposition 187 in California and the 1996 Welfare Reform Act, that restrict eligibility for social services and related insurance benefits have inhibited care seeking on the part of the foreign born. These effects are especially problematic for particularly vulnerable subpopulations of the foreign born, such as abused or pregnant women, children, the elderly, and the mentally ill (Brown, Wyn, & Ojeda, 1999; Fenton, Catalano, & Hargreaves, 1996; Friedland & Pankaj, 1997; Ivey & Kramer, 1998; Michael & Gany, 1996; Minkhoff, Bauer, & Joyce, 1997; Moss, Baumeister, & Biewener, 1996).

Many documented and undocumented immigrants find themselves among the working poor, who are employed in low-paying jobs but have no health insurance for themselves or their families. Those who work may be in a catch-22 situation: they do not have insurance coverage provided through their place of employment and yet are earning too much to qualify for Medicaid.

Uninsured undocumented immigrants in particular tend to seek care at free neighborhood clinics, staffed by volunteer providers, or on a cash-only basis from private or clinic providers who are willing to deliver services on this basis. Uninsured immigrants make greater use of hospital outpatient departments and emergency rooms than do people with private insurance. Undocumented immigrants are more likely to use emergency rooms than outpatient departments, mainly because they seek care either principally or solely in emergencies (Rumbaut, Chavez, Moser, Pickwell, & Wishik, 1988).

The availability and affordability of services, particularly the ability to pay for them, greatly affect whether immigrants and refugees seek care at all. The quality of the care provided is affected by its adequacy, as well as its acceptability, to those who are eventually served.

Conclusion

Vulnerable populations confront a welter of organizational and financial barriers to care. Organizational barriers include problems with the initial availability or accessibility of services, as well as discontinuities that result due to the lack of coordination and integration of services. This and the previous chapter document that the system of financing care for vulnerable populations has neither parity nor equity, meaning there is little equivalence across services or groups. Chapter Eight reviews the evidence regarding the costs and Chapter Nine the effectiveness of the care currently being provided to the vulnerable to assess the appropriateness and affordability of existing organizational and financial arrangements to serve them.

CHAPTER EIGHT

HOW MUCH DOES THEIR CARE COST?

Little uniformity exists in how the costs of caring for the vulnerable are defined or in the types of data available across studies or groups. In some studies, costs refer to the direct dollar expenditures by an agency or program. In others, true economic costs are estimated, based on assigning values to the amount of resources used or lost in a defined population as a result of illness. Direct costs in this case refer to those resources used in providing services (such as hospital, physician, or other treatment services), and indirect costs refer to lost productivity (due to absenteeism, death, or imprisonment, for example). In some cases, the out-of-pocket costs (or cash outlays) of the affected individuals or their families are an important component of the financial burden of care.

Cost-benefit and cost-effectiveness analyses are used to evaluate which programs yield the best outcomes relative to what they cost. In cost-benefit analysis, both costs and benefits are expressed in dollar terms; in cost-effectiveness analysis, benefits are expressed in nonmonetary units, such as days of hospitalization, numbers of physician visits, level of functioning, or quality-adjusted life-years.

This chapter reviews the evidence regarding the costs of care (however defined) for each group, as well as cost-benefit and cost-effectiveness studies that seek to determine which programs yield the best outcomes relative to their cost.

Cross-Cutting Issues

For some groups and programs, clear conclusions can be drawn. For others, the evidence is mixed, and for still others it is nonexistent.

Overall Costs

Sophisticated efforts to estimate the economic costs of mental illness, alcohol, and drug abuse have yielded relatively clear-cut findings regarding the major resources used or lost due to these problems. The bulk of the economic costs resulting from mental illness and alcohol abuse are the indirect costs of lost productivity, as well as the direct institutional, provider, and other treatment expenses; the social costs associated with crime-related expenditures and losses comprise the bulk of the economic costs of drug abuse.

True economic costs of other problems are not known. However, the evidence suggests that the economic and social consequences of infant deaths and those resulting from suicides and homicides, reflected in years of productive life lost, are substantial, as are the medical care and related expenses of caring for persons living with HIV/AIDS and victims of family abuse and neglect.

The financial burden on many of the vulnerable, as well as the institutions that care for them, is clearly reflected in the substantial out-of-pocket outlays assumed by the chronically ill and disabled and their families, as well as the disproportionate share of uncompensated expenditures borne by public hospitals in caring for persons living with HIV/AIDS.

Scant evidence of the costs of care for homeless and immigrant and refugee populations exists beyond reports of the expenditures and budgets of programs and agencies most directly involved with these populations.

Cost Benefit and Cost-Effectiveness

Even fewer data are available regarding the cost benefits or cost-effectiveness of alternative programs for caring for the vulnerable.

The clearest evidence of cost-beneficial effects exists for selected prevention-oriented services. The cost benefits and cost-effectiveness of prenatal care and other primary prevention–oriented services for high-risk mothers and infants have been clearly demonstrated. Studies of child abuse and neglect services also confirm that early interventions, such as parenting skills education and peer support, are much more cost-effective than programs that attempt to deal with treating these problems once they occur.

Cost-benefit and cost-effectiveness analyses of case management or noninstitutional alternatives for the chronically physically or mentally ill have yielded mixed results. In a number of cases, the costs of these alternatives were higher than those for institutional care. The outcomes were better according to some indicators and unchanged according to others.

Research on the costs of alternative programs relative to outcomes is either quite limited for certain groups, such as persons living with HIV/AIDS or alcohol or substance abusers, and virtually nonexistent for others, including suicide or homicide victims, homeless persons, and immigrant and refugee populations. In many cases, the objectives of the programs serving these populations are mixed or ill defined, as are the political or theoretical perspectives on the origins (or causes) of the problems underlying the design of these programs. (See Table 8.1.)

Population-Specific Overview

The overall costs and cost benefit and cost-effectiveness of programs to serve the vulnerable will be reviewed.

High-Risk Mothers and Infants

Prenatal care and related primary prevention–oriented services are much more cost-effective investments than inpatient neonatal intensive care for low birthweight or high-risk births.

Overall Costs. The overall expenditures for maternity care and delivery continue to increase due to the overall rise in health care costs, greater use of neonatal intensive care units, rising malpractice fees and claims, and the growing burden of uncompensated care.

The average cost of maternity care for a normal delivery is much lower than for cesarean delivery, and hospital-based birthing centers, including practitioners' fees, as well as midwives' fees for normal delivery, are substantially lower than those for physician deliveries. The costs for low birthweight and other high-risk infants are much higher than for normal deliveries. Data from the 1996 Healthcare Cost and Utilization Project documented that the average charges for a hospital stay for infant respiratory distress syndrome ($56,600), often resulting from premature births, as well as low birthweight births ($50,300), as being the second and third most expensive hospital diagnoses, respectively, following spinal cord injury ($56,800) (Agency for Healthcare Research and Quality, 1996).

The costs associated with low birthweight also include the costs of special education, early intervention, and other support services consumed disproportionately by low birthweight children. Based on 1988 national survey data, Lewit, Baker, Corman, and Shiono (1995) estimated that the incremental costs of the total medical and other resources used to care for the 3.5 to 4.0 million children born with a low birthweight from birth to age fifteen cost between $5.5 and $6.0 billion more than if they had been born normal birthweight. Low birthweight was estimated to account for 10 percent of all health care costs for children, an issue of increasing concern in employer-sponsored health plans as well (Chollet, Newman, & Sumner, 1996).

Cost Benefit and Cost-Effectiveness. A number of studies have documented the cost benefit and cost-effectiveness of programs to reduce teenage pregnancy, low birthweight births, and infant mortality. Burt (1986) calculated that in 1985, the American public paid an average of $13,902 per family over a twenty-year period for each first birth to a teenager, principally through Aid to Families with Dependent Children, food stamps, and Medicaid program support for these mothers, many of who drop out of school and are unemployed. If all teenage births were delayed until the mother was twenty or older, the cost per family would be $8,342, a net savings of $5,560 per birth.

A 1988 Office of Technology Assessment report, *Healthy Children: Investing in the Future*, estimated that for each low birthweight birth that was prevented, from $14,000 to $30,000 could be saved in the costs of newborn hospitalization, re-hospitalizations in the first years, and the long-term costs of institutional care, foster care, early intervention, special education, and services for individuals from one to thirty-five years of age. Based on California claims data for babies born in 1986 and 1987 who were eligible for Medicaid, Rogowski (1998) confirmed that a weight increase of 250 grams (.55 pounds) at birth saved an average of $12,000 to $16,000 in medical care costs during the first year of life, and a 500 gram (1.09 pounds) increase yielded approximately $28,000 in savings.

A 1985 Institute of Medicine (IOM) study documented that for mothers from high-risk socioeconomic groups on public assistance, every additional dollar spent on prenatal care would result in savings of $3.38 in the medical care costs of low birthweight infants. The IOM study was based on achieving the 1990 objective of 9 percent low birthweight births. A study in New Hampshire projected a savings of $2.26 for every dollar spent on prenatal care for mothers with less than a high school education. Target rates in that study were the actual low birthweight rates for New Hampshire women who received adequate prenatal care (Gorsky & Colby, 1989). These savings are unlikely to be realized unless the effectiveness of prenatal care in reducing preterm and low birthweight births is enhanced (Shiono & Behrman, 1995).

Joyce, Corman, and Grossman (1988) established an infant health production function across large counties in the United States, to compare the cost-effectiveness of various health programs, including prenatal care, neonatal intensive care units, and the Special Supplemental Food Program for Women, Infants and Children (WIC), in reducing race-specific neonatal mortality rates. Early initiation of prenatal care was found to be the most cost-effective means of reducing neonatal mortality rates. Neonatal intensive care saved more newborn lives but cost substantially more than the other programs, and hence was found to be the least cost-effective. With few exceptions, WIC was the second most cost-effective program, followed by abortion, family planning, community health center programs, and finally neonatal intensive care. In general, the most successful programs were even more cost-effective for African Americans than for whites.

Chronically Ill and Disabled

The out-of-pocket burden of care is substantial for many chronically ill and disabled, principally because of the limited coverage available for long-term care services. Cost-benefit and cost-effectiveness studies of home- and community-based

TABLE 8.1. PRINCIPAL COSTS OF CARE FOR VULNERABLE POPULATIONS.

Vulnerable Populations	Overall Costs	Cost Benefit/Cost-Effectiveness (CB/CE)
High-risk mothers and infants	The costs for low-birthweight and high-risk infants are substantially higher than for normal deliveries.	Every dollar spent on prenatal care could save as much as two to three dollars in the medical care costs of low-birthweight infants.
Chronically ill and disabled	The out-of-pocket cost burden is high for many of the chronically ill and disabled due to the lack of coverage for long-term care services.	CB/CE studies of home and community-based alternatives to institutionalized care have yielded mixed results regarding program costs and outcomes.
Persons living with HIV/AIDS	The monthly costs of care for persons with AIDS are estimated to range from $3,000 to $4,000, with antiretroviral therapy drugs assuming an increasing share of the costs.	Little data exist on the CB/CE of alternatives for organizing and delivering care to persons living with HIV/AIDS.
Mentally ill and disabled	About half of the economic costs of mental illness are due to the indirect costs resulting from lost productivity.	CB/CE studies of case management and other community-based alternatives for long-term care for the mentally ill and disabled do not clearly confirm that costs are less (offset) under these arrangements.
Alcohol or substance abusers	The vast majority of the economic costs of drug and alcohol abuse are due to the indirect costs resulting from lost productivity, impaired productivity, premature death, impaired productivity, institutionalization, incarceration, or being the perpetrator or victim of crime.	Both the availability and findings of CB/CE studies of substance abuse treatment alternatives vary across types of programs and public versus private tiers of service.

Suicide or homicide prone	In addition to direct expenditures by the criminal justice, social service, and other sectors, and major personal and societal costs of homicides and suicides are the years of potential life lost.	CB/CE studies of alternatives for preventing suicide or homicide or treating the perpetrators or victims of intentional violence are a largely neglected area of research.
Abusing families	Although a paucity of data are available on the costs of the array of categories of family abuse, the available evidence suggests that both the personal and social costs are high.	CB/CE studies of child abuse and neglect in particular suggest that primary prevention–oriented services provide a much greater prospect for savings and success than do programs to treat families in which abuse has already occurred.
Homeless persons	The direct and indirect costs of homelessness have not been estimated directly, though the burden of caring for them has fallen disproportionately on local and state governments and voluntary, nonprofit providers.	Homeless persons typically have unmet needs for medical care and substance abuse and mental health treatment that can lead to an exacerbation of these problems and to higher costs in caring for them.
Immigrants and refugees	The costs of caring for immigrants and refugees are borne principally by federal agencies charged with their entry, resettlement, and support; programs to which they seek entitlement; state and local agencies that assume responsibility for their care; as well as families.	Anti-immigrant policies that restrict immigrants' access to preventive and primary care services may result in greater overall costs of care for these populations.

alternatives to long-term institutionalized care have yielded mixed results regarding program costs and outcomes.

Overall Costs. Treatment and long-term care represent the lion's share of expenditures related to chronic illness and disability. A survey of the Association of State and Territorial Chronic Disease Program Directors asking about 1994 fiscal year expenditures, conducted by the Centers for Disease Control and Prevention, found that although chronic diseases are the major causes of death, disability, and medical expenditures in the United States, the total expenditure for chronic disease–control activities was around $287.3 million and the per capita expenditure was only $1.21 in the forty-one states reporting. The most frequently cited funding priorities were directed toward cancer, tobacco use, and youth (Centers for Disease Control and Prevention, 1997).

Particularly significant components of the costs of long-term care for the chronically ill and disabled are nursing homes, home health care, and associated community and supportive services. The nation spent $82.8 billion on nursing home care and $32.3 billion on home health care services in 1997. Nursing home residents and their families paid around one-third (31.1 percent) of the costs. The other payers were Medicaid (47.6 percent), Medicare (12.3 percent), private insurance (4.9 percent), and other private sources (1.9 percent). The average annual cost of a nursing home stay was around $40,000, and the average daily rates were higher for private pay than for Medicaid patients (National Center for Health Statistics, 1999d).

A particular concern in evaluating the costs of care for the chronically ill and disabled is the direct and indirect economic burden on the individuals themselves and their families. On average, Medicare beneficiaries spend 19 percent of their income on out-of-pocket health care costs: cost sharing for Medicare-covered services, out-of-pocket payments for noncovered services (such as prescription drugs), Medicare Part B premium, and supplemental health insurance premiums. Beneficiaries with incomes below the federal poverty level are estimated to pay an even higher proportion (over a third) of their income on health care (American Association of Retired Persons, 1997). The out-of-pocket costs of care for chronically ill children, particularly those who are technology assisted, are one of the major stressors on families in caring for these children at home (Aday, Aitken, & Wegener, 1988; Jacobs & McDermott, 1989).

Based on analyses of data from managed care providers, the costs of medical care for children and adults with chronic health conditions are estimated to be at least twice that of patients in general. A relatively few individuals with chronic illness account for the majority of expenditures (Fishman, Von Korff, Lozano, & Hecht, 1997; Ireys, Anderson, Shaffer, & Neff, 1997).

Cost Benefit and Cost-Effectiveness. Providing less restrictive alternatives to long-term stays in acute care hospitals or nursing homes has been hypothesized to reduce costs and enhance the well-being of the chronically ill elderly or disabled.

Experimental or quasi-experimental studies that assessed the costs and impact of home or community alternatives to nursing homes (case management or an extended package of services such as adult day care, homemaker services, and home health care) have found that home and community-based care appears to have had little or no impact on mortality, patient functioning, or nursing home placement. Some studies have shown improvements in participants' levels of satisfaction with care, social interaction, and quality of life as a whole. The costs of care were not reduced, however, and may have been greater by as much as 15 percent when home or community-based care services were used. Any reductions in nursing home costs were offset by the increased costs of providing expanded services to those who were likely at low risk of entering nursing homes, in the absence of these services. The studies concluded that improved targeting of high-risk elderly patients (particularly to avert hospitalization) and better controls on utilization could lead to more efficient service provision. Limitations of research include the quasi-experimental nature of the research designs, inadequate sample sizes, and rival hypotheses (sample subject attrition and selection, for example). These have created serious problems with interpreting and generalizing study results (Hedrick, Koepsell, & Inui, 1989; Vertrees, Manton, & Adler, 1989; Weissert & Cready, 1989a).

Persons Living with HIV/AIDS

The total cost of HIV/AIDS care and the distribution among types of costs have shifted over the course of the epidemic as a function of changes in patterns of care and the increased importance of drugs in treating the disease. HIV prevention interventions represent a cost-effective approach to reducing HIV/AIDS-related costs.

Overall Costs. Estimates of the average lifetime medical care costs of AIDS have varied widely, from a high of $147,000 for the United States as a whole for the period from 1981 to 1985, to a low of $27,000, based on a 1984 study done in San Francisco (Fox & Thomas, 1989; Hellinger, 1988a, 1988b, 1990, 1991, 1993a; Scitovsky & Rice, 1987; Scitovsky, 1988, 1989a, 1989b). A number of factors have contributed to variations in these estimates across studies, including differences in the time period on which the analyses are based, the case mix and components of services included, the use of costs in some studies versus charges in others, as well as changes in the methods of treatment over time, particularly the greater use of antiretroviral therapies and a shift to outpatient or community-based services (Green, Oppenheimer, & Wintfeld, 1994; Tolley & Gyldmark, 1993). Estimates of lifetime costs in 1996 after the approval of protease inhibitors ranged from $71,143 to $424,763. Trends related to the greater use of antiretroviral therapies and the increased length of survival of persons with AIDS nonetheless serve to increase the lifetime cost of caring for persons living with HIV/AIDS (Hellinger, 1998).

Due to these trends, the estimated monthly cost of treating a person with AIDS rather than lifetime costs may be a more informative figure for tracking changes in the overall total and mix of HIV/AIDS services delivery costs. Estimated costs per month between 1992 and 1996 ranged from $1,885 to $2,764. Estimates based on 1997 data were from $3,274 to $4,084. As with the lifetime costs of AIDS care, the proportion of monthly costs attributable to hospitalization fell and the proportion related to drug therapy increased from the early 1990s (Hellinger, 1998).

The cost of hospital care for persons with AIDS remains high, however, particularly in the last months of life (Fleishman, Mor, & Laliberte, 1995; Hellinger, Fleishman, & Hsia, 1994; Hurley et al., 1995). Home and community-based services offer an alternative to inpatient care, particularly in the context of a continuum of care for reducing the chance of hospitalization and enhancing the quality of life for persons living with HIV/AIDS. The provision of these services through state Medicaid programs in the United States was authorized through Section 2176 waivers under the Omnibus Budget Reconciliation Act of 1985. Research in states providing such services has documented that they are at least budget neutral in increasing the overall costs of care and may in fact result in some savings, particularly among groups, such as minorities, that might have had poorer access to such services prior to the waiver (Anderson & Mitchell, 1997; Dunn, 1997). Preliminary evidence comparing the care and costs for persons with AIDS in health maintenance organization (HMO) and fee-for-service arrangements suggests that HMOs may further reduce spending on inpatient care without observable decrements in functional outcomes or satisfaction. More research is needed in this area, particularly as persons with AIDS and disabled populations increasingly are enrolled in such arrangements through state Medicaid programs (Wilson, Sullivan, & Weissman, 1998).

Other important components of the costs of care for persons living with HIV/AIDS are direct nonpersonal costs, such as research, screening, health education, and support services, as well as indirect costs, such as lost output due to illness and premature death. The magnitude of nonpersonal direct cost outlays is largely dependent on future policies to support these services. Most of the indirect costs result from lost earnings due to premature death. This may differ, however, for different risk groups (homosexual white males versus minority intravenous drug users, for example) (Scitovsky, 1988, 1989a, 1989b).

Cost Benefit and Cost-Effectiveness. A variety of HIV prevention strategies have been implemented in both developed and developing countries, which vary significantly in overall program costs. These include mass media campaigns, peer education programs, sexually transmitted disease treatment, condom social marketing, safe blood provision, and needle exchange and bleach provision programs (Söderlund, Lavis, Broomberg, & Mills, 1993). Community-level interventions to prevent HIV transmission that use existing social networks appear to be particularly cost-effective strategies (Pinkerton, Holtgrave, DiFrancesico, Stevenson, & Kelly, 1998). Net reductions in the medical costs of care and treatment and net increases in quality-adjusted life-years resulting from HIV prevention in general make it a relatively cost-effective strategy (Guinan, Farnham, & Holtgrave, 1994; Holtgrave & Pinkerton, 1997).

Cost-effectiveness and related research also offer promising and important alternatives for evaluating the clinical and economic relevance of treatments for HIV-infected patients, such as zidovudine (Oddone et al., 1993). The lifetime medical and social costs of caring for pediatric AIDS cases are significant. Routine HIV screening of pregnant women offers a promising cost-effective alternative through permitting early intervention to inhibit the maternal-infant transmission of the disease (Havens, Cuene, & Holtgrave, 1997; Muller et al., 1996; Oldenettel, Dye, & Artal, 1997; Stoto, Almario, & McCormick, 1999).

Mentally Ill and Disabled

Almost half of the economic costs of mental illness have been estimated to be due to the indirect costs resulting from lost productivity, with most of the rest being due to direct institutional, provider, and related treatment expenses. The results of studies of the cost benefit and cost-effectiveness of case management and other alternatives for integrating the financing and delivery care of the mentally ill and disabled document that other (medical care) costs are less (or offset) under these arrangements.

Overall Costs. The magnitude of the costs of mental illness and the methods for estimating these costs have varied over time and across studies (Frank & Kamlet, 1985; Levine & Levine, 1975; Levine & Willner, 1976; McKusick et al., 1998; President's Commission on Mental Health, 1978b; Rice, Kelman, Miller, & Dunmeyer, 1990).

A 1990 study by Rice and others (1990) that estimated the direct and indirect costs of mental illness documented $103.7 billion in economic costs to the U.S. economy in 1985. For 1988 the total cost was estimated to have been $129.3 billion. Direct costs, which included the personal health care costs for institutional and provider services, and prescription drugs, as well as costs for support services, such as research and training for providers and administration, were 41.0 percent (or $42.5 billion) of the costs (in 1985).

Indirect costs include the illness (morbidity) and death (mortality) resulting from mental illness. Indirect costs due to morbidity, measured by the value of reduced or lost productivity, accounted for almost half— 45.7 percent (or $47.4 billion)—of the $103.7 billion in total economic costs. A total of 39,707 deaths were estimated to have been due to mental disorders, representing more than 1 million person-years lost (a loss of 26.4 years of life per person) and a loss of $9.3 billion to the economy (8.9 percent of total costs). The balance of the total economic costs (4.3 percent or $4.5 billion) was for other related costs, particularly the amounts spent by caregivers in providing care to mentally ill family members ($2.5 billion), as well as criminal justice–related expenses ($1.3 billion).

A 1996 study estimated $66.7 billion of expenditures for formal health care services used to diagnose and treat mental health conditions, representing about 84 percent of total mental health and substance abuse expenditures. Approximately 42.3 percent of the expenditures were for general service providers (community hospitals and physicians, for example) and the balance (57.7 percent) for specialty mental health providers. More than half (52.6 percent) of the expenditures were funded through public sources. The average annual growth in spending for the treatment of mental illness between 1986 and 1996 was lower (7.3 percent) than for personal health care experiences in general (8.3 percent). The increasing role of managed care in providing mental health and related behavioral health care services, particularly through declines in inpatient care, is credited with reducing the costs of such care over this period (Hay Group, 1999; Mark, McKusick, King, Harwood, & Genuardi, 1998; McKusick et al., 1998; RAND, 1998b).

For those covered by public or private plans, the out-of-pocket share of the cost for mental health care is higher than for general medical care, and publicly supported institutions are particularly likely to bear a disproportionate burden of caring for those who have no resources to pay for it themselves.

Cost Benefit and Cost-Effectiveness. The cost-effectiveness of mental health care services is enhanced in provider arrangements that emphasize quality improvements and comprehensive, coordinated care for the mentally ill. RAND researchers documented that the marginal cost of eliminating one functional limitation due to depression under conditions of improving the quality of care for such patients was around $1,000 to $2,000, which was one-fourth of the average cost of the outcome improvement under care as usual (RAND, 1998c). Effective case management of individuals who are dually diagnosed with substance abuse or other comorbid conditions among the mentally ill can also enhance outcomes and reduce long-term treatment costs (Clark et al., 1998; Croghan, Obenchain, & Crown, 1998; Dickey & Azeni, 1996; Jerrell & Hu, 1996; Salkever et al., 1999; Torrey, Bigelow, & Sladen-Dew, 1993).

An argument for providing third-party coverage for mental health services is the hypothesized medical offset effect, that is, the use of specialty mental health care services could result in a corresponding reduction in the use of and expenditures for physical health care services. Such savings have been documented in the cases of distressed medical inpatients, medical care outpatients with long-term somatization disorders, and clients receiving outpatient alcohol abuse treatment. Managed behavioral health care offers the potential for further improvements in the cost-effectiveness of mental health services through a closer integration and management of both medical and mental health care services. The precise impacts of these arrangements on patient quality and outcomes appear to be mixed, however (Olfson, Sing, & Schlesinger, 1999; Pallak, Cummings, Dorken, & Henke, 1993).

Alcohol or Substance Abusers

The productivity losses due to premature death, impaired productivity, institutionalization, incarceration, crime careers, or being victims of crime account for the bulk of outlays associated with drug and alcohol abuse. Cost-offset studies have documented significant cost savings from substance abuse prevention and early treatment programs.

Overall Costs. Smoking and related nicotine addictions were estimated to have cost the nation $91.3 billion in 1990 ($39.1 billion in direct costs and $52.1 billion in indirect costs). Tobacco use also contributes directly to the cost of other illnesses, such as heart disease and cancer (Committee to Identify Strategies to Raise the Profile of Substance Abuse and Alcoholism Research, 1997).

Alcohol abuse was estimated to have cost the nation $70.3 billion in 1985, $85.8 billion in 1988, and $148.0 billion in 1992. A further 12.5 percent increase to $166.5 billion was estimated between 1992 and 1995. Health care expenditures for alcohol abuse services ($5.6 billion) and the medical consequences of alcohol abuse ($13.2 billion) in 1992 accounted for $18.8 billion (12.7 percent). Around 107,400 persons died as a consequence of alcohol abuse. The productivity losses due to premature death, impaired productivity, institutionalization, incarceration, or being victims of crimes formed the largest proportion, as was the case with drug abuse ($107.0 billion, or 72.3 percent), of total costs. Societal costs, including crime, social welfare administration, motor vehicle crashes, and fire destruction, accounted for $22.2 billion (15.0 percent) (Harwood, Fountain, Livermore, & the Lewin Group, 1998; Rice, Kelman, Miller, & Dunmeyer, 1990).

A 1996 study estimated $4.9 billion of expenditures for formal health care services used to diagnose and treat alcohol abuse. Approximately 53.4 percent of the expenditures were for general service providers (community hospitals and physicians, for example) and the balance (46.6 percent) for specialty providers. More than half (57.6 percent) of the expenditures were funded through public sources. The average annual growth in spending for the treatment of alcohol abuse between 1986 and 1996 was lower (1.7 percent) than for personal health care experiences in general (8.3 percent) (Mark, McKusick, King, Harwood, & Genuardi, 1998; McKusick et al., 1998).

The total economic costs of drug abuse nationally were estimated to be $44.1 billion in 1985, $58.3 billion in 1988, and $97.6 billion in 1992. A further 12.5 percent increase to $109.8 billion was estimated between 1992 and 1995. Health care expenditures for drug abuse services ($4.4 billion) and the medical consequences of drug abuse ($5.5 billion) in 1992 accounted for $9.9 billion (10.1 percent). Underlying the cost of medical complications are the HIV/AIDS epidemics and related epidemics of tuberculosis and hepatitis B and C. Around

25,500 persons died in 1992 as a consequence of drug abuse. The productivity losses due to premature death, impaired productivity, institutionalization, incarceration, crime careers, or as a result of being victims of crimes was the lion's share—$69.4 billion (71.1 percent)—of total costs in 1992. Drug users experience more difficulty than nonusers in finding and holding a job, particularly in higher-skilled or higher-wage industries. Societal costs, including crime and social welfare administration, accounted for $18.3 billion (18.8 percent) (Harwood, Fountain, Livermore, & The Lewin Group, 1998; Rice, Kelman, Miller, & Dunmeyer, 1990).

A 1996 national study estimated $7.6 billion of expenditures for formal health care services used to diagnose and treat drug abuse. The vast majority (79.1 percent) of the expenditures were for specialty substance abuse treatment providers. Two-thirds (66.1 percent) of the expenditures were funded through public sources. The average annual growth in spending for the treatment of drug abuse between 1986 and 1996 (13.2 percent) was much higher than for personal health care expenditures in general (8.3 percent) (Mark, McKusick, King, Harwood, & Genuardi, 1998; McKusick et al., 1998).

Cost Benefit and Cost-Effectiveness. The focus of national drug policy has been primarily on supply-reduction strategies, such as source-country control, interdiction, and domestic enforcement, including the imposition of mandatory minimum drug sentences. RAND researchers have documented that treatment of heavy users is more cost-effective than supply-control programs and that mandatory minimum sentences are not as cost-effective as spending additional resources on either conventional enforcement or on drug treatment for heavy drug users (Caulkins, Rydell, Schwabe, & Chiesa, 1998; Rydell & Everingham, 1994). Evaluations in the drug abuse area have demonstrated that the benefits (in terms of clients' increased employment and lower involvement in crime) of methadone maintenance, residential therapeutic communities, and to some extent outpatient nonmethadone treatment programs equaled or exceeded the costs of these programs. Both drug use and criminal behavior among adult clients are reduced following inpatient, outpatient, and residential treatment for drug abuse (Gerstein & Harwood, 1990; Substance Abuse and Mental Health Services Administration, 1998e).

Substance abuse is associated with higher rates of emergency room and inpatient medical care utilization and related costs (Cartwright & Ingster, 1993; el-Guebaly, Armstrong, & Hodgins, 1998; Fox, Merrill, Chang, & Califano, 1995; French & Martin, 1996; Ingster & Cartwright, 1995; Nelson & Stussman, 1994). An important focus of research on the cost benefits of substance treatment programs has been medical offset effects, that is, whether the overall costs of medical care associated with alcohol problems are lessened when treatment for the underlying problem is provided. Failure to provide treatment programs can lead to a ramping effect, that is, health care costs increase at a higher rate as the length of time to treatment increases. Reviews of the literature in this area have demonstrated that for groups of employed individuals and those enrolled in private insurance or prepaid health plans, savings in medical care costs do result and are sustained over the long term. For publicly insured populations (those with Medicaid or Veterans Administration coverage, for example), for whom the ramping effects may be significant, savings tend to be less. These groups are much more likely to be low income, to have deferred seeking treatment until the medical complications of alcohol abuse have become severe, and bring fewer personal and social resources (self-esteem, less secure social networks or family support) to the treatment and recovery process. For such populations, more significant investments are required for effective treatment (Institute of Medicine, 1990; Langenbucher, 1994a, 1994b; Luckey, 1987; Substance Abuse and Mental Health Services Administration, 1999a).

The cost-offset literature suggests that primary prevention may hold promise for significant reductions in the costs of alcohol and substance abuse through avoiding the high costs of treatment. Furthermore, less costly interventions can be used at early stages of substance abuse when the prognosis is more favorable. Smoking cessation is also an extremely cost-effective intervention (Cromwell, Bartosch, Fiore, Hasselblad, & Baker, 1997; Kim, Coletti, Crutchfield, Williams, & Hepler, 1995; Substance Abuse and Mental Health Services Administration, 1999a). Research on the cost and benefits of prevention-oriented interventions for the use of alcohol and tobacco has demonstrated that higher excise taxes and minimum age provisions decrease adolescents' consumption of these substances that may serve as gateways for more serious drug use later (Bach & Lantos, 1999; Becker, Grossman, & Murphy, 1994; Chaloupka & Wechsler, 1997; Chaloupka, Grossman, & Saffer, 1998; Grossman & Chaloupka, 1998).

Suicide or Homicide Prone

In addition to expenditures by the criminal justice, social service, and other sectors that deal with the effects of suicide and homicide, other major personal and societal costs include the years of potential life lost (YPLL) due to early death, the direct costs of hospitalization and associated medical costs for severe injury, and the resulting impact on the quality of life of the family and community.

Overall Costs. In 1997, homicides accounted for 368.9 years of potential life lost per 100,000 people under age seventy-five. The YPLL rate per 100,000 persons was highest for black males (2,251.2) and lowest for white, non-Hispanic females (92.0). The years of potential life lost due to suicide were 378.0 per 100,000 in 1997, with the highest rates being for Native American males (913.0) and the lowest for Hispanic females (66.7) (National Center for Health Statistics, 1999d).

Gunshot injuries have been estimated to cost around $2.5 billion in lifetime medical costs. The indirect costs to families and society of violent deaths resulting from suicide and homicide are also substantial. Children who are victims of or witnesses to violence often suffer delays in physical, social, and emotional development and posttraumatic stress disorders. Battered women are at greatly elevated risk of alcoholism, drug abuse, attempted suicide, child abuse, rape, and mental health problems. The death of a wage-earning spouse can also result in serious economic deprivation for the surviving spouse and dependent children.

Surviving family members of suicide victims often experience shame and guilt, as well as fears regarding the prospect of other family members' making such attempts. Suicide can result in an inability to collect life insurance benefits or, in the instance of suicide attempters, increased financial burdens resulting from mental health or medical care treatment costs.

The "suicide contagion" that appears to be precipitated in some communities in response to a suicide and the movement of middle-class residents and businesses out of neighborhoods that have high rates of violent crime are examples of broader community or societal costs that result from suicide- and homicide-related violence (Rosenberg et al., 1987).

Cost Benefit and Cost-Effectiveness. Cost-benefit and cost-effectiveness analyses of alternatives for preventing suicide and homicide or treating the perpetrators and victims of these intentional acts of harm have documented that early childhood intervention programs and school-based drug prevention programs reduce the likelihood of poor developmental outcomes, initiating drug use, or the pursuit of criminal careers among at-risk children and adolescents (RAND, Institute for Civil Justice, 1999).

Abusing Families

Little systematic data are available on the direct, indirect, and related social costs of the array of categories of family abuse and neglect. The evidence that does exist, however, suggests that the human and personal costs of family abuse and neglect are substantial and that primary prevention–oriented services (such as home visiting, parenting education, educational and skills development, and peer support) provide a greater promise of savings and success than do programs to provide treatment in families in which abuse has already occurred.

Overall Costs. The socioemotional and physical impacts on both adult and child victims of abuse and neglect have been documented to be substantial. Daro (1988) estimated both the immediate and longer-term financial costs of child maltreatment. The immediate costs are hospitalizations for injuries associated with serious maltreatment, such as skull or bone fractures, internal injuries, and burns ($20 million); rehabilitation and special education services ($7 million); foster care ($460 million); and other immediate costs of educational, juvenile court, and private therapeutic services. Longer-term financial costs are those associated with juvenile court and detention ($14.8 million), long-term foster care ($646.0 million), loss of future earnings (from $658.0 million to $1.3 billion), and other costs associated with adult criminal court and detention, drug- or alcohol abuse–related treatment and potential welfare dependency.

Research on women seen in HMOs has documented that annual health care use and costs were greater among women who had experienced early childhood maltreatment. Women with sexual abuse histories had significantly higher primary care and outpatient costs and more frequent emergency room visits than did women without a history of such abuse (Walker et al., 1999).

Cost Benefit and Cost-Effectiveness. Studies examining the cost benefit and cost-effectiveness of alternative prevention and treatment services for child maltreatment have concluded that prevention-oriented services provide greater promise of both success and savings than do those that are oriented toward treating individuals and families in which abuse has already occurred (Chalk & King, 1998; Daro, 1988; Dubowitz, 1990).

Based on a review and synthesis of research in this area, Daro (1988) concluded that from a cost-effectiveness point of view, programs that provide parenting education, educational and skills development, lay therapy provided by individuals who have successfully gotten out of abusive situations, peer support groups, and group and family therapy yielded the greatest benefits relative to per client costs. Group or family therapy appeared to be a much more cost-effective treatment alternative than individual therapy, particularly because of the much higher costs and generally poorer outcomes associated with the latter intervention.

The costs of pediatric intensive care, as well as the rates of mortality and severe residual morbidity, are high for child and infant victims of abuse. Home health visitors and medical foster care represent much more cost-effective alternatives through preventing abuse among particularly at-risk infants and children (Dubowitz, 1990; Irazuzta, McJunkin, Danadian, Arnold, & Zhang, 1997).

Prevention services that are linked to existing universal service systems, such as public schools, public health care providers, community-based family service agencies, or churches, are much more likely to be cost-effective than those requiring new categoric institutions for dealing with the problem.

Homeless Persons

The burden of caring for homeless persons has largely fallen on local and state governments and voluntary, nonprofit providers. The total direct and indirect economic and social costs of homelessness have not been estimated directly. They are, however, likely to be substantial.

Overall Costs. One of the first major federal funding initiatives in this area, the Emergency Food and Shelter Program initiated in 1983, administered by the Federal Emergency Management Agency, provided funding for nonprofit groups and state governors, under the direction of a national board of representatives from major charitable organizations (the United Way, the Salvation Army, the National Council of Churches, and others). This funding was significant in catalyzing the establishment of a network of emergency shelters that became the backbone of the service system for homeless persons. The vast majority of the shelters are operated by private, nonprofit (particularly religious) organizations.

Subsequent federal initiatives for the homeless population have largely been encompassed within the provisions and amendments of the Stewart B. McKinney Homeless Act (Public Law 100–77) (General Accounting Office, 1990b). Among other federal programs serving homeless persons are nutritional programs within the Department of Agriculture; the Department of Defense surplus and food bank programs; Department of Health and Human Services programs for the homeless mentally ill, substance abusers, and runaway youths; the Veterans Administration health care programs for homeless veterans; and the Department of Housing and Urban Development initiatives to expand low- and moderate-income housing availability (U.S. Department of Housing and Urban Development, 1991).

The McKinney Act also catalyzed a larger role on the part of states and municipalities in caring for homeless persons. Because of limited resources in most states, the Council of State Governments has stressed the importance of designing preventive-oriented programs that attempt to address the root causes of homelessness (U.S. Commission on Security and Cooperation in Europe, 1990).

Based on the twenty-six cities surveyed in 1999 by the U.S. Conference of Mayors Task Force on Hunger and Homelessness, 96 percent of the cities reported using governmental funds (either locally generated revenues or federal or state grants). Approximately $225.5 million, including locally generated funds, state grants, McKinney Act funds, and Community Development and Community Services block grant funds, were expended by the survey cities during 1999 for homeless services (U.S. Conference of Mayors, 1999).

The total direct and indirect economic costs of homelessness have not been measured directly. These include the direct costs of medical care for homeless persons for conditions that in many cases are preventable or would be less likely to become serious with proper treatment. The burden of providing medical care for homeless persons also falls most heavily on institutions (such as county or inner-city teaching hospitals) that are already assuming a disproportionate burden of caring for those who cannot afford to pay for care. An estimated 26 percent of annual inpatient Veterans Administration mental health expenditures are spent on the care of homeless persons (Rosenheck & Seibyl, 1998; Salit, Kuhn, Hartz, Vu, & Mosso, 1998).

Growth in the direct and indirect costs of mental illness, substance abuse, HIV/AIDS, and family abuse is exacerbated by the growing number of homeless persons with these problems. As the number of children and women of childbearing ages continues to increase among the homeless population, the lost productivity and resulting burden of caring for vulnerable, multiproblem, homeless infants and children loom as a substantial, long-term societal, economic, and human cost. Dually diagnosed, as well as triply diagnosed, homeless persons (those with mental illness and substance abuse, and, in some cases, HIV/AIDS) represent both costly and difficult cases to treat (Martell et al., 1992; Salit, Kuhn, Hartz, Vu, & Mosso, 1998).

Cost Benefit and Cost-Effectiveness. Programs that serve the homeless population have a range of goals and objectives, including providing permanent housing, providing emergency shelter or food relief, reducing the prevalence of physical health problems, treating associated risks such as mental illness or substance abuse, or providing social support. The conduct of cost-benefit or cost-effectiveness analyses of programs to serve the homeless population requires a clear delineation of their major intended benefits.

Immigrants and Refugees

The costs of caring for immigrants and refugees are borne by the federal agencies charged most directly with their entry, resettlement, and support (such as the Immigration and Naturalization Service in the Department of Justice and the Office of Refugee Resettlement in the Department of Health and Human Services), the programs to which they seek entitlement (such as Medicaid, Medicare, Temporary Assistance for Needy Families, or Supplemental Security Income), the state and local institutions and providers that assume a large burden of their (often uncompensated) care, as well as the families and individuals themselves who seek to pay for care out of their own (often limited) resources.

Overall Costs. The long-term fiscal impact of immigrants on the U.S. economy varies by educational level and working status of the immigrant. Under some plausible assumptions, the net present value of the fiscal impact of an immigrant with less than a high school education is −$13,000; in contrast, the net present value for an immigrant with more than a high school education is +$198,000. Under most scenarios, the long-run fiscal impact of immigrants to the United States as a whole is positive at the federal level but negative at the state and local levels, especially in states with high concentrations of new immigrants (Smith & Edmonston, 1997).

Immigrants and refugees who do not have insurance coverage are much less likely to seek medical care than those with coverage. The mortality and morbidity associated with the resultant failure to treat what are often preventable or curable diseases among foreign-born men, women, and children is substantial. Denial of preventive and primary care services can lead to higher costs of caring for the foreign born, as well as the spread of contagious diseases such as tuberculosis (Ahearn & Athey, 1991; Bean, Vernez, & Keely, 1989; Fallek, 1997; Kulig, 1990; Loue, 1998; Rumbaut, Chavez, Moser, Pickwell, & Wishik, 1988; Siddharthan & Ahern, 1996; Toole & Waldman, 1990).

Cost Benefit and Cost-Effectiveness. Research has suggested that restricting immigrants' access to care may lead to greater rather than lower overall system costs. A cost-benefit analysis of policies eliminating the public funding of prenatal care for undocumented immigrants in California, for example, estimated that the program could save the state $58 million in direct prenatal care costs but could cost taxpayers as much as $194 million more in postnatal care costs, due to substantial corollary increases in low birthweight and prematurity (Lu, Lin, Prietto, & Garite, 2000).

As with the homeless population, cost-benefit or cost-effectiveness or other studies of programs to serve immigrants and refugees must take into account their complex health and social service needs, as well as recognize that many of the health and health care problems they experience have roots in other social or political domains.

Conclusion

Both the direct costs (such as hospital, physician, or other treatment services) and indirect costs due to lost productivity (due to absenteeism, death, or imprisonment, for example), as well as the out-of-pocket costs (or cash outlays) of affected individuals or their families, in caring for vulnerable populations are substantial. Prevention is probably one of the most cost-effective investments to ameliorate vulnerability, but the bulk of the resources consumed in caring for vulnerable populations are composed of the costs associated with treatment and the loss of human productive potential. Chapter Nine reviews how the effectiveness of programs and services to serve vulnerable populations relative to the investments made in them might be enhanced.

CHAPTER NINE

WHAT'S THE QUALITY OF THEIR CARE?

Considerations of the effectiveness of medical care have traditionally focused on the structure, process, and outcomes of the care provided. Structure refers to the characteristics of the institutions or providers delivering services. Process criteria relate to the treatment protocols or standards recommended or used by providers. Outcomes refer to the actual health consequences of the care delivery process for patients.

The measurement of outcomes and particularly the relationship of the structure and process of care to outcomes are increasingly important considerations in evaluating the effectiveness of medical care, as well as related programs and services. Furthermore, the issues of access and quality are often intertwined, in that considerations of access increasingly are tempered by considerations of whether gaining access to selected services would make a difference in terms of health outcomes.

This chapter reviews what is known and what still needs to be learned about the effectiveness of care provided to the vulnerable in the context of structure, process, and outcome criteria of effectiveness.

Cross-Cutting Issues

The results suggest that structure and process criteria have tended to dominate evaluations of the effectiveness of care being delivered for certain groups and in certain settings. The development of indicators of the outcomes of care and the linkage of structure and process criteria to outcomes are on the emerging frontier of effectiveness-of-care assessment in general, as well as in programs and services to care for the vulnerable in particular.

Structure and Process

For some groups, structure and process criteria have been used to a considerable extent in assessing effectiveness. Such criteria have, for example, tended to dominate in assessments of the effectiveness of care being provided the chronically ill and disabled in nursing homes, primarily in response to licensure, reimbursement, or other external requirements. Evaluations of the effectiveness of care in the mental health, alcohol and substance abuse, and family abuse fields have often focused on the training and qualifications of providers.

Mental health professionals have attempted to promulgate treatment protocols and standards through the auspices of local provider groups or national agencies or associations. These standards have been variably accepted and implemented, however.

The strength of the relationship of prenatal care to birth outcomes varies for different racial and ethnic groups. Recently there have been efforts to specify the content of prenatal care (procedures or protocols) likely to be most effective for women with different profiles of risk.

Structure, and particularly process, criteria are either very poorly developed for certain populations (persons living with HIV/AIDS, homeless persons, and immigrants and refugees) or have a very mixed record of success in improving outcomes for others (alcohol or substance abusers and perpetrators and victims of suicide, homicide, and family abuse, for example). Cultural barriers and prejudices or misunderstandings on the part of providers may play an important role in the care that many of these groups receive. Furthermore, new standards and protocols are needed as new services and treatment modalities (such as home care or case management) come to be used.

Outcomes

Considerable ambiguity surrounds the specification of outcome criteria of effectiveness. One particularly problematic aspect for all of the groups examined here is the specification of the desired program or treatment outcomes (or objectives). These are relatively clear for high-risk mothers and infants (to reduce the incidence of low birthweight infants or the number who die) and the chronically physically or mentally ill (to maximize physical or cognitive functioning), for example, but are extremely ill defined or ambiguous for others (persons living with HIV/AIDS, victims of abuse or violence, or homeless persons). In addition, the theoretical and associated empirical underpinnings to guide the design of interventions in these areas are weak due to limited research or ambiguous or conflicting theories and findings regarding the origins (or causes) of the underlying problem being addressed.

Clarification of what outcomes are desired, how they should be measured, and which interventions are most likely to be successful in effecting these outcomes are much needed areas of research in evaluating the effectiveness of care being provided to the vulnerable. (See Table 9.1.)

Population-Specific Overview

The structure, processes, and outcome indicators of the effectiveness of care for vulnerable populations are discussed in the following paragraphs.

High-Risk Mothers and Infants

Structural considerations of the effectiveness of maternal and child health emphasize comparisons of perinatal outcomes across different types of prenatal care and birthing delivery sites. Process evaluations examine the relationship of prenatal care and the technologies and procedures associated with delivery and high-risk newborn care to perinatal outcomes. Evaluations of the effectiveness of interventions to improve birth outcomes have focused on overall infant mortality and low birthweight indicators, as well as more refined rates of birthweight-specific mortality and congenital or birth-related morbidity or disability. Two major questions are important in relating the structure and process of care to perinatal outcomes: what exactly should the content of prenatal care be, and what types and how much technology should be used at birth and particularly in trying to sustain extremely low birthweight infants?

Structure and Process. The recommendations of the Public Health Service Expert Panel on the Content of Prenatal Care extended beyond traditional measures of the number and timing of prenatal visits to the utility of preconception and postpartum visits, psychosocial assessment and follow-up, early and continuing risk assessment, health promotion interventions (to quit smoking, for example), as well as varying the number, timing, and content of visits based on the assessed risk of the mother and fetus (Public Health Service, 1989).

The wider availability of neonatal intensive care units (NICUs) is credited with the decline in birthweight-specific neonatal mortality rates (Office of Technology Assessment, 1987a). Furthermore, there is evidence that low birthweight infants born in hospitals with NICUs experience substantially lower mortality than those born in hospitals lacking these facilities (Mayfield, Rosenblatt, Baldwin, Chu, & Logerfo, 1990; Paneth, 1990).

The research on deliveries in maternity or birthing centers, compared to those in hospitals, suggests that these centers offer a safe alternative for many women

TABLE 9.1. PRINCIPAL QUALITY ISSUES FOR VULNERABLE POPULATIONS.

Vulnerable Populations	Structure/Process	Outcomes
High-risk mothers and infants	Two major issues regarding the structure and process of care for high-risk mothers and infants are what the content of prenatal care should be, and what and how much technology should be used at birth.	Though the magnitude of the relationship varies, prenatal care is generally associated with better birth outcomes. High-technology delivery and neonatal intensive care can further harm as well as help high-risk infants.
Chronically ill and disabled	Protocols and criteria for evaluating long-term care tend to focus on what regulating or accrediting bodies require.	Though not well developed, outcomes-oriented research focuses on the impact of long-term care arrangements on patient functioning and quality of life.
Persons living with HIV/AIDS	"Caring," not "curing," is the major focus of much HIV/AIDS–related care.	The desired clinical outcomes of care for persons with HIV/AIDS are ill defined.
Mentally ill and disabled	Because of the array of providers and facilities involved in providing mental health care, there is considerable variability in the standards and norms of practice in this area.	Standards and guidelines development in the mental health area has not adequately related program or therapeutic practices to hypothesized or desired outcomes.

Alcohol or substance abusers	Quality assurance and assessment procedures in the alcohol and substance abuse area are nonexistent, implicit, or limited in application.	As with the mental health care area, the nature of the alcohol and substance abuse treatment system exacerbates problems in clearly defining desired outcomes and how best to achieve them.
Suicide or homicide prone	There is no widely shared consensus regarding how best to prevent or treat intentional violence, primarily because of the lack of an integrated theoretical base regarding its causes.	Individually oriented interventions may have little overall effect on community suicide or homicide rates.
Abusing families	Medical, social service, and related personnel may be inadequately trained to detect and intervene in cases of family abuse.	A multitude of outcomes may be the focus of interventions in the area of family abuse: increased knowledge of situations that might prompt it, behavioral evidence of change, reduction in reported prevalence, or increase in underreports of abuse.
Homeless persons	The problem of establishing quality-of-care norms for the homeless is exacerbated by their overall lack of basic support, as well as medical care, services.	The precise outcome objectives for programs to serve the homeless must be specified in evaluating the extent to which they effectively deal with the origins and consequences of the problem.
Immigrants and refugees	The effectiveness of care obtained by immigrants and refugees is greatly affected by its accessibility, adequacy, and acceptability to these populations.	Knowledge of social and cultural factors in caring for foreign-born populations will enhance the prospect of better compliance and outcomes.

and may in fact be less likely to result in cesarean deliveries for women with comparable risk profiles (Baruffi, Strobino, & Paine, 1990; Rooks et al., 1989).

Increasing emphasis is being placed on evidence-based practice and the development of guidelines for practice, based on reviews of existing research. The Low Birthweight Patient Outcomes Research Team, funded by the Agency for Healthcare Research and Quality, as well as systematic reviews of research on the effectiveness of pregnancy-related services by the Cochrane Collaboration, represent substantial and important efforts to develop guidelines for the prevention and treatment of poor pregnancy outcomes (Agency for Healthcare Research and Quality, 1998; Enkin, Keirse, Renfrew, & Neilson, 1995).

Outcomes. Research on the effectiveness of prenatal care examines (1) observational studies based on birth and death records, from either vital statistics or clinical databases, (2) evaluations of programs offering enriched or augmented prenatal care services, and (3) comparisons of outcomes in alternative provider or payer arrangements.

The observational studies as a whole have found a positive relationship between the use of prenatal care and birth outcomes. The magnitude of the association varies, however, due to differences in the care and outcome variables used in each study. Specific programs that have been evaluated with respect to their impact on birth outcomes include federally sponsored initiatives, such as Maternity and Infant Care Projects, the Improved Pregnancy Outcome Projects, and the Special Supplemental Food Program for Women, Infants and Children, as well as private foundation–supported efforts, such as the Robert Wood Johnson Foundation Perinatal and Rural Infant Care Programs, among others. The findings from evaluations of specific programs are less consistent, one reason undoubtedly being that the programs themselves represent varying types of prenatal and associated perinatal interventions (Office of Technology Assessment, 1988).

The implicit assumption that more technology at birth necessarily means better care is being challenged. Shy, Luthy, Bennett, and Whitfield (1990) found that the use of electronic fetal monitoring was associated with a threefold greater risk of cerebral palsy compared to the conventional practice of a nurse's using a stethoscope to check the unborn infant's heart rate during delivery. Sophisticated NICU technology can also precipitate iatrogenic (care-induced) conditions, such as bronchopulmonary dysplasia (a chronic lung disease in newborns) resulting from prolonged exposure to mechanical ventilation and retinopathy of prematurity (which causes abnormal growth of blood vessels into the retina and nerve tissue in the back of the eye, often leading to blindness) associated with administering high concentrations of oxygen to premature newborns. The very tiniest newborns (those less than 750 grams, or 1.6 pounds) are least likely to survive neonatal intensive care and most likely to have long-term disabilities when they do (Office of Technology Assessment, 1987b). Rosenblatt (1989) has pointed out the perinatal paradox in the United States of ensuring high-cost neonatal intensive care to high-risk infants and their mothers but not to ensuring access to lower-cost, and more effective, prenatal care services.

With the expanded enrollment of individuals with either public or private coverage in managed care, there is a corresponding interest in the varying impacts of alternative payer and provider arrangements on outcomes. Evaluations of Medicaid managed care compared to fee-for-service arrangements have in general yielded mixed results, in some cases demonstrating improved outcomes and in others no difference, or somewhat poorer outcomes, especially for selected high-risk women (for example, those with gestational diabetes). Pregnancy outcomes in general remain poor for low-income women and those on Medicaid, compared to their higher-income and privately insured counterparts (Bienstock et al., 1997; Klinkman, Gorenflo, & Ritsema, 1997; Oleske, Branca, Schmidt, Ferguson, & Linn, 1998; Ray, Gigante, Mitchel, & Hickson, 1998). Since 1995 a majority of states and the federal government have passed laws requiring insurers to cover a minimum period of hospitalization for mothers and newborns following delivery, in response to increasingly limited lengths of stays mandated by managed care providers. The cost and effectiveness implications of these shortened lengths of stays, as well as the laws to address them, have not been fully examined (Raube & Merrell, 1999).

Chronically Ill and Disabled

The nature of long-term care (LTC) differs from acute care along a number of dimensions that create special difficulties in developing criteria of effectiveness: LTC has a longer time horizon and represents a series of interrelated rather than discrete events of care; the goals of care (maintenance versus enhanced functioning versus rehabilitation) are not well defined; LTC largely comprises low-technology services provided by lay caregivers or paraprofessionals rather than highly technical care provided by skilled professionals; and because of the likely transitions among a variety of providers, the effectiveness of care for LTC consumers lies outside the control of any one provider (Kane & Kane, 1988).

Structure and Process. Protocols and criteria for evaluating the effectiveness of long-term care for the chronically ill and disabled are not well articulated. Efforts to assess the effectiveness of LTC have focused most often on nursing homes and more recently on home health care providers and board and care homes. As with assessment activities in the acute care area, most efforts have focused on structure and process measures of effectiveness.

The principal quality assurance activities for nursing homes are regulation-oriented approaches, such as licensure by the states, focusing principally on safety and fire codes; certification as skilled nursing or intermediate-care facilities to meet Medicare and Medicaid program standards; annual inspections to ensure that all care reimbursed by Medicaid and Medicare is medically necessary and of acceptable quality; ombudsman programs, required by the Older Americans Act, that act as nursing home patient advocates; and the training, licensure, and regulation of personnel, such as nursing home administrators. The Omnibus Budget Reconciliation Act of 1987 mandated the development of a minimum basic data set for planning to improve the quality of care in nursing homes. The Resident Assessment Instrument can, for example, be used as a tool to build a minimum database and set of indicators of the quality of care provided in nursing homes (American Association of Retired Persons, 1991; Kane & Kane, 1988; Phillips, Zimmerman, Bernabei, & Jonsson, 1997).

Standards for evaluating the structure and process indicators of effectiveness for other major categories of long-term care, such as home care, case management, and board and care homes, are even less well developed than those for nursing homes. Studies have documented considerable variability in the training and experience of employees of home health agencies providing high-risk infusion therapies, for example, and a range of quality problems in board and care homes, including physical abuse, unsanitary conditions, and the lack of medical attention to meet residents' needs (General Accounting Office, 1989a).

Outcomes. There is an increasing interest in specifying and measuring outcome indicators of effectiveness for LTC. An outcomes approach to assessing nursing home effectiveness would focus on actual, relative to possible, improvements in patients' status, given their level of functioning, such as enhanced personal satisfaction, participation in enjoyable activities, improved mobility, and rates of discharge home. In this context, structure and process measures of effectiveness (such as inadequate medical supervision of patients' health status; low levels of training and high turnover among the principal immediate caregivers, nurses' aides; the overuse of medications, especially psychoactive drugs; and lack of stimulating social or recreational activities) become relevant as points of intervention to produce improvements in patient outcomes (Kane, 1990; Kane & Kane, 1988).

Outcomes research on the effectiveness of home care and other community-based services has principally been undertaken in the context of evaluating the cost-effectiveness of these programs. There is a need to develop more formal, conceptual frameworks for understanding the correlates and outcomes of home care, as well as more explicit outcome and process measures of the effectiveness of care being provided to people at home (Kramer, Shaughnessy, Bauman, & Crisler, 1990). The Outcome-Based Quality Improvement for measuring outcomes across a continuum of home care and the Outcomes and Assessment Information Set functional status assessment tool mandated by Medicare represent useful approaches for assessing outcomes for home care patients (Neal, 1998; Shaughnessy, Crisler, Schlenker, & Arnold, 1997).

Evidence from the Medical Outcomes Study has suggested that elderly and poor chronically ill patients have poorer outcomes in health maintenance organizations than in fee-for-service systems (Ware, Bayliss, Rogers, Kosinski, &

Tarlov, 1996). The National Committee for Quality Assurance, a joint organization of health plans and purchasers, has developed the Health Plan Employer Data and Information Set, a set of indicators for monitoring and enhancing the effectiveness and appropriateness of care. Expansions of the core set of indicators have been recommended to assess better the care of chronically ill adults and children and, in particular, the relationship between the process and outcomes of care (Kuhlthau et al., 1998; McGlynn, 1996). The development of a broader continuum of care for the chronically ill, disabled children, and the elderly argues for the conceptualization and implementation of a population-based, multilevel systems approach for assessing the structure, process, and outcomes of medical and nonmedical programs and services required to address the needs of this population (DuPlessis, Inkelas, & Halfon, 1998).

Persons Living with HIV/AIDS

Persons living with HIV/AIDS require long-term care entailing a complex array of social and medical services, and caring, not curing, is the major focus of the caregiving process itself (Benjamin, 1989). A comprehensive, coordinated continuum of care is available only in fragments for persons with AIDS in many U.S. communities. The traditional problems of measuring structure, process, and outcome indicators of effectiveness are then made worse when the structures are ad hoc, the norms for the process of care are evolving, and the desired outcomes of the caregiving process are ill defined.

Structure and Process. Because of the difficulty of specifying and standardizing the desired outcomes of HIV/AIDS, care assessment has focused primarily on the structure and process rather than the outcomes of care and in particular on clinical criteria for determining "necessary and appropriate" care for such patients (Bozzette & Asch, 1995).

Higher survival rates and better outcomes have been found in hospitals and clinics that have more experience in caring for persons living with HIV/AIDS (Bennett, 1990; Kanouse, Mathews, & Bennett, 1989; Laine et al., 1998; Sandrick, 1993). Basic HIV preventive and primary care may not be adequately performed by many primary care physicians. Although knowledge of care guidelines and proficiency in providing care for persons who have HIV/AIDS according to these guidelines tend to be higher on the part of physicians who have more experience, this expertise does not necessarily translate into more appropriate screening and counseling of patients who may be at higher risk of contracting the disease. More extensive multidisciplinary efforts to educate primary care providers regarding guidelines for the prevention of HIV and the care of persons living with HIV/AIDS are needed (Curtis, Paauw, Wenrich, Carline, & Ramsey, 1995; Heath et al., 1997; Macher et al., 1994).

Studies examining the success of various public health interventions in increasing levels of knowledge and reducing the behavioral risks associated with

HIV/AIDS have provided evidence of success (Hardy, 1990; Moran, Janes, Peterman, & Stone, 1990). Evaluations of interventions to reduce high-risk behaviors among groups most at risk (such as homosexual and bisexual men and intravenous drug users) have demonstrated either increased awareness of risks or reductions or modifications of high-risk behaviors in general, though not necessarily for particularly at-risk demographic subgroups, such as adolescents, young heterosexual adults, those with less education, and minorities (Becker & Joseph, 1988; Dengelegi, Weber, & Torquato, 1990; Solomon & DeJong, 1989; Stephens, Feucht, & Roman, 1991).

Outcomes. Outcome assessments of AIDS patient care have focused on the efficacy and effectiveness of particular therapies, such as zidovudine and azidothymidine or routine immunizations of persons with AIDS.

Good access to HIV/AIDS services has been found to be associated with a higher quality of life and levels of satisfaction on the part of persons living with HIV/AIDS. Enhanced prenatal care services for high-risk pregnant women can lead to improved outcomes. Comprehensive, coordinated care by a multidisciplinary team of care providers offers a particularly cost-effective model of care for persons living with HIV/AIDS (Cunningham et al., 1998; Lê, Winter, Boyd, Ackerson, & Hurley, 1998; Newschaffer, Cocroft, Hauck, Fanning, & Turner, 1998; Stein, Fleishman, Mor, & Dresser, 1993).

The Agency for Healthcare Research and Quality has addressed HIV/AIDS-related effectiveness of care issues through its AIDS Medical Care Effectiveness Program and associated clinical guidelines development activities. Three major clinical issues need to be considered in developing a research agenda to evaluate the effectiveness of care of persons with AIDS (Agency for Healthcare Research and Quality, 1990b; Kanouse, Mathews, & Bennett, 1989):

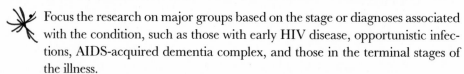 Focus the research on major groups based on the stage or diagnoses associated with the condition, such as those with early HIV disease, opportunistic infections, AIDS-acquired dementia complex, and those in the terminal stages of the illness.

- Conduct research on a range of alternative therapies to establish their effectiveness.
- Encompass both inpatient and outpatient components of care in the process.

Mentally Ill and Disabled

Quality assessment activities in the mental health care sector have been fragmented and reactive. The development of standards or quality review procedures has often been in response to external demands for accountability from insurers, program funders, or institutional accrediting bodies, such as Professional Standards Review Organizations, the Joint Commission on the Accreditation of

Healthcare Organizations, or state funding agencies. Standard setting has tended to emphasize structure and process indicators, while the linkage of these factors to outcomes remains poorly documented.

Structure and Process. Effectiveness issues relating to the structure of mental health services focus on the characteristics of the providers and facilities from which services are received. An array of providers with widely varying educational and licensure credentials deliver mental health care services, including M.D.-trained psychiatrists, master's- and Ph.D.-level psychologists, M.S.W.-level social workers, psychiatric nurses, as well as bachelor's-level counselors and therapists, or associate degree–level certified alcohol and drug abuse counselors, among others.

A great deal of mental health care is rendered by primary care physicians in general medical care settings. Controversy exists regarding the adequacy of training and the quality of care delivered by this array of mental health care providers. Furthermore, no well-developed, uniform standards exist for what types of services should be in place within particular mental health care delivery sites (psychiatric hospitals, residential treatment centers, outpatient treatment settings, and so on) to ensure high-quality care in those discrete facilities, much less in relationship to a comprehensive, integrated continuum of care for the mentally ill (Glied, 1998; Parikh, Lin, & Lesage, 1997).

The Joint Commission on the Accreditation of Healthcare Organizations, the National Committee for Quality Assurance, the Institute of Behavioral Healthcare, and the American Managed Behavioral Healthcare Association, among others, have developed quality indicators and measurement systems for the behavioral health care industry (Bickman & Salzer, 1997). The quality assessment systems for mental health care services have, however, been criticized as being dominated by a medical rather than a systems-oriented model, which, it is argued, fails to consider the family and community contexts and programs needed to meet the needs of the mentally ill most effectively (Kurland, 1995; U.S. Department of Health and Human Services, 1999). Substantial unmet needs for mental health care services and quality problems have been documented in nursing homes and correctional facilities in particular (Burns et al., 1993; Elliott, 1997).

Outcomes. Based on a comprehensive meta-analysis of more than three hundred studies, Lipsey and Wilson (1993) concluded that the efficacy of well-developed psychological, educational, and behavioral treatments for mental illness has been well established. According to Lyons, Howard, O'Mahoney, and Lish (1997, p. 1), it is the effectiveness of mental health services that is now of concern: specifically the questions of "what services work for whom, under what conditions, when should they be offered, and by which providers?" As with general medical care delivery, structure and process standards development activities have not adequately linked program guidelines to patient outcomes. Additional research is needed on the effectiveness of the care delivered in specific delivery settings (Edmunds et al., 1997).

Research findings on the effectiveness of behavioral managed care are mixed. A study of a Medicaid managed care demonstration in Minnesota found no difference in outcomes between managed care and fee-for-service enrollees. On the other hand, the Medical Outcomes Study found that although there were no differences in mental health outcomes for nonpsychiatric patients, among those with major depression seen by psychiatrists, the outcomes were poorer for those in health maintenance organizations (Christianson & Osher, 1994; Colenda, Banazak, & Mickus, 1998; Dana, Conner, & Allen, 1996; Mechanic, 1996c; Wells, Keeler, & Manning, 1990; Wells, Manning, & Valdez, 1989). Reductions in mental health care services as a function of caps on covered services or utilization review have been found to be associated with higher rates of hospital readmissions and increased costs for selected conditions (Popkin et al., 1998; Soumerai, McLaughlin, Ross-Degnan, Casteris, & Bollini, 1994; Wickizer & Lessler, 1998).

Psychopharmacological treatment of mental disorders has been one of the major developments supportive of the deinstitutionalization of the mentally ill. Individual variations in compliance, absorption, metabolism, side effects, and the interpersonal aspects of medication management can, however, greatly influence the overall effectiveness of these regimens.

Clinicians, clients, and families may tend to focus on somewhat different aspects of mental health, that is, the disease process, illness experience, or caregiving burden, respectively. Emerging systems for assessing the outcomes of mental health care services have attempted to encompass patients' and families' perceptions into assessments of the quality of and overall satisfaction with mental health care services (Björkman, Hansson, Svensson, & Berglund, 1995; Dickey & Wagenaar, 1994; Gardner, Nudler, & Chapman, 1997; Hermann, Ettner, & Dorwart, 1998).

As with outcomes and effectiveness research on medical care in general, improved specification is needed of the desired outcomes themselves, the precise treatment or program elements expected to affect these outcomes, and the costs of the therapies or interventions relative to any benefits achieved (Aday et al., 1999; Hargreaves & Shumway, 1989; Wells & Brook, 1989).

Alcohol or Substance Abusers

The fragmentation of treatment for substance abuse disorders across a variety of clients, settings, providers, and modalities exacerbates and compounds the problems in setting uniform and systematic standards for structural, process, and outcome indicators of effectiveness. To reflect the state of the art of substance abuse treatment better, an Institute of Medicine report on the treatment of alcohol problems suggested that the question, "Does treatment work?" should actually be rephrased as, "Which kinds of individuals, with what kinds of . . . problems, are likely to respond to what kinds of treatments by achieving what kinds of goals when delivered by what types of practitioners?" (Institute of Medicine, 1990, p. 143).

Structure and Process. A major problem in setting uniform and systematic standards within this field is the fact that there is a diverse array of practitioners providing services, with widely varying professional norms and expectations regarding the appropriate focus and outcomes of care. Alcohol and drug abuse counselors are, for example, important components of treatment in many settings. In some programs (particularly methadone maintenance or residential therapeutic community treatment programs), former or recovering addicts or alcoholics serve as the principal caregivers or counselors. In other instances (such as private chemical dependency programs), master's-level or Ph.D.-trained therapists or medical doctors may be the principal providers or overseers of care. Furthermore, for many individuals in recovery, volunteer self-help programs employing the twelve-step philosophy (such as Alcoholics Anonymous or Narcotics Anonymous) or those sponsored by community service agencies (such as the Salvation Army)—each of which has its own unique treatment or rehabilitation philosophy—may be important components of the aftercare process. The National Institute on Drug Abuse Collaborative Cocaine Treatment (Project Match) Study documented that well-trained and experienced drug counselors employing twelve-step recovery principles and focusing directly on stopping drug use can be successful in reducing cocaine use among drug-dependent clients (Crits-Christoph et al., 1999).

Process factors that have been identified in contributing to successful chemical dependency programs include providing timely and convenient access to services; flexible treatment interventions that match the treatment to salient client variables; inviting collateral involvement from family members, employers, or other informal client support systems; having caring and knowledgeable therapists, as well as motivated clients, who are held accountable for their sobriety; and following up with dropouts and graduates (Waltman, 1995). The length of time in treatment and frequent counseling have also been found to be positively associated with higher long-term abstinence rates (Ershoff, Radcliffe, & Gregory, 1996; Fiorentine & Anglin, 1997; Hser, Joshi, Anglin, & Fletcher, 1999; Simpson, Joe, Fletcher, Hubbard, & Anglin, 1999).

To the extent that certain institutions, agencies, or professionals engaged in substance abuse treatment seek to obtain licensing, accreditation, or third-party reimbursement from relevant public or private agencies, they are likely to undertake efforts to conform to those groups' standards. Interest in and compliance with such standards are, however, variable across types of providers and settings (Gerstein & Harwood, 1990; Institute of Medicine, 1990).

There is an increasing emphasis on linking the structure and process of treatment to outcomes and in developing more standardized systems of accountability for provider performance. The Center for Substance Abuse Treatment within the Substance Abuse and Mental Health Services Administration has convened a number of consensus panels to develop and disseminate treatment improvement protocols—best practices guidelines for the treatment of different substance abuse disorders. The Office of National Drug Control Policy, the Center for Substance Abuse Treatment, and the National Association of Alcohol and Drug Abuse Directors, among others, have developed related effectiveness indicators and measurement systems for substance abuse treatment programs. These systems and related performance report cards are intended to permit comparisons of performance, relative to accepted indicators and standards, across managed care plans and other provider groups (Gustafson & Darby, 1999).

Outcomes. A particularly problematic issue in outcomes-oriented assessments of substance abuse services is that the desired outcomes are not well defined. Alternative outcomes include primary aims, such as reducing or eliminating the actual intake of the substance or diminishing the prospect of death or disability or associated social costs such as substance abuse-related crime or motor vehicle deaths, as well as secondary aims, such as improving individual or family social functioning, locating employment, or attaining educational or job-related skills. Neither the priorities nor the means for achieving them are well defined. Furthermore, clients with the most difficulties in all of these areas of functioning are most likely to be served by programs in the public or voluntary service sector, which tend to have the smallest per capita levels of investment (Gerstein & Harwood, 1990; Institute of Medicine, 1990).

A National Academy of Sciences Panel on Performance Measures and Data for Public Health Performance Partnership Grants has formulated a framework for identifying and gathering data around relevant and related performance indicators for public health substance abuse and mental health programs. These indicators include: (1) health status outcomes related to changes in physical or mental status, social functioning, and consumer satisfaction; (2) intermediate outcomes related to changes in risk status; (3) process measures regarding what to do to, for, with, or by defined individuals or groups as a part of the delivery of services; and (4) capacity, reflected in the ability to provide specific services, such as clinical screening and disease surveillance. Much more work needs to be done in developing indicators for specific substance abuse program goals and identifying relevant data sources for operationalizing these measures (Perrin & Koshel, 1997).

Suicide or Homicide Prone

No well-developed or widely shared standards regarding appropriate and effective prevention- and treatment-oriented interventions regarding suicide and homicide are available, principally because of the purported multifactorial etiology of these problems and the corollary lack of integrated, multidisciplinary, theory-based research and evaluations of program effectiveness to guide the development of such standards.

Structure and Process. The principal implicit structural considerations of effectiveness in the areas of suicide and homicide prevention and treatment concern the competency of gatekeepers and other personnel who might be in a position of identifying or treating at-risk individuals, the availability of case finding or outreach programs for particularly high-risk subgroups (such as the isolated or institutionalized elderly or teenage school dropouts), and the adequacy and accessibility of treatment programs and services for the perpetrators, as well as survivors, of acts of intentional personal or interpersonal injury (such as suicidal attempters and their families or individuals incarcerated for assaultive violence).

The prevention of violent behavior may lie in deeper changes in the social structure to address the differential social status and associated investments in social and human capital available to individuals and communities most vulnerable to such violence (Gurr, 1989).

Outcomes. There are major interventions available to prevent youth suicide (Eddy, Wolpert, & Rosenberg, 1989):

- Affective education, to help young people understand and cope with problems that lead to suicide
- Early identification and treatment of those most at risk
- School-based screening programs
- Crisis centers and hot lines
- Improved training of professionals
- Restriction of access to the three main methods of suicide (firearms, medications, and high places)

There are no conclusive studies demonstrating that one type of treatment—psychotherapeutic, behavioral, or psychopharmacologic—is clearly superior in treating adolescent suicide attempters (Trautman, 1989). Interventions that limit the availability of options to harm oneself (such as the regulation of handguns or prescription medications) may be more effective than those that rely primarily on individuals' deciding to change their behavior (education or counseling) (Starfield, 1989).

The major types of interventions to prevent or diminish the inal careers and associated crimes of violence are strategies to p ticipation in such activities, strategies to modify the criminal c and collective or selective incapacitation (incarceration) of fenders. More well-designed demonstrations and evaluati sess the effectiveness of these alternatives. Research has

childhood intervention and enrichment programs such as Head Start and programs to train parents and teachers in methods of communicating with and supervising children to modify antisocial behaviors resulted in lower rates of subsequent criminal activity (RAND, Institute for Civil Justice, 1999).

Attempts to modify criminal careers through behavioral modification approaches have met with some success with small samples of delinquents followed for short periods of time. Indirect approaches to career modification through intensive drug abuse surveillance and treatment appear to be most successful in reducing the frequency of serious offenses by criminals addicted to hard drugs (Blumstein, Cohen, Roth, & Visher, 1986a). Programs to upgrade employment skills have been documented to be successful in modifying offenders' careers in the United Kingdom.

Incapacitation (or incarceration) principally attempts to reduce crime by removing offenders from the community. Collective incapacitation seeks to lengthen the period of incarceration for groups of offenders (those who committed violent crimes, for example), while selective incarceration focuses on individuals who are deemed to be at most risk of being continued offenders. Considerable ethical controversy surrounds the use of selective incapacitation, principally related to imposing a punishment on an individual before a crime is committed and the fact that certain individuals or subgroups (such as racial and ethnic minorities) are more likely to be targeted for lengthened periods of imprisonment using this approach.

In either case, the impact of these methods is likely to be small relative to the number of individuals who would need to be imprisoned to offset criminal activity in the community. Furthermore, these methods do not address the fundamental issue of whether "replacements" may continue to be produced for those who are removed from circulation, since the underlying sources of the problem remain unaddressed (Blumstein, Cohen, Roth, & Visher, 1986a).

Abusing Families

As with a number of other categories of vulnerable populations just reviewed, the standards of appropriate and efficacious care for victims of intimate abuse are not well developed.

Structure and Process. Structural considerations of effectiveness focus on the training and availability of personnel to treat victims of abuse. Some child protective services caseworkers, for example, have caseloads of thirty to fifty (or even more) families, although many experts believe that caseworkers can effectively serve no more than twenty such cases. In some states, child protective services workers have fewer than forty hours of training, and a number of states do not require that they hold a professional degree (Gelles & Cornell, 1990).

The development of standards and educational interventions to teach general parenting and child-rearing skills may be effective means of preventing child abuse and neglect, particularly among young parents (Browne, Davies, & Stratton, 1988; Knudsen, 1988).

The medical model of training tends to reinforce a detached stance that inhibits physicians' asking questions to determine whether injuries to patients whom they see in their practice result from abuse (Randall, 1990). The Joint Commission on the Accreditation of Healthcare Organizations and the American Medical Association Council on Scientific Affairs, among others, have developed and promulgated protocols for identifying, treating, and properly referring victims of abuse and neglect. These standards remain poorly implemented in practice, primarily due to failing to incorporate requisite training regarding these protocols in undergraduate, graduate, and continuing medical education training programs (Abbott, 1997; Cohen, De Vos, & Newberger, 1997; Conti, 1998; Feldhaus et al., 1997; Hayden, Barton, & Hayden, 1997; Reiniger, Robison, & McHugh, 1995; Tilden et al., 1994; Wright, Wright, & Isaac, 1997). Research examining the impact of programs to improve the identification of and management of domestic violence by primary care and emergency room physicians has, however, documented increased case finding and documentation of domestic violence on the part of providers (Public Health Service, 1990; Thompson, 1998).

Outcomes. The results of the Minneapolis Police Experiment (MPE), published in the mid-1980s, documented lower recidivism rates in which mandatory (presumptive) arrest was used when abuse was suspected, compared to other approaches to dealing with domestic disturbances (separation and advice and mediation). Major problems existed with the internal and external validity of the MPE study design, however, and a replication of the experiment in Omaha yielded more mixed results (Gelles & Cornell, 1990).

As with these studies, attempts to assess the desired outcomes of prevention and treatment programs in the family abuse area are plagued with a number of methodological difficulties. A major problem concerns the lack of a clear specification of the desired outcome of a given intervention. Is it an increased knowledge on the part of the family regarding identifying events or actions that might precipitate violence and the means for dealing with them, behavioral evidence regarding changes in the family members' patterns of interaction, a reduction in the reported prevalence of abuse, or an increase in the reported rates of abuse that were previously unreported?

Other major methodological problems in documenting the best means to improve the outcomes for this population include the lack of well-developed theories for guiding the design of experimental interventions, the absence of randomized designs, and the lack of replicative evidence of program success across a variety of communities or population groups (Chalk & King, 1998; Dubowitz, 1990).

Homeless Persons

The problem of establishing quality-of-care norms for homeless persons is exacerbated by the fact that most have inadequate access to care of any kind, and even when they do get care, it may be virtually impossible for them to carry through with recommended treatment or follow-up regimens given the circumstances of their lives on the street. Major publicly and privately supported projects concerned with the delivery of health care services for the homeless population (Robert Wood Johnson Foundation Health Care for the Homeless, Health Resources and Services Administration Health Care for the Homeless, Veterans Administration Homeless Chronically Mentally Ill [VA-HCMI], and Veterans Affairs–Health Care for Homeless Veterans [VA-HCHV], among others) have attempted to tailor programs to take into account the unique needs and circumstances of homeless persons.

Structure and Process. One focus of improving the effectiveness of care to homeless persons is more appropriate training for the personnel who care for them: public and community health nurses; family physicians, pediatricians, and other physicians who see homeless persons in their practices; hospital emergency room or outpatient service providers; and the important cadre of health professional volunteers who provide care to homeless persons in shelters, free clinics, and other places where homeless persons gather (Berne, Dato, Mason, & Rafferty, 1990; Weinreb & Bassuk, 1990). Case managers are an important component of the major health and mental health care programs serving the homeless population. The roles and qualifications of these case managers are, however, neither clearly nor uniformly defined (Institute of Medicine, 1988c; Stephens, Dennis, Toomer, & Holloway, 1991).

Data gleaned from the Robert Wood Johnson Foundation Health Care for the Homeless program and other studies provide an informational base for designing better targeted and more effective interventions for addressing the unique and multifaceted needs of homeless persons. In particular, the integration of mental health, substance abuse, dental, optometry, and podiatry services with primary care is useful in addressing the multifaceted health needs of homeless persons (Brickner, Scharer, Conanan, & Scanlan, 1990; Wright & Weber, 1987). Quality assurance activities for programs serving homeless persons must take into account that different processes or procedures (additional follow-up activities) may be required to obtain desired standards (child immunization levels) that might be achieved with less effort in other types of practice (Altamore, Mitchell, & Weber, 1990).

Programs that incorporate outreach and case management components appear to have been successful in getting many homeless persons in for needed services. These are intensive and expensive services that are still largely unavailable to homeless persons in most U.S. cities and localities, however. Adequate discharge planning and the availability of residential treatment options are significant gaps in addressing the long-term needs of multiproblem homeless individuals (Drake, Wallach, & Hoffman, 1989; Institute of Medicine, 1988c). An evaluation of the VA-HCMI program showed that veterans who completed a prescribed length of stay in residential treatment postdischarge had the best long-term mental and physical outcomes compared to those who dropped out or left the program early (Rosenheck, Gallup, Leda, Gorchov, & Errera, 1990).

Outcomes. As with other categories of vulnerable populations, the desired outcomes of treating homeless persons are not well specified in a policy or program sense. Perhaps the best and most desirable outcome is for no one to be homeless in the first place.

Immigrants and Refugees

The effectiveness of care that immigrants and refugees obtain is greatly affected by its accessibility, adequacy, and acceptability—that is, what type of care they are able to get, whether it is enough as well as appropriate for their needs, and whether they are able or willing to follow the plan recommended for treating their complaint.

Structure and Process. The financial and institutional barriers that inhibit immigrant and refugee populations' seeking care were discussed in Chapter Seven. The lack of bilingual providers or translators can influence whether people feel comfortable going to a particular facility, as well as the effectiveness of the care they receive there. Sometimes impromptu interpreters, such as janitors or orderlies, are called on to translate, which may result in inaccurate information being conveyed, as well as reluctance on the part of the patient to be forthcoming. Providers who do not clearly understand the symptoms or complaints being presented by patients are more likely to diagnose the problem inaccurately or prescribe inappropriate therapies. Similarly, patients may not fully understand the diagnosis and the instructions they are subsequently given to treat the problem (Downs, Bernstein, & Marchese, 1997; Rumbaut, Chavez, Moser, Pickwell, & Wishik, 1988).

The delivery of high-quality medical care to immigrant and refugee populations is also inhibited by providers' limited knowledge of how to treat their special health problems and needs and patients' limited knowledge of public health or health promotion practices. Health care workers who are not aware of the higher prevalence of genetic-related disorders, such as Cooley's anemia, lactose intolerance, or other problems among ethnic or racial subgroups, are less likely to screen for them and more likely to misdiagnose or misprescribe as a result. Providers may also be unfamiliar with how to diagnosis or treat diseases that are common in certain foreign-born populations but relatively rare in general U.S. medical practice, such as parasitic infestations or congenital malaria. The special anatomical and physiological characteristics (lighter body weight or eye conformation) of certain ethnic subgroups (such as Asians) may require adaptations of medications or surgical procedures (dosages or lens implantation in cataract surgery), which providers should take into account in treating these patients (Lin-Fu, 1988).

Cultural beliefs and practices affect immigrant and refugee populations' willingness to seek and comply with Western medical practices. Mexican immigrants, particularly those residing along the border, can easily buy and self-administer antibiotics and other medications without prescriptions from Mexican pharmacies or may use folk healers (*curanderos*) who understand the folk illnesses and diagnoses common in Mexico. Many Hmong and Khmer refugees adhere to traditional healing methods, especially those practiced by shamans (the Hmong *txi neng*, the Khmer *krou*). The traditional home healing practice used in Southeast Asia called *kos khyal* ("coining" or applying warm coins) can create burns or bruises on a child's stomach, back, arms and legs that look similar to those inflicted by intentional abuse. Toxic lead and arsenic are components of some Chinese folk remedies. The prevalence of smoking has been found to be high and the level of knowledge of the risk factors associated with cancer and heart disease low among Southeast Asian refugee and immigrant groups.

Religious and cultural beliefs and attitudes toward the unborn child, women's roles, and the role of family members in making decisions come into play as well in different groups' willingness to accept and adhere to Western medical practices. Many refugees suffer from serious mental health problems that require a culturally sensitive process of diagnosis and treatment (Chen, Kuun, Guthrie, Li, & Zaharlick, 1991; Jenkins, McPhee, Bird, & Bonilla, 1990; Lee, 1988; Lin-Fu, 1988; Loue, 1998; Rumbaut, Chavez, Moser, Pickwell, & Wishik, 1988).

Outcomes. Knowledge of the social and cultural factors that play an important role in the life of foreign-born populations can facilitate the development of a more acceptable, adequate, and effective care plan from both the provider's and patient's points of view.

Conclusion

This chapter has documented essentially three areas of assessment, focusing on the structural, process, and outcome indicators of effectiveness. The questions posed have moved from a consideration of what is in place and what is done, to the outcomes for those who are the recipients of service, and what contributes to these outcomes and why. The development of measures and designs, as well as the very definitions of the questions to pose in the area of evaluating outcomes for assessing the effectiveness of care in general and for vulnerable populations in particular, are nonetheless in their infancy in many ways. The next chapter reviews these and other research questions that need to be addressed to understand and address the health and health care needs of vulnerable populations.

CHAPTER TEN

WHAT DO WE STILL NEED TO KNOW?

As with the system of providing and paying for services for the vulnerable, the conduct of related research is often categorical, fragmented, and not linked to other relevant bodies of research. Moreover, it fails to identify the issues that cut across different professional or service delivery domains. For example, policymakers, providers, and researchers concerned with the chronically ill elderly or chronically ill children or the mentally ill or persons living with HIV/AIDS or homeless persons, respectively, may be interested in the utility of case management for improving the delivery of services to the population group of most concern to them, but have little or no knowledge of the experiences in implementing particular case management models with other populations.

Three major types of research needs and priorities can be identified:

- Descriptive research, which focuses on the methods and measures for identifying who are the vulnerable, how many there are, and who is most likely to be vulnerable
- Analytic research, directed more toward understanding why some groups are more vulnerable than others, and the program or policy alternatives that are therefore most relevant for preventing vulnerability or caring for those who are already in need
- Evaluative research, concerned with assessing how well the programs and services that have been developed and implemented, based on previous descriptive and analytic research, have done in addressing or mitigating the needs of the groups they were most intended to serve

Examples of descriptive, analytic, and evaluative research needed to identify, understand, and address the health and health care needs of vulnerable populations are highlighted in the summary of cross-cutting issues and discussion of each group that follows.

Cross-Cutting Issues

The review confirmed that further research is needed to characterize more clearly who the vulnerable are, understand the origins of their vulnerability, and evaluate which programs are most likely to be successful in either meeting or ameliorating their needs. Following is a summary of major cross-cutting research difficulties.

Descriptive Research

- Ambiguity in the definitions of the population
- Variability in the quality or completeness of information available on the population across data sources
- Changes in the definitions of the population or the availability of information on it over time
- Lack of demographic identifiers or detail (on race and ethnicity, for example) for the comparison of subgroups within the population

Analytic Research

- Lack of well-developed, integrated, multidisciplinary theoretical perspectives and associated empirical research on the origins of the problem
- Paucity of longitudinal research—within the life span of individuals or in the aggregate—on the origins, incidence, and consequences of the problem
- Paucity of comparative data—on rare or hard-to-locate at-risk subpopulations or cross-nationally—on the origins, prevalence, and consequences of the problem

Evaluative Research

- Lack of well-articulated program and policy goals
- Lack of formal state-of-the-art review and assessment of existing research on program performance
- Lack of clearly articulated short-term and long-term research agendas for assessing probable program performance
- Lack of well-designed small-scale and large-scale demonstration projects for evaluating program performance
- Need to build the capacity and knowledge base through training researchers, replicating studies, and disseminating current research on program performance

- Need to develop comprehensive, coordinated interagency-oriented research agendas to address cross-cutting programmatic needs for vulnerable populations

Descriptive Research

A fundamental problem in identifying who and how many are vulnerable is ambiguity in the definitions of the vulnerable populations themselves. High-risk mothers and infants have been variously identified using predictors and indicators of both morbidity and mortality (such as rates of teen births, low or very low birthweight infants, and maternal and infant deaths). The chronically ill and disabled have been defined based on diagnoses, disability, and functional status, as well as quality-of-life measures. The case definition of HIV/AIDS has been revised three times since it was first published in 1982. At least four generations of studies in the mental health field can be identified, all of which used different approaches or different instruments for defining cases of mental illness.

The measurement of alcohol or substance abuse is made more difficult by the fact that there are different stages in the development of the addictive behaviors themselves: nonaddictive use, excessive use (abuse), addictive dependency, and recovery or relapse. Accurate reports of homicides and suicides depend on discerning the intent of the perpetrators of the acts resulting in these deaths. Maltreatment can encompass both acts of commission (abuse) and omission (neglect), as well as a variety of types of harm or endangerment (physical, sexual, or emotional). The condition of homelessness can be assessed with respect to time (temporarily, episodically, or chronically homeless) or location (living on the streets, in temporary housing, or with relatives). Immigrants and refugees encompass those who are in the United States legally as well as those who are not, and among the latter, settlers, who intend to reside in the United States permanently; sojourners, who plan to return to their country of origin; and commuters, who live in Mexico or Canada, for example, and regularly cross the border to work in the United States, are all included.

Different studies tend to use different definitions or focus on different aspects of need for these groups. Often data are not available in a timely fashion or vary a great deal in quality and completeness across studies and sources. Cutbacks in funding, as well as changes in definitions of cases over time (which may be warranted to capture the changing dynamics of the problem, such as HIV/AIDS), can jeopardize the availability of longitudinal data to trace changes in the incidence or prevalence of these problems. The lack of relevant demographic identifiers or detail (by race and ethnicity, for example) can also limit the ability to look at differences among groups for whom the risk or magnitude of problems is most likely to vary.

Researchers in a particular area need to work toward identifying common definitions of terms, the content and timing for collecting information for a minimum basic data set on a given population of interest, and uniform standards for evaluating and reporting data quality.

Analytic Research

A major limitation in adequately understanding the origins of many of the problems examined here is the absence of well-developed or -integrated theoretical perspectives. Practitioners and researchers tend to focus on explanations rooted in their own disciplinary frameworks (of medicine, psychiatry, psychology, sociology, or social work, among others). Biological, psychological, and sociological explanations have all been used to understand the origins of suicide and interpersonal violence, for example. However, the complexity of these and other problems points to the need for broader, multidisciplinary theory development and research, and a corresponding expansion of the types of information gathered to conduct research adequately, based on this perspective.

Longitudinal studies best illuminate the causes and consequences of vulnerability. For an individual, the development of chronic illness, suicidal tendencies, HIV/AIDS, or substance abuse may be a product of a life course of experiences (being in a particular family, living a certain lifestyle, or working in a stressful or high-risk job). Similarly, at a national and local level, the magnitude and risks of these and other problems (such as homicide, family violence, or homelessness) may be affected by social, economic, or political changes (such as the loss of jobs in certain sectors of the economy, diminished federal or local commitments to maintaining the stock of low-income housing, or a declining tax base for the support of public education and related social services). Currently there is a paucity of longitudinal research looking at the correlates and consequences of vulnerability—either within the life span of individuals or in the aggregate, over time, at the local and national levels.

Comparative studies are also useful in addressing the question of why some groups are more vulnerable than others. Collecting data on rare or hard-to-locate at-risk populations (such as drug users, runaways, pregnant homeless women, and elderly women living alone) is often costly and complex; nevertheless, these data are valuable for generating and testing hypotheses regarding the probable causes and consequences of vulnerability. Cross-national comparative studies are also useful in exploring the impact of political, social, cultural, economic, and related factors on the prevalence or incidence of addictive behavior or family abuse, for example.

Evaluative Research

A limited amount of research has been conducted evaluating the costs and benefits of many programs and services designed to care for the vulnerable. The desired outcomes of these programs are often ambiguous or ill defined, and the research that has been done has not been summarized or integrated in a coherent fashion.

A first step in developing a more solid foundation for designing new programs is to review and systematically evaluate research on the success or failures of existing programs and how these outcomes were measured, based on formal meta-analysis procedures or consensus conferences of experts. This process should lead to the formulation of a research agenda focusing on programs and services to address both immediate and pressing needs, as well as to ameliorate or eliminate these problems over the long term. An aspect of the dilemma in dealing with certain issues (such as substance abuse or family violence) is the previous lack of investment or a diminished continuation of investment in research to understand what works and what does not.

Given the paucity of funding for research in most areas, small-scale demonstration and evaluation studies could be conducted to establish a basis for deciding whether to proceed with larger-scale demonstration projects. Program evaluations should, however, attempt to apply sound tenets of experimental design in order to maximize the internal validity (accuracy) and external validity (generalizability) of what is learned from these efforts.

An important aspect of this agenda-setting process would be to build the capacity and knowledge base in an area through providing support to train researchers, replicate previous studies, and integrate and disseminate findings.

Building a coordinated and comprehensive research agenda also requires cooperation among agencies in the design, implementation, and evaluation of programs, where none has traditionally existed. The multifaceted mosaic of needs of many of the vulnerable (such as homelessness, substance abuse, family abuse, and HIV/AIDS) does not fit neatly into existing agency or governmental divisions of categorical program responsibility.

Population-Specific Overview

The descriptive, analytical, and evaluative research priorities for vulnerable populations are summarized in the discussion that follows.

High-Risk Mothers and Infants

More information is needed to identify demographic (particularly ethnic) subgroups, behavioral risks, and appropriate care protocols for high-risk mothers and infants.

Descriptive Research. Birth and death certificates are the major sources of data on high-risk mothers and infants, yet the information recorded in these sources is often inaccurate or incomplete (Brunskill, 1990; Hexter et al., 1990; Kirby, 1997;

McDermott, Drews, Green, & Berg, 1997). Particular problems with vital statistics data include the unavailability and misclassifications of detailed racial and ethnic group breakdowns. National data on births of Hispanic parentage are available in only selected states and the District of Columbia in selected years, which makes it difficult to track changes in Hispanic birth-related statistics nationally. Low birthweight data on births of Asian parentage were first published in 1984. Data on Native American populations are limited to those who live in states with reservations. The revolving door of Mexico-U.S. migration patterns has also given rise to concerns about the serious underreporting of Hispanic infant deaths in the border regions of the United States. Furthermore, there is a three- to four-year time lag in the availability of national natality and mortality estimates (Kennedy & Deapen, 1991).

Analytic Research. More analytic studies are needed to examine the risk factors associated with poor pregnancy outcomes. Data on income, behavioral, and medical risks, program eligibility, and medical care use have not traditionally been available from vital statistics sources. The National Center for Health Statistics has conducted a number of studies to provide comprehensive information on the correlates and outcomes of pregnancy. These include the development of expanded standardized birth, death, and fetal death certificates; linked birth and death record files; and the National Maternal and Infant Health and Longitudinal Follow-up Surveys.

Expanded birth certificates collect additional information on the medical and behavioral risk factors associated with pregnancy and the technologies used at birth. Revised death certificates collect more detailed information on causes of death. Linked birth and death records permit a direct examination of the association between infant mortality and various maternal risk factors and whether these associations are changing. These data sources constitute rich mines of information for examining the impact of risk and related care factors on pregnancy outcomes cross-sectionally and over time.

Evaluative Research. Studies to examine the impact of particular programs on perinatal outcomes are often based on weak evaluation research designs. A critical review and synthesis of studies of the effectiveness of programs to improve pregnancy outcomes pointed out that in many of these studies, history, differential selection, and experimental mortality are powerful alternatives to concluding that any particular program (such as the Special Supplemental Food Program for Women, Infants and Children or Maternity and Infant Care Projects [MICP]) had an impact on reducing infant mortality rates (Shadish & Reis, 1984).

There is also a paucity of research on the probable impact of many of the expanded components of prenatal care, recommended by the Public Health Service expert panel, such as preconception visits, behavioral risk assessment and intervention, and psychosocial counseling, on actual birth outcomes (Alexander

& Korenbrot, 1995; Public Health Service, 1989). Technology assessment studies are also needed to estimate the costs and effectiveness of high-technology prenatal care and birthing procedures, particularly for high-risk newborns (Horbar & Lucey, 1995).

The Institute of Medicine (1988d) panel on prenatal care concluded that there is a surfeit of research documenting the financial and institutional barriers to prenatal care. Subsequent research should focus on the cost and effectiveness of specific mechanisms for removing these barriers to prenatal care services and in sustained support for research evaluating the impact of public or private-supported demonstration projects in this area.

Chronically Ill and Disabled

Descriptive research should focus on the development of uniform definitions and data sets for identifying the chronically ill and disabled, and more analytical and evaluative research is needed to guide the formulation of a cost-effective long-term care policy for this population.

Descriptive Research. One of the principal problems in conducting research on the chronically ill and disabled is the considerable variability that exists in the definitions and criteria that have been used to describe this population. Fundamental conceptual questions concern which type of indicators—diagnoses, disability, functional status, quality-of-life measures or others—are most relevant for describing the chronically ill and disabled, and why. Furthermore, the measurement of child health status must take into account the unique developmental needs of children and the key interface of biological, family, and social factors that influence children's health and well-being (Bergner, 1989; Spilker, Molinek, Johnston, Simpson, & Tilson, 1990; Stewart et al., 1989; Szilagyi & Schor, 1998; Thompson-Hoffman & Storck, 1991).

Disability and functional status-related measures, such as activities of daily living and instrumental activities of daily living, are often-used indicators of the chronically ill and disabled elderly, although the operational definitions of these measures vary across studies. This becomes particularly problematic in estimating the numbers of individuals in need of home care services and in establishing subsequent program eligibility. Different magnitudes of those in need may be estimated depending on the criteria and cutting points applied (Interagency Forum on Aging-Related Statistics, 1989; Spector, 1990; Stone & Murtaugh, 1990).

The National Center for Health Statistics National Health Interview Survey child health and disability supplements have provided invaluable information on the characteristics of chronically ill and disabled children and nonelderly, as well as elderly, adults (National Center for Health Statistics, 1999f). The Research Archive on Disability in the United States represents a compilation of data from national surveys addressing a variety of topics on the disabled population in the United States (Lang, 1998).

The long-term focus of care for the chronically ill and disabled compels a look at whether their status improves or declines over time. Longitudinal data are needed to facilitate forecasting changes in the profile of needs and probable case mix of services (Habib et al., 1988).

Formal and informal caregivers are a particularly important component of care for the chronically ill and disabled. Research on caregiving, however, has been plagued by inadequate attention to who exactly is included in the definition of caregivers, the extent of patient needs as they influence variability in caregiver demands, the generalizability and representativeness of study samples, the omission of the patients' own perspectives on their functional ability, and failure to consider the presence of an extended support network in addition to the primary providers of care (Barer & Johnson, 1990).

Analytic Research. Analytic questions of interest with respect to the chronically ill and disabled include considerations of models to predict rates of utilization or expenditures for nursing home, home care, or related long-term care services. Such models are useful, for example, in computing the actuarial risk of service use in formulating long-term care insurance policies, determining the importance of knowledge or other access barriers to care seeking, and the influence of community or political factors on public expenditures for long-term care (Liu, Manton, & Liu, 1990; Lowe, 1988; McCaslin, 1988; Williams, Phillips, Torner, & Irvine, 1990).

Federal agencies, such as the National Center for Health Statistics (1988b) and the National Institute on Aging (1989), have provided recommendations for the minimum basic data set and types of analyses needed to guide the development of policy on long-term care and aging. These include identifying the characteristics of both the providers and recipients of long-term care, the assumptions that underlie and the factors that affect their interaction, and methodological approaches for studying these relationships. Of particular concern are how to reduce the need for and associated costs of long-term care, how to improve the effectiveness and efficiency of long-term care, how to monitor its changing supply and demand, and what are the special problems of subpopulations, such as the oldest old, women, and older rural people.

Population-based research regarding the predictors of chronic illness must attend to conceptualizing the multilevel environmental, social, and individual determinants of disease occurrence and the use of more sophisticated methodological tools, such as hierarchical or multilevel modeling or geographic information systems, for empirically measuring the relative contributions of these respective types of predictors (McKinlay & Marceau, 1999).

Evaluative Research. Numerous studies have been conducted on the cost and effectiveness of alternative models of long-term care delivery. Investigations in this area have tended to suffer from deficiencies in the development of theory to guide the conduct of the research, the strength of the evaluation designs, and the specification and measurement of program outcomes (Hughes, 1985; Shaughnessy, 1985; Toseland & Rossiter, 1989). Research is also needed examining the impact of policy initiatives, such as prevention-oriented programs, managed care, and related financing and cost-containment options, on the health and well-being of the chronically ill and disabled (Halfon, Schuster, Valentine, & McGlynn, 1998; Wagner, 1997).

Persons Living with HIV/AIDS

Changes in definitions, the dynamic nature of the epidemic, and constrained research and service delivery funding have complicated efforts to understand the origins and consequences of HIV/AIDS.

Descriptive Research. Identifying who has, as well as who is likely to develop, HIV/AIDS is one of the fundamental research questions in tracking the epidemiology of the epidemic. The case definition for AIDS has been revised three times (in 1985, 1987, and 1993), since it was first published in 1982 (Centers for Disease Control and Prevention, 1985, 1987). The 1987 revision allowed for the presumptive diagnosis (without laboratory evidence of HIV infection) of AIDS-associated diseases and expanded the spectrum of HIV-associated diseases reportable as AIDS. These changes affected the comparability of case reports over time and differentially increased the rates and case mix severity for certain subgroups (such as minorities and intravenous drug users) when compared with earlier definitions (Payne, Rutherford, Lemp, & Clevenger, 1990; Selik, Buehler, Karon, Chamberland, & Berkelman, 1990). A study of AIDS deaths in San Francisco found that the numbers of deaths for minorities (especially Hispanics) was even higher than reported due to the misclassification of Hispanics as whites (Lindan et al., 1990). The Centers for Disease for Control and Prevention proposed another approach to identifying AIDS cases, based on whether a person had 200 or fewer CD4 cells per cubic milliliter of blood (American Public Health Association, 1991). This revised definition, which took take effect in 1993, resulted in an earlier diagnosis of women and children who have AIDS. Careful consideration of the definitional and measurement issues in identifying persons with AIDS is essential in accurately describing and forecasting the future of this dynamic epidemic.

HIV seroprevalence surveys are a particularly important tool for this purpose, since they provide an idea of who and how many people are likely to develop AIDS over time. The sensitivity and specificity (accuracy) of the HIV antibodies tests developed for population-based screening are generally very good, although the ethical implications of disclosing test results, particularly inaccurate (either positive or negative) results for any given individual, may be problematic (Burke et al., 1988; Khabbaz, Hartley, Lairmore, & Kaplan, 1990). The Centers for Disease Control and Prevention family of HIV seroprevalence surveys conducted in purposively selected sentinel sites—clinics for sexually transmitted diseases, drug treatment centers, and selected hospitals, among others—is, however, not representative of the population as a whole or at-risk subgroups within it (Centers for Disease Control and Prevention, 1998b).

The National Research Council Committee on AIDS Research and the Behavioral, Social, and Statistical Sciences, as well as others, have strongly endorsed the conduct of more extensive methodological research on designing high-quality seroprevalence and other surveys of persons most at risk of HIV/AIDS, who may also be the hardest to locate and interview (such as intravenous drug users). They also pointed out the need for strong experimental and quasi-experimental designs of the studies in this area and urged the formulation of a rigorous research agenda focusing on the structure, process, and outcome of major public health interventions to prevent the spread of HIV/AIDS (Coyle, Boruch, & Turner, 1991). This research agenda would include approaches to designing probability samples of rare populations, reducing nonresponse bias, and enhancing the validity and reliability of the data obtained from these respondents (Laumann, Gagnon, Michaels, Michael, & Coleman, 1989; Miller, Turner, & Moses, 1990; Watters & Biernacki, 1989).

Analytic Research. The first generation of federal funding for health services research on HIV/AIDS (1986–1991) focused on the cost and financing of HIV/AIDS care. The research agenda has subsequently been expanded to encompass more studies of the effectiveness and accessibility of HIV/AIDS care (Rudzinski, Marconi, & McKinney, 1994; Weissman et al., 1994).

An array of analytic epidemiological, behavioral, and social science research is needed, however, to understand better the correlates and consequences of the epidemic (Allen & Curran, 1988; Henry, 1988; Van Devanter, 1999). Basic social and behavioral science research on the sexual behavior of subgroups who may be most at risk—homosexual and bisexual males, teenage heterosexuals, male and female prostitutes—or those for whom the risks may increase over the course of the epidemic, such as the elderly, is needed. National survey data on the prevalence and correlates of HIV risk-taking behaviors among high-risk populations, as well as clinical data on the pathogenesis and disease progression of HIV/AIDS related to mental health and substance abuse problems in these populations, would be particularly helpful to assist in designing effective interventions (Auerbach, Wypijewska, & Brodie, 1994; Institute of Medicine, 1991a; Riley, Ory, & Zablotsky, 1989; Turner, Miller, & Moses, 1989).

Statistical models for estimating and comparing risks among groups, examining the prognosis at different stages of the disease, and projecting subsequent rates of survival postdiagnosis are needed for evaluating the process and outcome of care for persons living with HIV/AIDS (Feinstein, 1989; Justice, Feinstein, & Wells, 1989; Redfield & Tramont, 1989; Sechrest, Freeman, & Mulley, 1989).

Comprehensive and valid methodologies for estimating and projecting the rates of survival and costs of HIV/AIDS care are essential for evaluating the probable price tag and economic impact of the epidemic (Begley, Crane,

& Perdue, 1990; Bilheimer, 1989; Scitovsky, 1988, 1989a, 1989b; Thompson & Meyer, 1989).

Strategies for the design and conduct of research related to HIV/AIDS should ideally employ a variety of contrasting (quantitative and qualitative) methods of sampling, data collection, and measurement, as well as protocols for evaluating the biases of each method throughout the course of the study (Shadish, 1989).

Evaluative Research. There is a need for wider use of randomized field experiments or, if randomization is not possible, the application of carefully conceived quasi-experimental or related designs, to control for the array of alternative explanations besides the program itself (such as who chooses to use it, who drops out of it, and what other things are going on in the community) that may account for any changes observed for persons living with HIV/AIDS that are the target of such interventions (Coyle, Boruch, & Turner, 1991; DiFranceisco et al., 1998; Miller, Turner, & Moses, 1990; Turner, Miller, & Moses, 1989).

Evaluations of major HIV/AIDS prevention programs—media campaigns, health education and risk reduction, and testing and counseling—should address the extent to which they become operational (formative evaluation), how well they work (process evaluation), and whether they achieve their intended goals (outcome evaluation). Better specification of the desired outcomes of these programs is also needed, particularly in terms of the behaviors they are intended to influence (Agency for Healthcare Research and Quality, 1990a).

Participatory action research acknowledges the importance of the participation of those being studied directly in the design and evaluation of HIV/AIDS prevention or treatment programs (Ferreira-Pinto & Ramos, 1995; Huby, 1997). A particular area of need is the effect of HIV/AIDS on families, including the design and evaluation of family-centered services, who gives care and what they do, and the effectiveness and outcomes of family caregiving (Brown, 1997).

Mentally Ill and Disabled

Significant methodological issues surround how best to identify and collect data on the mentally ill and disabled.

Descriptive Research. The design of methodologies for studies of the prevalence and distribution of mental illness has been and continues to be a challenge for the field of psychiatric epidemiology. At least four generations of epidemiological studies, with varying methodologies, can be identified. The first generation, prior to World War II, used record sources and key informants to define cases of mental illness. The second generation, post–World War II, typically used a single psychiatrist or a small team headed by a psychiatrist, in which community residents were interviewed, and in some cases standardized protocols were used. The Epidemiological Catchment Area (ECA) program and National Comorbidity

Surveys, using lay interviewers and standardized survey sampling and data collection procedures, typify the third generation of studies. A fourth generation of psychiatric surveys focuses more explicitly on the social functioning of those identified as mentally ill, as a more informed basis for planning programs to meet the needs of this population (Bebbington, 1990; Kessler et al., 1994; Robins, 1990; Robins & Regier, 1991; Willis, Willis, Manderscheid, Male, & Henderson, 1998).

A continuing methodological concern in psychiatric surveys is the definition of "caseness"—that is, how individuals come to be classified as mentally ill. This problem is rooted in philosophical disputes regarding the appropriateness of assigning primacy to psychiatric diagnoses in making these judgments, as well as the validity and reliability of specific instruments used for this purpose, such as the Diagnostic Interview Schedule and Composite International Diagnostic Interview applied in the ECA survey and National Comorbidity Survey, respectively (Dingemans, 1990; Helzer, Spitznagel, & McEvoy, 1987; Kessler et al., 1994; Klerman, 1989; Kovess & Fournier, 1990; Mirowsky & Ross, 1989a, 1989b; Swartz, Carroll, & Blazer, 1989; Tweed & George, 1989). A related problem is the design of culturally sensitive and appropriate approaches to measuring the prevalence of disorders in different racial and ethnic groups and cross-nationally (Neighbors, Jackson, Campbell, & Williams, 1989; Robins, 1989; Rogler, 1989).

Furthermore, the need for mental health services has variously been measured indirectly through social indicator–type community profiles reflecting correlated risks of mental illness (such as income and racial distributions), as well as rates of mental illness under treatment or the proportion of cases receiving or not receiving mental health services (Cleary, 1989; Goldsmith, Lin, Bell, & Jackson, 1988).

Analytic Research. Mental health services research is an increasingly important field of study. This type of research has focused on the organization and financing of the mental health care services system and its associated impact on the access, cost, and effectiveness of care. There is, however, a need to enhance the capacity for health services research in state mental health agencies and managed care organizations through committing funds, building databases, and hiring staff trained to conduct such research (Bevilacqua, Morris, & Pumariega, 1996; Mechanic, 1996b; Norquist & Macgruder, 1998).

Prevention intervention research is a promising and important new emphasis in mental health care. The concept of risk reduction, and particularly the design and testing of interventions to ameliorate the risks of mental illness, are at the heart of prevention research. Components of a research agenda in this area include identifying causal risk factors that may be altered through interventions, analyzing the interplay between risk and protective factors in developing mental disorders, and testing the effects of these interventions through rigorous prevention intervention trials. The Institute of Medicine Committee on Prevention of Mental Disorders has identified the need for a federal research infrastructure to support a more fully developed prevention intervention research agenda through interagency coordination and collaboration regarding projects and funding, in training researchers to work in this area and in enhancing means for disseminating the results of this research to the field of practice (Mrazek & Haggerty, 1994).

Evaluative Research. There is a paucity of systematic, well-designed evaluations of the operation and impact of mental health treatment and services delivery programs. Meta-analyses (that is, systematic, quantitative syntheses and critiques) of the findings from existing evaluations of various programs (such as case management or other aftercare options) provide a foundation for understanding what can be validly concluded from existing research, as well as formalize and focus an evaluative mental health services research agenda (Hargreaves & Shumway, 1989). Such analyses have documented the efficacy of well-developed psychological, educational, and behavioral treatments for mental health and substance abuse disorders, as well the effectiveness of primary prevention mental health programs for children and adolescents (Durlak & Wells, 1997; Lipsey & Wilson, 1993).

As with evaluations of the impact of health care programs in general, a better specification is needed of the outcomes the programs are expected to accomplish, such as those developed in the RAND Medical Outcomes Study for comparing the physical, social, and role functioning of depressed patients seen in a variety of delivery settings (Ware, 1989; Wells, Manning, & Valdez, 1989; Wing et al., 1998). Evaluative research also needs to link the structure and process of care delivery to patient outcomes more effectively. Comparisons of outcomes between different types of managed care organizations, as well as the specification of the mechanisms (such as the financial incentives or practice norms that guide providers) that give rise to identified differences among plans, would also importantly add to the body of knowledge regarding the performance of behavioral managed care (Edmunds et al., 1997; Leff & Woocher, 1998; van der Feltz-Cornelis et al., 1997; Yuen, 1994).

There is a need for sound, full economic evaluations of mental health care. Program evaluations often fail to measure costs or do so in an incomplete or inappropriate way. Most have been restricted to analyses of direct costs only, and few have used quality-of-life assessment and utility methods central to cost-effectiveness analyses (Evers, Van Wijk, & Ament, 1997; McCrone & Weich, 1996).

Alcohol or Substance Abusers

The knowledge base on alcohol and substance abuse is characterized by considerable variability across data sources and disciplines.

Descriptive Research. A variety of data sources and approaches are used in estimating the prevalence and distribution of substance abuse problems. These include more behaviorally oriented social surveys, such as the National Household Survey on Drug Abuse and the Monitoring the Future survey of high school seniors; epidemiologically oriented studies of problem prevalence, such as the ECA and National Comorbidity Survey; surveillance systems, such as the Drug Abuse Warning Network; facilities-based sources, such as the Substance Abuse and Mental Health Services Administration's (SAMSHA) Drug and Alcohol Services Information System, composed of the National Master Facility Inventory, Uniform Facility Data Set, and the Treatment Episode Data Set; and outcomes-oriented studies such as SAMSHA's Services Research Outcomes Study.

These studies measure different aspects of the problem or focus on different subgroups of the population. As a result, they may point to somewhat conflicting conclusions about the patterns of drug dependence—for example, a decreased prevalence of the problem based on national household- and school-based surveys, but higher rates of drug-related deaths reported through the routine surveillance systems. The data obtained from different sources may, however, be capturing different stages of the development of the addictive behavior: non-addictive use, excessive use (abuse), addictive dependency, recovery, or relapse (Collins & Zawitz, 1990; Rouse, 1996; Westermeyer, 1990). A problem with these data systems, as well as conventional screening procedures in primary care clinical practice, is that they may fail to identify and thereby underestimate the actual drug-using population (Brookoff, Campbell, & Shaw, 1993; Johnson et al., 1995; Johnson, Gerstein, & Raskinski, 1998).

The major areas of need with respect to improving and enhancing the usefulness of these disparate data-gathering activities include information on the nature and extent of drug abuse (particularly for at-risk populations such as pregnant women, persons living with HIV/AIDS, prisoners, and homeless persons), the morbidity and mortality associated with drug abuse, data on the capacity and utilization of the prevention and treatment systems, the costs and financing of care, and treatment outcomes. Better integration and validation of existing data-gathering efforts are also needed—through, for example, using common core questionnaire items and determining the extent of overlap across sampling frames, as well as conducting more analytic and integrative analyses across the array of existing data sets to address drug policy issues (Haaga & Reuter, 1991; Public Health Service Task Force on Drug Abuse Data, 1990).

Analytic Research. Documented needs for analytic research on the prevention and treatment of alcohol and drug abuse problems include more theory-driven research; the integration of the theoretical perspectives and findings of biomedical, social science, and behaviorally oriented research in understanding and designing interventions to address the multiplicity of causes of the disorders; the integration of long-term, life span, and developmental as well as comparative (including cross-national) research perspectives; the clarification and quantification of desired treatment or prevention outcomes; the support of long-term community trials; and studies to evaluate both the cost and effectiveness of prevention and treatment-oriented interventions (Committee to Identify Strategies to Raise the Profile of Substance Abuse and Alcoholism Research, 1997; Fillmore, 1988; Fulco, Liverman, & Bonnie, 1996; General Accounting Office, 1990a; Gerstein & Harwood, 1990; Institute of Medicine, 1987, 1989c, 1990; Lamb, Greenlick, & McCarty, 1998).

The field of drug abuse services research has focused in particular on the organization and financing of drug abuse services and methods for assessing the access, cost, and effectiveness of care. Of increasing interest is consideration of services outside the specialty treatment sector, especially the impact of managed care arrangements and the utility of health insurance claims, as well as other large-scale databases, in assessing system performance (Garnick, Horgan, Hendricks, & Constock, 1996; Kelly, 1997; Weisner & Schmidt, 1995). Drug abuse services researchers have developed the Drug Abuse Treatment Cost Analysis Program and other procedures for more uniform approaches to estimating program costs and associated outcomes that could be practically and easily applied across an array of program settings (French, Dunlap, Zarkin, McGeary, & McLellan, 1997; French, Mauskopf, Teague, & Roland, 1996; French & McGeary, 1997).

Evaluative Research. The support of federal research for mental and addictive disorders through the major constituent institutes of the Alcohol, Drug Abuse, and Mental Health Administration (ADAMHA)—the National Institute of Mental Health, National Institute on Drug Abuse, and National Institute on Alcohol Abuse and Alcoholism—declined in real purchasing power from 1966 to the mid-1980s. The Drug Abuse Reporting Program, which tracked a sample of clients in treatment from 1969 to 1973, and the Treatment Outcome Prospective Study, which tracked clients from 1979 to 1981, as well as the Client Oriented Data Acquisition Process to collect data on clients in drug abuse treatment, begun in 1972, were effectively terminated. During the 1980s, when the drug problem was growing in importance, the availability of research funds for the generation of knowledge for addressing the problem was declining.

Since 1986, the research budgets of these agencies have grown. The Minimum Treatment Client Data Set, Drug Abuse Treatment Outcome Study, and Treatment Outcome and Performance Pilot Studies, Services Research Outcomes Study, and the Cooperative Agreement for AIDS Community-Based Outreach/Intervention Research Program, among others, have been developed with support from the National Institute on Drug Abuse and/or National Institute on Alcohol Abuse and Alcoholism to evaluate program effectiveness (Coyle, 1998; Gustafson & Darby, 1999; Haaga & Reuter, 1991).

Existing knowledge about the prevention of alcohol and drug abuse is limited by the following problems: inadequate information about program integrity (the degree to which a program was implemented as planned) or a rush to pass judgment on a program before it is stable enough to be evaluated; weak or imprecise measures of outcomes; poor research designs; and an emphasis on statistical significance to the neglect of policy or programmatic significance. Traditionally most prevention programs have focused on educational or psychosocial interventions with individuals in an effort to remedy deficiencies of knowledge, coping skills, and behavior. The causes of substance abuse include a variety of social and environmental, in addition to individual, correlates. More recently, prevention research has begun to focus on the individual in the context of peers, families, schools, and communities and on appropriate multilevel analytic strategies for estimating these respective influences (Dane & Schneider, 1998; Fulco, Liverman, & Bonnie, 1996; Gerstein & Green, 1993; Lamb, Greenlick, & McCarty, 1998; Palmer, Graham, White, & Hansen, 1998).

Suicide or Homicide Prone

Longitudinal studies and demonstration projects are needed to better understand the origins of violence and how best to prevent or ameliorate it.

Descriptive Research. Information on completed (and, particularly, attempted) suicides and homicides is variable and incomplete. No common definition of what constitutes a suicide exists, and because of the social stigma that often results from suicides, other causes of death may be assigned to save the family or other survivors embarrassment. A survey of medical examiners yielded the estimate that the number of suicides reported may be half the true number. Furthermore, attempted suicides are not reportable through any vital statistics or epidemiological surveillance system. There is also generally at least a two- to three-year lag in the availability of data on completed suicides and homicides through the vital statistics system (Jobes, Berman, & Josselson, 1987; Moscicki, 1989; O'Carroll, 1989).

Major sources of data on homicide-related crime include the Federal Bureau of Investigation Uniform Crime Reports (UCR) (particularly its Supplementary Homicide Reports) and the National Crime Survey (NCS) of U.S. households. The UCR provides reports only on known assaults, and local police have a great deal of discretion with respect to whether and how to fill out such reports. Systematic and easy methods for amending or updating such reports once new information is obtained on the case are not in place.

The NCS is intended to elicit information on crimes that might not be reported formally to local police authorities. The NCS was revised to correct the major problems that had previously characterized that study (anomalous findings, inadequate measurement of revictimization, and sample attrition). NCS results are nonetheless affected by the problems that usually attend surveys addressing such topics, such as greater noncoverage or nonresponse of particularly at-risk groups or the underreporting of sensitive or personally traumatic events. Neither of these data sources captures good information on a particularly important correlate of homicide: interpersonal family violence and abuse (Rokaw, Mercy, & Smith, 1990; Skogan, 1990; Taylor, 1989; Whitaker, 1989).

Analytic Research. Insufficient information is available on death certificates that would facilitate studies of the correlates and causes of violent deaths due to homicide or suicide, such as a previous history of suicide or mental illness, substance abuse, family structure, or socioeconomic status. Psychological autopsies have been used to assess the reasons that a particular individual may have chosen to commit suicide. This procedure involves an intensive interview or series of interviews with persons who knew the victim to determine the social and psychological circumstances surrounding the incident. This methodology, along with other types of data, may be useful in generating meaningful theories and hypotheses regarding the etiology of suicidal acts (Brent, 1989).

Much more research is needed using life span and developmental and causal approaches to understanding suicidal and homicidal behavior. Theories of suicide have tended to emphasize cross-sectional, not longitudinal, analyses. Studying individual suicide and criminal careers, as well as the experience of historical demographic (age-gender-race) cohorts, may provide a better understanding of the etiology and evolution of violent behaviors at both the individual and societal levels. A better understanding is needed as well of the extent to which violent acts are contagious, that is, lead to other acts of individual or interpersonal violence.

There is also a paucity of multidisciplinary theory and research examining the array of biological, psychological, and social antecedents and correlates that have been identified from disparate bodies of research in this area, particularly for groups that might be most at risk (the elderly and minorities, for example). An important ethical question posed in estimating the cost of violent deaths in terms of years lost of life is the implicit devaluing of the elderly, for whom suicide rates are highest, by focusing on the estimated years of *productive* life lost, that is, those up to age sixty-five (Alcohol, Drug Abuse, and Mental Health Administration, 1989a, 1989b, 1989c, 1989d; Berlin, 1987; Blumstein, Cohen, Roth, & Visher, 1986a; Gibbs, 1988; Gould, Wallenstein, & Davidson, 1989; Grossman, Milligan, & Deyo, 1991; Leenaars, 1989; Stack, 1987).

Evaluative Research. Much more research is needed evaluating the cost and effectiveness of prevention and treatment-oriented interventions to address problems of personal and interpersonal violence. Such evaluations should focus on what types of services in particular might work best (hot lines, therapy, outreach, and so on) and for what groups (adolescents, elderly, minorities) (Rodriguez & Brindis, 1995). Designs, such as interrupted time series, that have been conventionally employed to trace the impact of policy changes (for example, gun control legislation) on violent deaths (for example, homicides) could be strengthened by choosing relevant control sites, considering a number of possible intervention times, and testing for the robustness of the intervention results using multiple data sets (Britt, Kleck, & Bordua, 1996).

An important strategy for beginning to fill the substantial gaps in knowledge in this area is to support small-scale demonstration projects, along with well-designed independent program evaluations, to see what works best. Based on the results of these studies, models could be selected for larger-scale demonstration projects and subjected to rigorous external evaluation as a basis for developing better-informed programmatic and policy priorities in this area (Alcohol, Drug Abuse, and Mental Health Administration, 1989a, 1989b, 1989c, 1989d; Blumstein, Cohen, Roth, & Visher, 1986a; Streiner & Adam, 1987).

Abusing Families

A deeper understanding of abusing families could be gained from more integrated, multidisciplinary theory development and research in this area.

Descriptive Research. Considerable variability exists in how abusing families are defined. Maltreatment can be designated by acts of commission (abuse) or omission (neglect); probable (endangerment) as well as actual injury (harm); professional reports of incidents of harm (cases) or family reports of actions that could result in harm (family violence); physical, as well as sexual or emotional, abuse; and by victim—child, wife, husband, sibling, parent, elderly, and so on. *Abuse* and *neglect* are often used interchangeably in the literature, although maltreatment is generally regarded as encompassing both. There are also varying opinions with respect to whether domestic violence is best defined in terms of discrete incidents of injury or the ongoing dynamics of power and control within intimate relationships (Cicchetti & Carlson, 1989; Flitcraft, 1997; Gelles & Cornell, 1990).

These varying definitions, as well as the differing methodologies used to gather data, lead to varying estimates of the incidence and prevalence of the problem. The major types of studies (and examples of each) are clinical studies of victims or perpetrators of abuse (Clinical Demonstration of Child Abuse and Neglect), official reports to protective service agencies (National Study on Child Neglect and Abuse Reporting), interviews with abuse and neglect service providers (Study of the National Incidence and Prevalence of Child Abuse and Neglect), and surveys of U.S. families (National Crime Survey, National Surveys of Family Violence).

Clinical studies tend to be based on few cases and rely on clinician judgments of maltreatment. Official reports overrepresent certain groups (minorities, low income), double-count cases (due to more than one incident's being reported), and may or may not be substantiated by a fuller investigation. Middle-class professionals tend to label certain incidents as abuse or neglect that others would not as a function of their cultural referents and norms or particular disciplinary background. Family members may not feel comfortable in reporting sensitive events, such as acts of intrafamily violence or victimization in surveys.

The relative advantages and disadvantages of these various data-gathering approaches need to be weighed and understood in designing surveillance systems to monitor the prevalence and incidence of maltreatment (Cicchetti & Carlson, 1989; Gelles & Cornell, 1990).

Numerous methodological difficulties surround correctly identifying incidents of child sexual abuse in particular, through surveys (Edwards & Donaldson, 1989; Haugaard & Emery, 1989), the use of anatomical dolls in counseling or court (Freeman & Estrada-Mullaney, 1988), and medical examinations and screening tools (Kleinman, Blackbourne, Marks, Karellas, & Belanger, 1989; Krugman, 1989). More research is needed to refine the reliability and validity of methods of detecting this particularly sensitive type of abuse. The moral and ethical implications of false positives or false negatives are substantial for both the suspected victim and perpetrator of such acts (Haugaard & Reppucci, 1989).

Analytic Research. A major limitation of analytic research on maltreatment is the absence of a well-developed theoretical foundation. Investigators have used an array of micro- and macro-oriented theories. The theories have tended to focus on discrete dynamics or explanations of causality (psychopathology, learning behavior, or status inequality, among others), or have encompassed so many interacting components as to be virtually untestable empirically (systems theory). Furthermore, research based on these theories has tended to use cross-sectional or retrospective study designs, with all the attendant weaknesses of trying to attribute the causes of events after their occurrence (Cicchetti & Carlson, 1989; Gelles & Cornell, 1990).

Subsequent research in this area should focus on developing a multidisciplinary theoretical foundation and prospective (or longitudinal) analytic (in addition to descriptive) databases. Research should seek to uncover and understand the commonalities, as well as the discrete causes, of the array of acts encompassed within the concepts of maltreatment (or family violence). Professionals from different disciplines (psychiatry, psychology, sociology, and medicine, among others) must engage in dialogue that invites a multidisciplinary look at the problem and be willing to discard disciplinary prejudices (or paradigms) when the empirical evidence consistently fails to support those perspectives.

Furthermore, the problem must come to be viewed in a developmental context and the research designed accordingly to look over time (or longitudinally) at why and how these patterns emerge. Analytic models that examine the geographic and community-level correlates of domestic violence are also important in developing a sound foundation for predicting who is most likely to be at risk and the design of prevention or treatment interventions that work because they fundamentally address the root causes of the problem (Browne, Davies, & Stratton, 1988; Cicchetti & Carlson, 1989; Finkelhor, Hotaling, & Yllo, 1988; Fryer & Miyoshi, 1995; Gelles & Cornell, 1990; Hotaling, Finkelhor, Kirkpatrick, & Straus, 1988a, 1988b; Maiuro & Eberle, 1989; O'Campo et al., 1995; Schene & Bond, 1989; Straus, 1988).

Evaluative Research. Reviews of the results and methodological problems associated with evaluations of family abuse primary prevention programs in general, specific primary prevention programs focusing on hospital-based interventions during the perinatal period or school-based interventions for older children, and evaluations of the overall effectiveness and cost-effectiveness of treatment programs for individuals and families in which maltreatment has already occurred point to a number of steps that should be taken to improve the design and conduct of such evaluations. These include the following recommendations (Chalk & King, 1998; Cohn & Daro, 1987; Crowell & Burgess, 1996; Daro, 1988; Dubowitz, 1990; Fink & McCloskey, 1990; National Research Council Panel on Research on Child Abuse and Neglect, 1993):

- Clarify and clearly operationalize program objectives.
- Specify the theoretical underpinning and key elements of the intervention, as well as the extent to which it was actually implemented.
- Randomly assign individuals or families to experimental and control conditions (or at least attend to the need for relevant comparison groups).
- Replicate the intervention across a number of different populations or communities.
- Select a sufficiently large sample size and relevant statistical procedures for ensuring the statistical conclusion validity of study results.
- Assess the extent to which program effects are sustained over the long term.
- Be sensitive to the unintended negative consequences (or side effects) of the intervention (such as fear arousal in children regarding abuse).

The results of program evaluations in this area suggest that prevention efforts to stop maltreatment before it begins are much more likely to be both effective and economical than the treatment of individuals or families for whom it has already emerged as a problem. Furthermore, total reform prevention, directed at underlying social and political inequities (structural unemployment, gender discrimination, and so on), may ultimately be more successful than patchwork prevention, which attempts to address categorically discrete pieces of the problem (such as sex abuse education or violence prevention) (Garbarino, 1986). Thus far, no substantial social or political interventions have sought to adopt the total reform prevention approach to maltreatment (however maltreatment is defined), and patchwork prevention in this area remains just that.

Homeless Persons

There is a paucity of data on the number and needs of the homeless throughout the nation and insufficient attention to examining the deeper social and economic roots of homelessness.

Descriptive Research. Homelessness is a difficult and dynamic concept to define and measure. It is perhaps most appropriately considered as a point along a continuum defined by both time and space, ranging from a complete absence of shelter to a stable home environment (U.S. Commission on Security and Co-operation in Europe, 1990).

People may be temporarily, episodically, or chronically homeless. That is, they may be displaced from their homes temporarily because of an economic or natural calamity (such as a loss of a job or fire), they may go in and out of homelessness (due to intermittent bouts of family violence or unstable aftercare arrangements postinstitutionalization), or they may be without a stable residence for extended periods of time (because of the lack of ties to family or institutional care arrangements) (Institute of Medicine, 1988c).

Homelessness may also be defined based primarily on the type of place in which people usually spend the night. The McKinney Act defined a homeless individual as someone who (1) lacked a fixed, regular, and adequate nighttime residence, or (2) who had a primary nighttime residence that was a supervised shelter that provided temporary living accommodations, an institution that provided a temporary residence for individuals intended to be institutionalized, or a public or private place not designed for, or ordinarily used as, a regular sleeping accommodation for human beings.

Some individuals may not be literally without a roof over their heads, but are nonetheless at considerable risk of being so. These people are doubled up with friends or family, living in accommodations they are renting by the day or week, or in jails or hospitals awaiting discharge but with no stable home to which to return (National Alliance to End Homelessness, 1988).

The methods that have been employed in generating national estimates of the homeless population are indirect estimation, one-time censuses, and household surveys. The indirect estimation method involves asking knowledgeable informants (such as shelter administrators or city officials) about the estimated number of homeless persons (Institute of Medicine, 1988c). Examples include the U.S. Conference of Mayors Task Force on Hunger and Homelessness (U.S. Conference of Mayors, 1999) and the U.S. Department of Housing and Urban Development National Survey of Shelters (U.S. Department of Housing and Urban Development, 1989).

The one-time census is conducted at one point in time in a given area where homeless persons are expected to gather, as did the 1990 U.S. Census Street and Shelter Night count and the Chicago Homeless Study (Rossi, 1989; Taeuber & Siegel, 1990).

The estimates yielded by these methods may differ as a function of when and where a particular study was done. Furthermore, estimates of the prevalence of homelessness at one point in time may differ from the number of incidents (incidence) of people being homeless in the course of a year. Point estimates, such as those based on indirect estimation and one-time censuses, characterize the number of individuals who are homeless at a given point in time, such as a typical day. Period prevalence estimates are intended to reflect those who have experienced homelessness during a given period of time, such as the past year or past five years. Household surveys have been conducted to estimate the period, rather than the point, prevalence of homeless adults and youths, thereby providing more insight into the process by which individuals enter or exit from homelessness. The surveys on which such estimates are based, however, typically exclude institutionalized populations and those living in group quarters (such as single-room-occupancy hotels) (Link et al., 1994; Ringwalt, Greene, Robertson, & McPheeters, 1998).

Estimates of categories of the homeless population (such as the homeless mentally ill or substance abusers, among others) are equally or even more difficult to obtain (General Accounting Office, 1988a). The paucity of adequate state, local, and national data, and particularly the number and characteristics of subgroups of the homeless population, complicate efforts to plan programs and services to meet their needs adequately.

Analytic Research. A place to start in designing the next generation of more explanatory studies of homelessness is to synthesize systematically what is known already. A 1986 National Institute of Mental Health conference attempted to synthesize the first generation of largely descriptive studies of the homeless mentally ill, to provide a foundation for subsequent analytic research in this area (Morrissey & Levine, 1987). A 1988 Institute of Medicine report (1988c) provided an overview and synthesis of research on the health and health care of homeless persons. Some members of the Institute of Medicine panel that produced that report, however, filed a supplementary statement, asserting that the report did not go far enough in examining the deep political, social, and economic root causes of the problem (Holden, 1988).

There is a paucity of longitudinal research on the homeless population, tracing their movement in and out of homelessness, and the physical, psychological, and social correlates and consequences of homelessness—particularly for the burgeoning number of children numbered among the homeless population— however defined.

Evaluative Research. Lessons for developing policies and programs to address homelessness should be drawn from the failures of deinstitutionalization, in which a large-scale social experiment was rapidly put into place in the absence of supporting scientific evidence of its likely consequences (Wyatt, 1986).

Special data collection problems exist in conducting evaluations of programs for homeless persons. Services are often delivered in nontraditional settings, such as public shelters, churches, or soup kitchens, that do not permit either confidential or comfortable contexts for interviewing clients. The transiency of homeless clients and their unwillingness or inability to provide an accurate location for follow-up data collection results in missing outcome data. Since delivery of care is primary in the often resource-strained environments in which homeless persons are served, resources and staff support for the conduct of the research are often limited. Furthermore, data systems in such settings may be nonexistent, incomplete, or difficult to access (Hunter, Crosby, Ventura, & Warkentin, 1997). Research on the predictors of shelter utilization is useful in predicting the likely demand for and management of shelter services (Culhane, Averyt, & Hadley, 1997; Culhane & Kuhn, 1998; Culhane, Lee, & Wachter, 1996).

A number of the major programs to serve the homeless population (such as the Robert Wood Johnson Foundation Health Care for the Homeless, Veterans Administration Homeless Chronically Mentally Ill, and McKinney Act programs) have had accompanying evaluations of their implementation, if not their impact. More interagency cooperation and coordination is needed in reviewing the results of evaluations conducted to date in this area and in developing demonstrations and evaluations of alternatives for caring for particularly vulnerable subgroups of the homeless population, such as the chronically and mentally ill and disabled, substance abusers, persons living with HIV/AIDS, and children.

Both short-term alternatives for addressing the consequences of homelessness and long-term options for ameliorating its causes must be elements of research, demonstrations, and policy in this area.

Immigrants and Refugees

Research on immigrant and refugee populations presents special challenges regarding finding hard-to-locate populations (particularly undocumented persons), designing culturally sensitive research protocols, and discerning the unintended and intended consequences of health and social policies.

Descriptive Research. No precise counts exist of the number of undocumented persons residing in the United States. Research to derive such estimates has been conducted by the Census Bureau, the Immigration and Naturalization Service (INS), and the Program for Research on Immigration Policy (a joint effort of the RAND Corporation and the Urban Institute), among others, based on special surveys done expressly for that purpose or on projections derived from data on the number of undocumented persons apprehended (Bean, Edmonston, & Passel, 1990; Bean, Vernez, & Keely, 1989).

Undocumented residents have been conceptualized as belonging to three major groups based on their intended duration of residence in the United States: settlers, sojourners, and commuters. No precise estimates of the number in each group, much less their varying needs, demands, and contributions to U.S. society, exist (Bean, Edmonston, & Passel, 1990; Bean, Vernez, & Keely, 1989).

Individual case studies or local patient or community surveys have been conducted to document the needs of discrete categories of immigrants or refugees. The INS, Current Population Survey, and census provide general demographic and socioeconomic status information on the foreign born. Annual surveys of refugees conducted by the Office of Refugee Resettlement have focused primarily on issues of their economic adjustment: employment and labor force participation and use of public assistance or services. No comprehensive data on the health and mental health needs of major categories of recent immigrants and refugees are available at the state or national level (Ahearn & Athey, 1991; Haines, 1989; Hernandez & Charney, 1998; Rumbaut, Chavez, Moser, Pickwell, & Wishik, 1988).

Analytic Research. More formalized epidemiological surveillance methods in refugee camps, as well as in immigrant and refugee communities in the United States, are needed to identify the reasons for and rates of illness outbreaks in these populations (Elias, Alexander, & Sokly, 1990; Rumbaut, Chavez, Moser, Pickwell, & Wishik, 1988).

Both longitudinal surveys and ethnographic studies are needed to measure the physical and psychological development and the range of contextual factors influencing the development of children and youth in immigrant families. More research is needed to understand the relative importance of the availability, affordability, and acceptability of services, among other factors, that affect different immigrant and refugee subgroups' access. This research needs to be designed in a culturally sensitive fashion, with keen attention to the beliefs and practices that are likely to influence their behavior and how best to design studies to capture these influences accurately (Edmonston, 1996; Hernandez & Charney, 1998).

Evaluative Research. Epidemiological as well as access data would be useful in evaluating the impact of public health and medical care interventions to address the needs of the foreign born.

Unintended, as well as intended, consequences have resulted from U.S. immigration policies and programs. For example, the Immigration and Reform Control Act of 1986 has been credited with reducing the immigration of the undocumented foreign born (intended), as well as increase employer discrimination against the foreign born in general (unintended) (Bean, Edmonston, & Passel, 1990; Bean, Vernez, & Keely, 1989). Research is also needed examining the health and mental health impact of policies, such as the scattering or separation of refugee families, or the loss of benefits for legal immigrants due to the enactment of the Welfare Reform Act.

Conclusion

This book illuminates the cross-cutting insights that can be gained from reviewing the efforts and experiences in identifying, understanding, and addressing a wide array of vulnerable populations. Much is known, but much still needs to be learned in this area from a variety of contributors. Clinicians can contribute to a fuller understanding of how best to enhance the quality and effectiveness of care. Social scientists can contribute to identifying the social determinants of significant health disparities across groups and the interventions that would work best to ameliorate them. Economists can assist in illuminating which interventions are most efficient, relative to the investments made to implement them. The final chapter reviews the principles and parameters of a community-oriented health policy to address the health and health care needs of vulnerable populations, based on the information and analyses presented in this and previous chapters.

CHAPTER ELEVEN

WHAT PROGRAMS AND POLICIES ARE NEEDED?

An important policy recommendation, based on the analyses of the health and health care needs of vulnerable populations in this book, is that to illuminate the origins and remedies of vulnerability most clearly, the "second" language of community (reciprocity, interdependence, and the common good), in addition to the "first" language of individualism (autonomy, independence, and individual rights), must be more widely understood and used in social and political discourse surrounding these issues.

Critics of contemporary U.S. society have argued that developing the primordial (primary, personal), as well as purposive (secondary, task-oriented), ties between individuals in families and small social or community groups can be a powerful social and organizational alternative for enhancing individual and collective well-being (Bellah, Madsen, Sullivan, Swidler, & Tipton, 1985; Putnam, 1995).

Most large-scale contemporary institutions concerned with enhancing individual or community well-being (such as medical care, social services, and education) are characterized by increasingly bureaucratized and centralized models of social organization, with hierarchical forms of management by specialized experts (or technocrats). This form of organization tends to mediate the interpersonal social ties among the individuals working within them, the intersectoral linkages and cooperation among the diverse institutions, and the interdisciplinary collaboration and communication among the dominant professional groups within each (Coleman, 1993). The design of more effective and culturally sensitive programs and services for the most vulnerable must be grounded in more effective communication and collaboration between those intended to benefit and those charged with developing such programs.

Revisiting and Revivifying a Long-Standing Policymaking Paradigm: Community Participation and Empowerment

Community participation and empowerment have ostensibly been central components of the design of social and health programs in the United States as well as other countries (Aday, Begley, Lairson, & Slater, 1998).[1] The extent to which individuals affected by these initiatives have been fully involved in shaping them has, however, often been less than fully realized in practice. Public health and health promotion professionals have often imposed interventions they deem selected target communities or populations need, without either soliciting or fully taking into account what the affected groups and individuals may want or argue that program developers may claim that communities have been involved in shaping such interventions when there has actually been little or only token participation on the part of affected groups (Israel, Schulz, Parker, & Becker, 1998; Rissel, 1994; Robertson & Minkler, 1994; Wallerstein & Bernstein, 1994).

The discourse theory of contemporary German philosopher Jürgen Habermas (1995, 1996) provides a template for examining the nature of these exchanges and the aims and actions of the institutional and individual actors involved in them. For Habermas, communication directed toward mutual understanding among affected parties can best establish the foundations of trust and collaboration needed for solving the problems with which each is concerned, but perhaps from different points of view.

Habermas's discourse theory is most directly concerned with the extent to which those likely to be affected by decisions participate in shaping them (Habermas, 1996). The defining normative underpinning for Habermas's theory is grounded in his discourse principle: "Only those norms are valid to which all affected persons could agree as participants in rational discourse(s)" (Habermas, 1996, p. xxvi). "Rational discourse" in this case refers to communication directed toward mutual understanding rather than strictly ends-oriented or instrumental (technical-rational or strategic) aims. Habermas's discourse principle is grounded in fundamental democratic ideals, in which the power to govern is ultimately vested in the people and exercised by them directly or indirectly through a system of representation, involvement in a public political sphere, and free elections.

The discourse principle characterizes policy or development activities that are oriented toward gaining a reasonable consensus about the definition of the problem and how best to proceed to address it on the part of the stakeholders most likely to be affected by the resulting policy. Communication grounded in mutual respect between stakeholders is essential to ensuring the realization of this principle in the formulation of policy at both the micro- and macrolevels. For Habermas, the foundations of trust and collaboration required to be successful in addressing more instrumental aims are established through such "communicatively rational" discourse. These norms of deliberative justice would be attended to at the microlevel in forging effective patient-physician relationships, in shaping culturally sensitive service provision at the institutional level, and in ensuring the full participation of affected populations in the design of health policies and programs at the system and community levels (such as environmental justice or HIV/AIDS advocacy) (Charles & DeMaio, 1993; Labonte, 1993, 1994; Waitzkin, Britt, & Williams, 1994).

This philosophical and programmatic thrust as well as the parallel participatory action research agenda based in the writings of Brazilian social activist Paulo Freire (1970) are intended to listen to and learn from communities more fully. Communication with and the involvement of affected parties in the design and implementation of programs are essential. This emphasis acknowledges that by giving voice to concerns in their own syntax and semantics, they learn together how best to address them. This perspective is manifest in the formulation and implementation of community-based health education and health promotion initiatives (Wallerstein, 1992; Wallerstein & Bernstein, 1994).

Norman Daniels (1996, p. 10) has argued for incorporating the norms of "deliberative democracy" in developing managed care policies and procedures. He means that participation on the part of affected parties (such as patients and providers) must be ensured in decision making regarding how to protect normal functioning for a given population within defined resource constraints. This perspective would, for example, oppose the gag rule that inhibits physicians from providing full information to patients about their treatment options, make explicit and provide an opportunity to discuss the rationale for decisions about covering new technologies, and streamline patient grievance and dispute resolution procedures and make them less adversarial.

Empirical indicators of deliberative justice attempt to express the type and extent of involvement of affected groups' participation in formulating and implementing policies and programs. Arnstein (1969) conceptualized a ladder of citizen participation, with the respective rungs representing a gradient running from nonparticipation, to tokenism, to increasing levels of citizen power and control. Charles and DeMaio (1993) incorporated this and other dimensions (reflecting the perspective being adopted, that of a user versus a policymaker, as well as the decision-making domain, individual treatment, overall service provision, or macropolicy formulation) in constructing a framework for assessing lay participation in health care decision making. Promoting lay participation and empowerment has been a particular focus of health education and health promotion activities in the United States and Canada, as well as other countries (Labonte 1993, 1994; Robertson & Minkler, 1994). Related indicators, of particular relevance in the managed care context, would focus on the nature and quality of communication between patients and providers, the extent to which norms of deliberative democracy guide the development and organizational policies and procedures, and the magnitude of trust of health care providers or organizations on the part of consumers (Daniels, 1996; Mechanic, 1996a; Waitzkin, Britt, & Williams, 1994).

Community-oriented health policy would focus on the importance of affected groups' participation in the development of programs and resources to ameliorate the risks and consequences of vulnerability to poor physical, psychological, or social health at the patient-provider, institutional, and community levels.

Social and Economic Policy: Investing in Individuals and the Ties Between Them

Community-oriented health policy also acknowledges the central role that community-oriented social and economic, as well as medical care and public health, policies play in attenuating the risks and consequences of vulnerability through investing in individuals and the supportive ties among them.

Social Status

Employment opportunities and associated wage rates, particularly in the top-earning positions, continue to be more limited for women and minorities than for white males. Children are not in a position to organize and advocate as are adults or the elderly. The overt or covert use of violence is sanctioned in many families to reinforce the power-dominance relationships between males and females or parents and children.

Social and economic policy to ameliorate vulnerability would focus on mitigating the socially and legally sanctioned power and status differentials, based on age, gender, and racial or ethnic group membership. In the absence of a responsive social and legal infrastructure for addressing these claims, community-oriented social action is likely to be manifested in grassroots social movements (the civil rights and women's movements, for example) and related nonviolent (marches on Washington) and violent (the Los Angeles riots) public protests to bring attention to these claims.

Social Capital

The increase in the number of families in which infants and children are being raised by a single parent, young and elderly adults living alone, and new (or at least increasingly visible) forms of emotional and sexual intimacy manifest in relationships between "mingles" (individuals who are not married but are living with a sexual partner) or "long-time companions" calls for a renewed look at how social and economic policy might serve to enhance, rather than diminish, the prospect for social capital formation within such arrangements.

Family-centered policies represent a step toward this objective, whereby families could be defined to encompass the array of primary social units or households concerned with the mutual care and support of members. The strengthening of these units and the caring and nurturing functions they serve would be the focus of family-centered public policy. State and federal legislation to promulgate parental leave, child care, family preservation–oriented child welfare legislation, family-centered care for children with special needs, and caregiver respite alternatives are examples of more family-oriented social and economic and associated health care policies.

Related community-based efforts include attempts to build cooperative bridges between the variety of human and social services agencies and programs (such as schools, child welfare agencies, adult protective services, correctional systems, mental health, drug or alcohol treatment, and related domains) to address the needs of multiproblem families. Such initiatives recognize the importance of a holistic and multifaceted approach to the multidimensional functions of the family unit.

The initiatives that offer the greatest promise of success are ones in which neighborhood residents are directly involved in the needs identification and program development process. Having this grassroots investment is most likely to lead to programs that match community needs and catalyze the greatest measure of local ownership and participation. Perhaps equally or more important, the act of participation itself may serve to generate, discover, or strengthen informal networks of support (for child care, transportation, or respite, for example) between neighborhood residents to lighten their individual and collective burdens.

Human Capital

The availability of social capital directly affects the level of investments in human capital. Family or other social support is important in encouraging children to stay in school or assisting with child care, to facilitate individual family members' participation in the workforce. Household and per capita incomes are directly affected by the number, as well as earning power, of the individuals contributing to those revenues. Families and intimate social networks help to ensure that members have a home or a place to live.

Community-oriented social and economic policy acknowledges the importance of investing in community institutions and resources that are both indirectly and directly supportive of the generation of human capital. Recent decades have, however, seen a diminished, rather than enhanced, federal policy commitment in many of these domains, such as schools, jobs, housing, and associated family and individual economic safety nets.

Certain school-oriented investments may greatly increase social and human capital generation. Early childhood education programs, particularly those that encourage parental involvement and skills development, such as Head Start, have demonstrated significant short-term and long-term educational and social successes (in terms of better school performance, reduced dropout rates, and fewer teen pregnancies, for example). School-based clinics and associated parent-

and family-oriented multiservice programs (where mothers can get parenting or family planning advice or earn their general equivalency diploma, for example) offer opportunities to support young and single-parent families in developing parenting, educational, and job-related skills. The reform of federal, state, and local financing of public education could help to minimize the widely varying levels of investments in children in different communities. Per capita expenditures tend to be the least in those economically and socially segregated neighborhoods in which the children (low-income minorities) can least afford the diminished opportunities resulting from poor educational preparation.

Well-paying jobs sufficient to support themselves and their families are an increasingly illusive possibility for many Americans. Young, single-parent families and minority males have been most adversely affected by these trends. However, the experiences of college-educated married couples, both of whom must work to fulfill the American dream their parents accomplished on a single breadwinner's salary, as well as the high school graduate working full time whose earnings still fail to lift her family out of poverty, provide pervasive evidence of the impact of the changing nation's economy on U.S. families. States and municipalities could be encouraged to forge and strengthen partnerships for economic development among neighborhood organizations, local businesses, and governmental agencies. With support from federal and state sources, depressed communities and neighborhoods could organize community improvement and development councils to attract and retain new businesses. The design of these initiatives must take into account the norms of deliberative justice and the extent to which local governmental, business, and community interests are fully involved in the decision-making process more effectively than has been the case in the past.

Social and economic trends and policies have served to increase rather than diminish disparities in the distribution of income and wealth in U.S. society. Economic development efforts and initiatives to create new jobs would assist in remedying these disparities. The reduction of blocked opportunities to equal pay and positions in higher-paying sectors on the part of women and minorities could also be undertaken, as could human capital investments in education and jobs training for particularly at-risk groups. The minimum wage, unemployment, and transfer program benefits must be routinely assessed with respect to which they provide adequate economic safety for individuals and families. Expanding the earned income credit for families, as well as improving the enforcement of child support payments, would also contribute directly to enhancing the economic well-being of families with dependent children.

Renewed federal, state, and local governmental support, as well as encouragement of private sector involvement in developing low-income housing alternatives, would help to ameliorate the burgeoning crisis of homelessness. Community participation is essential in planning such initiatives, so that the integrity of existing neighborhoods, as well as the cooperation of adjoining ones, is ensured. Tearing down buildings in deteriorating areas by eminent domain and constructing either expensive high-rise middle-class or public welfare brick-and-mortar ghettos in their place will not necessarily solve the problem of affordable and habitable domiciles for low-income community residents. Supportive housing alternatives for many of the vulnerable populations examined here, such as the chronically ill elderly, the mentally ill, persons living with HIV/AIDS, and homeless persons, are urgently needed in many U.S. communities. Both local advocates and opponents must be encouraged to engage in dialogue about these options around the norm of community responsibility, to balance the voices of "NIMBY"-ism (that is, the not-in-my-backyard view) that are likely to characterize the response of residents in many U.S. neighborhoods.

Medical Care and Public Health Policy: Paying for the Future—A Shared Responsibility

The current array of programs and services to address the health and health care needs of vulnerable populations (such as high-risk mothers and infants, persons living with HIV/AIDS, substance abusers, and victims of family abuse) is underdeveloped and poorly integrated and poses substantial organizational and financial barriers to access in many U.S. communities. Furthermore, current methods of private and public third-party reimbursement tend to exacerbate rather than ameliorate these difficulties.

Sharply divided tiers of service exist for the vulnerable seen in publicly versus privately supported service sectors. This is particularly the case in the mental health and substance abuse fields, but is also increasingly the experience of persons living with HIV/AIDS and others for whom distinctly different doors are opened (or closed), based on how they intend (or, more important, whether they can afford) to pay for care.

Many face an imposing jungle of conflicting requirements and application procedures to establish eligibility for needed programs and services. Categorical funding streams and related financial incentives have tended to encourage the formation of competitive agencies or programs, operating in discrete noncollaborating sectors, rather than an integrated system of care for individuals in need of services from a variety of agencies or institutions.

A more community-oriented set of norms would attempt to encourage interagency cooperation around population- or client-centered goals. A number of programs focusing on different groups of the vulnerable (such as the Robert Wood Johnson Foundation and the Health Resources and Services Administration Health Care for the Homeless projects; National Institute of Mental Health Community Support Program and Child and Adolescent Service System Program; and the Robert Wood Johnson Foundation AIDS Health Services Program, among others) have encouraged the formation of community consortia of agencies and providers to facilitate the development of more integrated systems of caring for the most vulnerable. These initiatives may be viewed as bureaucratic surrogates, or in some cases, catalysts for the development of local, grassroots efforts to assist and support vulnerable community members. These consortia and related programs and experiences should be evaluated with respect to their success in developing these formal and informal community arrangements, as well as, and perhaps most important, whether outcomes were improved for the populations they were intended to serve.

Policy debates regarding reform of the U.S. medical care system have focused on alternatives for covering and paying for services. A plethora of proposals have emerged. Many attempt to reach near-universal coverage but differ primarily in the means for doing so. With the defeat of the Clinton health care reform initiative in the early 1990s, comprehensive health care reform was essentially stymied at the federal level. Nevertheless, a number of states have experimented with universal coverage strategies, including employer mandates or tax credits, and comprehensive cost containment strategies, such as statewide global budgets, single-payer systems, and managed competition. An increasing number of Medicaid-eligible individuals are enrolled in managed care arrangements. The Child Health Insurance Program has provided resources to states for extending Medicaid coverage and eligibility or facilitating the coverage of children and families who do not qualify under a state's Medicaid program.

Federal and state health care reforms can be evaluated with respect to the incentives or disincentives they provide for reducing or eliminating existing financial barriers to access, as well as for developing a more universal community-oriented continuum of programs and services to address the health and health care needs of vulnerable populations. Selected criteria proposed here relate to features of the plan itself, as well as the distribution of benefits and burdens between patients and providers.

Plan

Criteria for evaluating features of the plans are the universality of coverage, the provision of a decent basic minimum set of covered services, minimization of disparities between public and private tiers of payers, and the use of broad rather than narrow risk pools as a basis for determining premiums.

Plans that cover large population groups in a similar fashion and use a broad actuarial base in computing risks are most likely to ensure equity of access. The former minimizes the disparities in the type or extent of coverage provided, and the latter ensures that the burdens and benefits are spread more widely and evenly.

Need and effectiveness norms focus on whether certain procedures or services have been demonstrated in the aggregate to improve patient functioning or well-being. Such a perspective would underlie the entire range of preventive, treatment, and long-term care services for vulnerable populations. Existing and proposed models for providing and paying for care for the vulnerable should be evaluated in the context of their adequacy in providing a decent basic minimum set of services across this caregiving continuum.

Community rating refers to the fact that the basis for computing actuarial risks and the attendant impact on premiums is based on broad, rather than narrow, population groupings. Experience rating, in contrast, bases the rate setting on a narrowly defined group of eligibles. This latter strategy provides incentives to limit eligibility and enrollment to those who are likely to require the least or least expensive care, to keep the price of premiums down. The result is that those most in need (those with serious health problems or at risk of developing them, such as persons who are HIV positive) are likely to be excluded or charged very high rates for coverage. Carve-outs are a widely used option for covering and paying for services for groups that are likely to have disproportionately higher costs (such as those who are mentally ill or are being treated for substance abuse). The challenge is to determine rates of reimbursement that ensure adequate care to consumers, as well as reasonable coverage of costs to service providers.

Patients

The features to consider in minimizing financial barriers to access from the patient's point of view are the use of progressive (rather than regressive) methods for determining their contributions and limiting the amount that patients have to pay out of pocket. These are quite intimately linked, rather than discrete, criteria.

Health insurance premiums are relatively regressive methods of paying for medical care since they do not take into account the varying incomes or resources available to enrollees. Progressive taxation or related means of financing tied to ability to pay provide a more equitable basis for distributing the cost of coverage. The burden of out-of-pocket costs for medical care has traditionally fallen most heavily on those with the lowest incomes, for whom even a relatively small dollar outlay comprises a substantial proportion of their financial resources. Evidence from the RAND Health Insurance Experiment and Medical Outcomes Study suggest that increased cost sharing does reduce consumers' use of services (Brook et al., 1983; Ware et al., 1996). The findings also suggest that increased cost sharing may serve to ration more effective (preventive) rather than less effective (hospitalized) care. Restrictions, limitations, and managing care did not negatively affect the clinical outcomes of average patients, but the poor and elderly were adversely affected.

Provider

Plan features that serve to reduce the disincentives for providers to treat certain types of patients are using the same reimbursement rate regardless of who pays for the care (private versus public insurer, for example) and limiting or capping reimbursement across all providers.

One of the major dilemmas that has emerged with the current multitiered system of financing care is the widely varying rates of reimbursement to providers by different payers. The fact that the rates of Medicaid reimbursement in some states are lower than those of private insurers has resulted in a reduction in the number of providers who are willing to see Medicaid-eligible clients.

The maintenance of the usual and customary fee arrangements under Medicare and Medicaid have contributed significantly to the spiraling costs of medical care in the decades that followed. Diagnosis-related groups and physician relative-value-based reimbursement under Medicare are the major policy instruments that have been developed to deal with this issue in the public sector. These also represent means for standardizing the rates of reimbursement across providers seeing Medicare patients. Medical care systems in other countries, such as Canada, use more macro- rather micro-oriented approaches to limiting reimbursement, through negotiating global budgets and fee schedules with providers.

The assumption underlying these or other methods of capping provider reimbursement is that providers, not patients, are the main generators of demand for costly medical care services (hospitalizations, high-technology procedures, tests, pharmaceuticals, and so on). Cost-containment incentives need to be developed for these important medical care "consumers" as well. Capitation, negotiated fees, and carve-outs represent the principal means for limiting provider fees under managed care arrangements. The challenge in setting these rates is how to cover providers' aggregate costs effectively and not to introduce disincentives for providers to serve individuals whose care may not be fully reimbursed, many of who are the sickest and most vulnerable.

Synthesis of research on health maintenance organizations (HMOs) and other forms of managed care has confirmed that HMOs had lower hospital admission rates, shorter hospital lengths of stay, lower use of expensive procedures, and greater use of preventive services than traditional indemnity plans. Overall, enrollee satisfaction with services was lower in HMOs than traditional fee-for-service plans, but HMO enrollees reported greater satisfaction with costs (Blendon, Knox, Brodie, Benson, & Chervinsky, 1994; Mark & Mueller, 1996; Miller & Luft, 1994).

Growth in managed care and competition has dramatically altered economic incentives in health care. Providers have been induced to consider adopting more efficient means of production, reduce prices, and provide care demanded by consumers and payers. Physician practice continues to move toward more efficient personnel mix and scale, the average size hospital is increasing, very expensive and difficult services are being regionalized, and the number of HMO systems and their enrollments are increasing. These changes have reduced the rate of growth in cost, especially to employers. Other democratic, developed countries appear to have been more successful at controlling spending, insuring their populations, and achieving health outcomes in the past. Whether they are truly more efficient is impossible to determine from aggregate data. Even so, attaining cost control and access goals is an important social achievement. Emerging models of more community-oriented managed care, which point to a promising wedding of managed care and population health-oriented principles (described more fully in the discussion that follows), offer innovative alternatives for enhancing access, increasing efficiency, and improving health (Aday, Begley, Lairson, & Slater, 1998; Culyer, 1992; Lairson et al., 1997).

Community-Oriented Health Policy: Building a Community-Oriented Continuum of Care

Community-oriented health policy acknowledges that individuals' health and well-being are affected by the communities and families into which they are born and spend their lives, and it is to these social arrangements that people return after being discharged from the medical care system (Aday, 1997).[2] It attempts to bridge both the individual and community perspectives on vulnerability and to design programs and services to ameliorate the risks and consequences of poor physical, psychological, and social health.

A community-oriented health policy would encourage intersectoral linkages between the medical care and other human and social service resource development programs and services within a community; interdisciplinary collaboration between and among professionals in these institutions; and local leadership in developing and implementing programs to address the complex medical, psychological, social, and economic needs of the community. Features of such a policy are manifest in the formation of community-based organizations and consortia to develop programs and services for vulnerable populations, such as homeless persons, persons living with HIV/AIDS, and the chronically mentally ill; the promulgation of models of community organization and action for implementing the Public Health Objectives for the Nation; and the development of community or neighborhood health centers and community-oriented primary care models of service delivery. Client- or family-centered case management may also be a useful program component or complement to facilitate individuals' seeking and using relevant programs and services encompassed within a community-oriented continuum of care. Tables 5.1 through 5.9 in summarized the major types of programs and services that could be incorporated in such a continuum, including primary prevention-oriented, treatment-oriented, and long-term care services. Such a continuum provides a means for mitigating the risks that give rise to, as well as those that result from, being in poor health.

Primary prevention efforts include both community and public health programs and services. The risk of illness is greatest for those who have the fewest material and nonmaterial resources. Poverty and its associated deprivations and risks is a major correlate of poor birth outcomes in minority populations. The dramatic diminishment of low-income housing stock in many U.S. cities due to the combined policies of regentrification and the withdrawal of federal financial support are major contributors to homelessness. Lack of adequate family or social support compromises the ability of the chronically ill elderly to continue to live on their own. Addressing these fundamental correlates and consequences of vulnerability lies outside the traditional domain of medical care practice and policy. Their contribution to understanding the root causes of vulnerability, however, points to the broader policy and societal context in which vulnerability must be addressed.

The public health system has been the traditional focus of community interventions, particularly primary prevention-oriented programs (in the areas of lead paint abatement, HIV/AIDS education, and smoking cessation, among others), to address the health and health care needs of vulnerable populations. The Public Health Service's Health Objectives for the Nation define a comprehensive public health agenda that deals with a number of the vulnerable populations that have been the explicit focus of the book (such as high-risk mothers and infants, the chronically ill and disabled, alcohol or substance abusers, and suicide and homicide victims), as well those population subgroups most likely to be at risk (children, adolescents, elderly, and minorities).

Primary prevention efforts at the beginning of the care continuum are small relative to the resources devoted to the treatment of the physical, mental, and social consequences of poor pregnancy outcomes, chronic physical or mental illness, HIV/AIDS, alcohol and substance abuse, violence, and the conditions prevalent in particularly at-risk homeless and refugee populations. Similarly, at the other end of the continuum, long-term institutional and home and community-based care for vulnerable populations is an important but undeveloped and underfinanced component of needed programs and services.

The market-oriented approach to health care reform, which currently dominates state and federal health care reform, focuses on the management of and competition between discrete providers of services. It is manifest in the proliferation and consolidation of provider networks into integrated systems of delivering and financing medical care, which impose varying constraints on providers' fees and consumers' utilization of services. Applying community-oriented lenses to these developments would seek to illuminate the resultant distribution of and linkages among providers along a continuum of preventive, treatment, and long-term care services.

A community-oriented health policy to address the health and health care needs of vulnerable populations acknowledges the essential social origins and consequences of poor physical, psychological, and social functioning and the array of community-based, nonmedical social and community support services required to ameliorate both the risk and consequences of vulnerability. It also considers the distribution of programs and services across social and economic strata (defined by social status, social capital, or human capital resource differences) within the community. A broader set of goals and objectives is required to capture the full scope and impact of a community-oriented approach to health policy.

Such a policy seeks to surface and address the overt and covert attitudes and practices, reinforced by local and larger institutions (such as business, the media, governmental entities, and special interests), that constrain the regard, power, and opportunities accorded different age, gender, and racial and ethnic social status groups.

It simultaneously acknowledges, draws on, invests in, and generates the essential and important nonmaterial social capital resource by maximizing the participation of individuals and groups within the community in defining priorities and developing resources to address them.

It seeks to enlarge the human capital assets and investments (such as jobs, schools, housing, and other resources) that undergird and enrich the immediate and long-term productive potential of those who live, work, and raise and care for their families in those neighborhoods.

It envisions a blueprint and a team of architects, from the public and private sectors and affected communities, to undertake the design of a comprehensive, integrated, prevention-oriented continuum or system of programs and services accessible to all members of the community.

It embraces a comprehensive definition of health and well-being and embodies a restive, normative judgment of outcomes, motivated by assessments of the extent to which the health of the community as a whole, not just individual patients or clients within it, can be improved.

A central concern with the increasing dominance of the medical care environment by for-profit managed care entities is that the most vulnerable (especially those who are or are most likely to have the poorest health) are also most likely to be the ones these plans seek to exclude. The failure of federal health insurance reform and the diminished availability of employment-based coverage to many workers and their dependents raise serious concerns about the growing number of Americans without any form of private or public insurance coverage. Many of these individuals may be placed at substantial risk that providers' doors will be closed to them. Nonetheless, managed care–dominated reforms continue to transform the coverage and services provided to the employed and their dependents, as well as Medicaid- and Medicare-eligible individuals. The question then becomes what possibilities might exist for shaping them to serve the needs of the most vulnerable.

Evidence in more mature managed care–dominated markets suggests an increasing recognition on the part of managed care organizations that the entire community is their target population, as they increasingly penetrate these markets or experience high turnover in plan membership (Shortell, Gillies, & Anderson, 1994; Shortell, Gillies, Anderson, Erickson, & Mitchell, 1996). The Medicine/Public Health Initiative emanating from a historical national congress, sponsored by the American Medical Association and American Public Health Association in the spring of 1996, established an institutional foundation for developing fruitful collaborations between medicine and public health (Medicine/Public Health Initiative, 1999). An increased emphasis on population health also underlines the importance of upstream, primary prevention and the role of effective partnerships among managed care, public health, and other community entities and agencies in addressing the social determinants of health and ameliorating health risks (such as substance abuse or violence) that ultimately lead to increased health care costs (Kindig, 1997).

As public health departments and community providers come to define and redefine their unique role in these environments as well, the promise of a new form of medical care organization, representing a partnership between managed care and public health interests—community-oriented managed care—has emerged (Lairson et al., 1997; Starfield, 1996). Such entities begin to approximate what Showstack, Lurie, Leatherman, Fisher, and Inui (1996) have described as more "socially responsible managed care."

Community-oriented managed care has its counterpart in Canada, which has traditionally had a community health, but not a managed care, emphasis, as a comprehensive health care organization in selected areas in the province of Ontario. These entities have as a primary focus how the health of the population or community as a whole might be enhanced by an integrated array of medical and nonmedical programs and services. A central component of health care reform in Canada is involving affected individuals and subpopulations in the planning and management of the health system. The development of regional authorities is one of the main avenues used in the various provinces in translating the principle of participation into practice (Charles & DeMaio, 1993; Mhatre & Deber, 1992).

Managed care, and particularly for-profit managed care systems, are likely to dominate health care service provision increasingly in the public and private sectors in the United States. Models of managed care currently dominating the medical care marketplace cannot, however, be accurately characterized as being substantially leavened with essences of a more community- or population-oriented perspective on health and health care—in either the macrocosm of strategic planning and system design or the microcosm of practice. However, it may be that their success in a mature managed care environment might lie with attending to this perspective in their overall missions and designs. Undergirding such reforms may well be the development of innovative modes of state, local, and perhaps federal financing and risk-sharing arrangements, to ensure that the uninsured and the most vulnerable may also be desired and sought-after segments of the market. The charge to the public health and health services research communities that remains is nonetheless to monitor and evaluate the promises and outcomes of these dramatic changes for the health and health care of the most vulnerable (Aday, 1997).

Conclusion

The arguments and evidence presented throughout this book pose the question of what allocation of medical and nonmedical investments may be most beneficial for enhancing Americans' health and well-being. The answer provided here from the point of view of community-oriented health policy is that human and social capital and the families and communities in which these resources are both generated and consumed should be the primary focus of public and private investments in Americans' individual and collective well-being. It compels ensuring the full participation of U.S. families and communities in shaping their collective welfare. This perspective considers the universal investments to facilitate this developmental process, as well as the specific entitlements required to open more windows of opportunity for the most vulnerable. A community-oriented point of view reconsiders the extent to which hierarchical, bureaucratic, professionally dominated forms of organization are the best or most effective methods for addressing multifaceted human and social needs. It calls for an evaluation of needed preventive medical care and public health investments and scrutinizes the incentives and disincentives built into existing and proposed systems of organizing and financing medical care in the United States for reducing the risk of poor physical, psychological, and social health.

Ultimately this perspective argues that the remedies for our individual and collective vulnerability are found in the bonds of caring human communities.

Notes

1. Selected material in this section was drawn from Aday, Begley, Lairson, & Slater (1998). Used with permission from *Evaluating the Healthcare System: Effectiveness, Efficiency, and Equity, 2nd Edition*, by L. A. Aday, C. E. Begley, D. R. Lairson, & C. H. Slater (Chicago: Health Administration Press, 1998).
2. Selected material in this section was drawn from Aday (1997). "*Vulnerable populations: A community-oriented perspective.*" Used with permission from *Family and Community Health, 19*(4), 1–18 (Gaithersburg, MD: Aspen Publishers, 1997).

RESOURCE A

NATIONAL DATA SOURCES
ON VULNERABLE POPULATIONS

RESOURCE A. NATIONAL DATA SOURCES ON VULNERABLE POPULATIONS.

Agency and data source	Universe/sample	Vulnerable Populations								
		MCH	CHR	PWA	MEN	SAB	S&H	FAB	HOM	REF
Agency for Healthcare Research and Quality AIDS Cost and Services Utilization Survey (ACSUS)	Sample of AIDS providers and patients in different geographical locations (1992)			X						
HIV Cost and Services Utilization Study (HCSUS)	Nationally representative sample of people in care for HIV infection (1996–1999)			X						
National Medical Care Expenditure Survey (NMCES)	Sample of U.S. civilian noninstitutionalized population, plus physicians, facilities, and employers providing them care or coverage (1977–1979)		X		X					
National Medical Expenditure Survey (NMES)	Sample of U.S. civilian noninstitutionalized population, American Indians and Alaskan natives, plus physicians, facilities, and insurers providing them care or coverage (1987)		X		X					
Medical Expenditure Panel Survey (MEPS)	Sample of U.S. civilian noninstitutionalized population, plus providers, insurers, employers, and nursing homes providing them care or coverage (1996)		X		X					
American Humane Association and National Center on Child Abuse and Neglect National Study on Child Neglect and Abuse Reporting	Child maltreatment reports from state child protective service personnel (1976–1987)							X		
American School Health Association National Adolescent Student Health Survey (NASHS)	National sample of eighth- and tenth-grade students from public and private schools (1987)		X	X		X	X			
Centers for Disease Control and Prevention Behavioral Risk-Factor Surveillance System (BRFSS)	Sample of populations, initially in selected states (by 1994 all states, three territories) and Washington, D.C., with phones (1984–present)	X	X	X		X	X			

Survey	Description					
HIV/AIDS Surveillance System	All AIDS cases and deaths reported in 50 states, Washington, D.C., U.S. dependencies and possessions (1981–present); cases of HIV infection, not AIDS, reported by states with confidential HIV reporting systems, 32 reporting areas by 1999 (1991–present)		X			
HIV Seroprevalence Surveys	HIV seroprevalence tests in selected years and selected sentinel sites (such as STD clinics, drug treatment centers, women's health centers, and other) throughout the United States (1989–present)		X			
Pregnancy Risk Assessment Monitoring System (PRAMS)	Sample of new mothers in participating states, 18 in 1999 (1988–present)	X				
Youth Risk Behavior Surveillance System Alternative High School Youth Risk Behavior Survey (ALT-YRBS)	Sample of students in grades 9–12 who attend alternative high schools in the fifty states and Washington, D.C. (1998)		X		X	X
Household-based survey	National sample of youth and young adults aged 12–21 years, whether enrolled in school or not (1992)		X		X	X
National College Health Risk Behavior Survey (NCHRBS)	Sample of undergraduate students (1995)		X		X	X
Youth Risk Behavior Survey (YRBS)	Sample of students in grades 9–12 in public and private schools in the fifty states and Washington, D.C., at national level, and within some states, cities, and territories (1991–present, biennially)		X		X	X
Health Care Financing Administration National Long-Term Care Survey (NLTCS)	Sample of disabled Medicare population (baseline–1982, 1984, 1989, 1994, 1999)		X	X		
Medicare Current Beneficiary Survey (MCBS)	Representative national sample of the Medicare population (1991–present)		X			
International Center for the Disabled (ICD)	Sample of U.S. civilian noninstitutionalized disabled population 16+ (1986)		X			

RESOURCE A. *(Continued)*

Agency and data source	Universe/sample	Vulnerable Populations MCH	CHR	PWA	MEN	SAB	S&H	FAB	HOM	REF
National Center on Child Abuse and Neglect										
Study of National Incidence and Prevalence of Child Abuse and Neglect	Child maltreatment reports from community professionals in child protective services and other agencies in a sample of U.S. counties (1980, 1986, 1993)							X		
National Child Abuse and Neglect Data System (NCANDS)	Child maltreatment reports from state child protective service personnel (1990–present)							X		
National Center on Elder Abuse										
Survey of the States on Domestic Elder Abuse	Survey of adult protective service and state units on aging in fifty states, Washington, D.C., Guam, Puerto Rico, and Virgin Islands (1986–present)							X		
National Center for Health Statistics and Centers for Disease Control and Prevention										
Hispanic Health and Nutrition Examination Survey (HHANES)	Sample of Hispanics six months–seventy-four years in five states and two localities with large Hispanic populations (1982–1984)		X		X	X				
National Ambulatory Medical Care Survey (NAMCS)	Sample of nonfederal office-based physicians and visits (annually 1974–1981, 1985, 1989 to present, annually)		X		X	X				
National Health and Nutrition Examination Survey (NHANES)	Survey of selected age groups of U.S. noninstitutionalized population (1960–1962, 1963–1965, 1966–1970, 1971–1974, 1976–1980 with follow-up 1982–1984, and 1988–1994; annually, beginning in 1999)		X		X	X				
National Health Interview Survey (NHIS)	Sample of U.S. noninstitutionalized population (1957–present, annually)	X	X	X	X	X				
National Home and Hospice Care Survey (NHHCS)	Sample of health agencies and hospices in the United States (1992, 1993, 1994, 1996)		X							

Survey / System	Sample description				
National Hospital Ambulatory Medical Care Survey (NHAMCS)	Sample of visits by patients to hospital emergency rooms and outpatient departments (1992–present, annually)			X	X
National Hospital Discharge Survey (NHDS)	Sample of discharges from U.S. hospitals (1964–present)			X	X
National Immunization Survey (NIS)	Sample of children 19–35 months of age in households with phones, and vaccination providers in the United States (1994–present)		X		
National Linked File of Live Births and Infant Deaths	Linked birth and death records (birth cohort linked 1983–1991, period linked 1995–1996)		X	X	
National Maternal and Infant Health Survey and Longitudinal Follow-up Survey	Sample of death, birth, and fetal death records (1988) and follow-up (1991)		X	X	
National Nursing Home Survey	Sample of nursing homes, residents, and employees (1973–1974, 1977, 1985, 1995, 1997)		X	X	
National Survey of Family Growth	Sample of women 15–44 years of age—U.S. civilian noninstitutionalized population (1973, 1976, 1982, 1988, 1995)		X	X	
National Vital Statistics System					
Mortality Statistics	State death certificates	X	X	X	X
Natality Statistics	State birth certificates	X	X		
Survey of Children with Special Health Care Needs	Sample of children under 4–35 months of age in households with phones (2000)	X			
Survey of Families with Young Children	Sample of children under 18 years of age in households with phones (2000)	X	X		
National Center for Health Statistics and Centers for Disease Control and Prevention and Health Care Financing Administration					
National Medical Care Utilization and Expenditure Survey (NMCUES)	Sample of U.S. civilian noninstitutionalized population and Medicaid enrollees in California, Michigan, New York, and Texas (1980–1981)		X	X	

RESOURCE A. (Continued)

Agency and data source	Universe/sample	MCH	CHR	PWA	MEN	SAB	S&H	FAB	HOM	REF
				Vulnerable Populations						
National Institute of Child Health and Human Development										
National Longitudinal Study on Adolescent Health (Add Health)	School students, grades 7–12, from a nationally representative sample of high schools, and their feeder schools, and parents, peers, and school administrators (1994–1996)	X	X	X			X			
National Institute on Alcohol Abuse and Alcoholism, Division of Biometry and Epidemiology										
Alcohol Epidemiologic Data System (AEDS)	Surveillance data on alcohol consumption, alcohol-related condition and deaths (1977–present)					X				
National Longitudinal Alcohol Epidemiologic Survey (NLAES)	Sample of civilian, noninstitutionalized adults, age 18+ in the forty-eight contiguous states and Washington, D.C. (1992)					X				
National Institute on Drug Abuse										
Community Epidemiology Working Group (CEWG)	Surveillance of patterns and trends in drug abuse in major U.S. cities (1976–present)					X				
Drug Abuse Treatment Outcome Study (DATOS)	Sample of individuals in selected drug treatment programs in eleven cities (1991–1993)					X				
Monitoring the Future (MTF)	National sample of eighth-, tenth-, and twelfth-grade students and follow-up of subsamples of young adults (1975–present)					X				
National Institute of Mental Health										
Epidemiological Catchment Area (ECA) Program Surveys	Sample of population in mental health service catchment areas in New Haven, Connecticut (1980–1981), Baltimore (1981–1982), St. Louis (1981–1982), Durham, North Carolina (1982–1983), Los Angeles (1983–1984)				X	X	X	X		

Survey	Description					
National Youth Survey	National sample of juveniles 11–17 and their parents (1976) plus follow-up (1977–1980, 1983, 1987, 1994)	X	X	X		
National Surveys of Family Violence	Sample of members of U.S. families (1976, 1986)			X		
Office of Refugee Resettlement Annual Survey of Refugees	Sample of U.S. refugees (1975–present)					X
RAND Corporation Medical Outcomes Study (MOS)	Sample of physicians in four regions plus patients seen in five-day screening period and those with tracer conditions (1986–1989)	X	X			
Substance Abuse and Mental Health Services Administration Alcohol and Drug Services Study (ADSS)	National sample of substance abuse treatment programs—facilities, providers and clients (1997–1999)	X				
Client/Patient Sample Survey of Inpatient, Residential and Less Than 24-Hour Care Programs	Sample of clients admitted, readmitted, discharged, and transferred into and out of organized mental health settings (1997), plus those under active care as of May 1, 1997	X	X			
Drug Abuse Warning Network (DAWN)	Sample of nonfederal, short-stay, general hospitals that have a 24-hour emergency department in the coterminous United States, and medical examiner facilities in metropolitan areas throughout the coterminous United States (1972–present)	X				
Drug Services Research Survey (DSRS)	National sample of drug treatment providers and clients (1989–1990)	X				
Inventory of Mental Health Organizations and General Hospital Mental Health Services (IMHO/IGHMHS)	Complete enumeration surveys of all specialty mental health organizations (1986–present, biennially)	X				

RESOURCE A. *(Continued)*

Agency and data source	Universe/sample	Vulnerable Populations								
		MCH	CHR	PWA	MEN	SAB	S&H	FAB	HOM	REF
Substance Abuse and Mental Health Services Administration *(Continued)*										
National Household Survey on Drug Abuse (NHSDA)	Sample of U.S. civilian noninstitutionalized population, 12+ (1972–present)					X				
NHSDA Module on Mental Health	Sample of U.S. civilian noninstitutionalized population, 12+ (1994, 1996, 1997)				X					
Services Research Outcomes Study (SROS)	Follow up to the DSRS (1995–1996)					X				
State Alcohol and Drug Abuse Profile (SADAP)	Sample of alcohol and/or drug treatment programs in fifty states, Washington, D.C., and U.S. territories (1982–present)					X				
Treatment Episode Data Set (TEDS)	Data from the states on treatment admissions to substance abuse treatment facilities eligible for state and/or federal funding (1989–present, annually)					X				
Uniform Facility Data Set (UFDS) Survey	Sample of substance abuse treatment facilities and state-identified prevention and education facilities, and development of the National Drug and Alcoholism Treatment Unit Survey (annually, 1995–present)					X				
Substance Abuse and Mental Health Services Administration and National Institute of Mental Health										
National Comorbidity Survey (NCS)	Nationally representative sample of the U.S. civilian noninstitutionalized population, aged 15–54, living in the forty-eight conterminous states (1991)				X	X				
U.S. Bureau of the Census										
Census Count of the Homeless	Counts and characteristics of people at preidentified selected locations, where homeless persons usually gather, on "Shelter and Street Night" (March 20–21, 1990)								X	

Data source	Description							
Current Population Survey (CPS)	Longitudinal monthly survey of sample of U.S. civilian noninstitutionalized population						X	
Survey of Income and Program Participation (SIPP)	Longitudinal panel survey of U.S. civilian noninstitutionalized population (1984–present)						X	
U.S. Conference of Mayors City Surveys of Hunger and Homelessness	Surveys of city officials in cities on U.S. Conference of Mayors Task Force on Hunger and Homelessness (1982–present)	X					X	
U.S. Department of Defense Worldwide Surveys of Substance Abuse and Health Behaviors among Military Personnel	Sample of U.S. active duty military personnel in the army, navy, marines, and air force (1980, 1982, 1985, 1988, 1992, 1995, 1998)			X	X	X	X	
U.S. Department of Justice, Bureau of Justice Statistics National Crime Victimization Survey (NCVS)	Sample of U.S. civilian noninstitutionalized population, 12+ (1973–present, with major redesign in the early 1990s)		X	X	X			
Survey of Adults on Probation (SAP)	Nationally representative sample of adult probationers (1995)		X	X	X	X		
Survey of Inmates in Federal Correctional Facilities (SIFCF)	Nationally representative sample of inmates in federal prisons (1991, 1997)		X	X	X	X		
Survey of Inmates in Local Jails (SILJ)	Nationally representative sample of inmates in local jails (1978, 1983, 1989, 1996)		X	X	X	X		
Survey of Inmates in State Correctional Facilities (SISCF)	Nationally representative sample of inmates in state prisons (1974, 1979, 1986, 1991, 1997)		X	X	X	X		
U.S. Department of Justice, Federal Bureau of Investigation Uniform Crime Reports (UCR)/Supplementary Homicide Reports (SHR)	Arrest data from city, county, state law enforcement agencies (1930–present)			X	X			

RESOURCE A. *(Continued)*

Agency and data source	Universe/sample	Vulnerable Populations								
		MCH	CHR	PWA	MEN	SAB	S&H	FAB	HOM	REF
U.S. Department of Justice, Immigration and Naturalization Service										
Statistical Yearbook of the Immigration and Naturalization Service	Compilation of immigration statistics from entry visas and change-of-immigration-status forms (annual)									X
U.S. Department of Justice, National Institute of Justice, Bureau of Justice Assistance										
Arrestee Drug Abuse Monitoring Program (ADAM)	Sample of arrestees/detainees in twenty-three cities, and replacement and expansion of drug use forecasting (1997–present)				X	X				
Drug Use Forecasting (DUF)	Quota of male and female arrestees and juvenile arrestees/detainees in twenty-three cities (1986–1996)				X	X				

Note: MCH = high-risk mothers and infants; CHR = chronically ill and disabled; PWA = persons living with HIV/AIDS; MEN = mentally ill and disabled; SAB = alcohol or substance abusers; S&H = suicide or homicide prone; FAB = abusing families; HOM = homeless persons; REF = immigrants and refugees.

RESOURCE B

SOURCE NOTES ON THE DATA TABLES

Table 2.1

1. 1970, 1975, 1980, 1985, 1988–1996: NCHS, 1998c, Table 11 (p. 181). 1986–1987: NCHS, 1996b, Table 11 (p. 90). 1997: NCHS, 1999d, Table 11 (p. 119).
2. 1970, 1980, 1985, 1988–1996: NCHS, 1998c, Table 23 (p. 193). 1975, 1986–1987: NCHS, 1994c, Table 20 (pp. 82–83). 1997: NCHS, 1999d, Table 22 (p. 132).
3. 1970, 1975, 1980, 1985, 1988–1996: NCHS, 1998c, Table 6 (p. 176). 1986–1987: NCHS, 1996b, Table 7 (p. 86). 1997: NCHS, 1999d, Table 6 (p. 114).
4. 1970, 1980, 1985, 1990–1996: NCHS, 1998c, Table 2 (pp. 172–173). 1975, 1986–1989: NCHS, 1994c, Table 3 (p. 64). 1997: NCHS, 1999d, Table 3 (pp. 110–111).
5. 1970, 1980, 1985, 1990, 1993–96: NCHS, 1998c, Table 45 (p. 245). 1975: NCHS, 1979, Table 1–15 (p. 1–73). 1986, 1987: NCHS, 1993, Table 41 (p. 73). 1988, 1989, 1991, 1992: NCHS, 1995a, Table 45 (p. 128). 1997: NCHS, 1999d, Table 44 (p. 184).

Table 2.2

1. 1970, 1980, 1985, 1990, 1993–1996: NCHS, 1998c, Table 31 (pp. 203–206). 1991–1992: NCHS, 1996b, Table 30 (pp. 110–111). 1985–1989: NCHS, 1993, Table 28 (pp. 45–46). 1975: NCHS, 1983, Table 28 (pp. 105–106). 1997: NCHS, 1999d, Table 30 (pp. 142–145).
2. 1985: NCHS, 1986, Table 57 (pp. 82–83). 1986: NCHS, 1987, Table 57 (pp. 85–86). 1987: NCHS, 1988a, Table 57 (pp. 84–85). 1988: NCHS, 1989a, Table 57 (pp. 84–85). 1989: NCHS, 1990a, Table 57 (pp. 83–84). 1990: NCHS, 1991a, Table 57 (pp. 82–83). 1991: NCHS, 1992a, Table 57 (pp. 82–83). 1992: NCHS, 1994a, Table 57 (pp. 83–84). 1993: NCHS, 1994b, Table 57 (pp. 82–83). 1994: NCHS, 1996a, Table 57 (pp. 81–82). 1995: NCHS, 1998a, Table 57 (pp. 77–78). 1996: NCHS, 1999b, Table 57 (pp. 81–82).
3. 1975, 1980: NCHS, 1982, Table 27 (p. 80). 1985, 1990: NCHS, 1992b, Table 59 (p. 200).

1986, 1991: NCHS, 1993, Table 61 (p. 99). 1987, 1992: NCHS, 1994c, Table 69 (p. 153). 1988: NCHS, 1990b, Table 50 (p. 162). 1989: NCHS, 1991b, Table 52 (p. 121). 1993: NCHS, 1995a, Table 62 (p. 153). 1994: NCHS, 1997, Table 62 (p. 180). 1995: NCHS, 1998c, Table 60 (p. 271). 1996: NCHS, 1999d, Table 59 (p. 210).

4. 1991–1992: McNeil, 1999a. 1994–1995: McNeil, 1999b.

5. 1977: NCHS, 1995b, Table 3 (pp. 287–290). 1985, ADLs: NCHS, 1989c, Table 28 (p. 38). 1985, IADLs: NCHS, 1999g. 1995, ADLs and IADLs: NCHS, 1999h.

Table 2.3

1. Centers for Disease Control and Prevention, 1998a, Tables 1, 2 (pp. 310–311).

2. 1989: Centers for Disease Control and Prevention, 1990a (pp. 6, 8, 10, 12, 14, 15, 19, 20, 22, 23). 1990: Centers for Disease Control and Prevention, 1992 (pp. 7, 9, 12, 14, 19, 22, 23, 24, 26, 27). 1992: Centers for Disease Control and Prevention, 1994b (pp. 17, 20, 27, 32). 1993: Centers for Disease Control and Prevention, 1995 (pp. 8, 9). 1997: Centers for Disease Control and Prevention, 1998b (pp. 5, 6).

3. Total number, under 13, 13+. 1986–1989, 1991: NCHS, 1993, Table 53 (p. 89). 1985, 1990, 1992–1996: NCHS, 1998c, Table 55 (p. 265). 1997: NCHS, 1999d, Table 54 (p. 204). 1998, Cumulative total: Centers for Disease Control and Prevention, 1999b, Table 5 (p. 14). Number by transmission category, 13+: 1986–1989, 1991: NCHS, 1993, Table 55 (pp. 91–92). 1985, 1990, 1992–1996: NCHS, 1998c, Table 56 (pp. 266–267). 1997: NCHS, 1999d, Table 55 (pp. 205–206).

4. 1985–1997, counts of death in persons with HIV/AIDS: Centers for Disease Control and Prevention, 1998c, Table 13 (p. 19). 1993–1998, estimated deaths of persons with AIDS: Centers for Disease Control and Prevention, 1999a, Table 28 (p. 37).

5. 1997, death rates for HIV infection: NCHS, 1999d, Table 43 (pp. 182–183). 1987–1996, death rates for HIV infection: NCHS, 1998c, Table 44 (pp. 243–244).

Table 2.4

1. 1991: Kessler et al., 1994, Table 2 (p. 12). 1994: Substance Abuse and Mental Health Services Administration, 1996, Table 3A.2 (p. 67). 1996: Substance Abuse and Mental Health Services Administration, 1998b, Table 12.4 (p. 177). 1997: Substance Abuse and Mental Health Services Administration, 1999c, Table 13.5 (p. 189).

Table 2.5

1. Rouse, 1998 (p. 112).

Table 2.6

1. NCHS, 1999g. NCHS, 1999h.

Table 2.7

1. Age 12+, 1979, 1985, 1991–1998: Substance Abuse and Mental Health Services Administration, 1999e, Table 4B (p. 65), Table 5B (p. 67). Age 12+, 1982, 1988, 1990: Substance Abuse and Mental Health Services Administration, 1998b, Table 2.3 (p. 30), Table 2.4 (p. 31).
2. Ages 12–17, 18–25, 26–34, 35+, 1997, 1998: Substance Abuse and Mental Health Services Administration, 1999e, Table 7 (p. 69), Table 8 (p. 70), Table 9 (p. 71), Table 10 (p. 72). Ages 12–17, 18–25, 26–34, 35+, 1979–1996: Substance Abuse and Mental Health Services Administration, 1998b, Table 2.6 (p. 33), Table 2.7 (p. 34), Table 2.8 (p. 35).
3. Johnston, O'Malley, & Bachman, 1999, Tables 5.2, 5.3, 5.4 (pp. 129–131).
4. 1985–1993: Indian Health Service, 1998, Table 4.29 (p. 96). Indian Health Service, 1999.
5. 1985–1988: Substance Abuse and Mental Health Services Administration, 1994 (p. 50). 1989–1990: Substance Abuse and Mental Health Services Administration, 1998a, Table 2 (p. 32). 1997–1998: Substance Abuse and Mental Health Services Administration, 1999f, Table 2 (p. 58).

Table 2.8

1. 1950, 1970, 1980, 1985, 1990, 1994–1997: NCHS, 1999d, Tables 46 and 47 (pp. 189–194). 1989, 1991–1993: NCHS, 1996b, Tables 46 and 47 (pp. 149–154). 1986–1988: NCHS, 1991b, Tables 34 and 35 (pp. 97–100). 1975: NCHS, 1980, Table 14 (p. 137).

Table 2.9

1. 1980–1987: American Humane Association, 1989, Figure 1 (p. 5), Figure 2 (p. 6). 1990–1996: Administration for Children, Youth and Families, National Center on Child Abuse and Neglect, 1999. 1997: Administration for Children, Youth and Families, Children's Bureau, 1999, Table E-2 (p. E-4).
2. Sedlak & Broadhurst, 1996, Table 3–1 (p. 3–3), Table 3–3 (p. 3–18).
3. 1986–1996: Tatara & Kuzmeskus, 1997 (p. 12).
4. Greenfeld et al., 1998 (p. 37).

Table 2.10

1. U.S. Department of Housing and Urban Development, 1984 (p. 19).
2. Burt & Cohen, 1989, Table 2.3 (p. 29), p. 32.
3. Burt & Aron, 2000, slides 9, 10.
4. National Alliance to End Homelessness, 1988 (p. 2).

Table 2.11

1. 1961–1970, 1971–1980, immigrants and refugees: U.S. Bureau of the Census, 1991, Tables 7 and 10 (pp. 10–11). 1981–1990, 1991–1997, immigrants; 1981–1990, 1991–1996,

refugees: U.S. Bureau of the Census, 1999e, Tables 8 and 9 (pp. 11–12). 1997, 1998, refugees; 1998, immigrants: U.S. Bureau of the Census, 1999b, Table 1 (p. 7), Table 2 (p. 8).

Table 3.1

1. Age groups, 1985: NCHS, 1988c, Table 1–39 (p. 65), Table 1–81 (pp. 237–238). Age groups, 1997: NCHS, 1999a, Table 45 (pp. 75–76). Race, 1985, 1997: NCHS, 1999d, Table 11 (pp. 119).
2. Race, black and white, 1985, 1997: NCHS, 1999d, Table 22 (p. 132). Race, Native American, 1985: Indian Health Service, 1998, Table 3.9 (p. 50). Race, Native American, 1997: Indian Health Service, 1999. Race, Hispanic, 1997: NCHS, 1998b, Table 26 (p. 82).
3. Age groups, 1985: NCHS, 1988c, Table 1–44 (pp. 70–72). Age groups, 1997: NCHS, 1999a, Table 33 (pp. 60–61). Race, 1985, 1997: NCHS, 1999d, Table 6 (p. 114).
4. Race: NCHS, 1999d, Table 3 (pp. 110–111).
5. Race—white, black, Hispanic: NCHS, 1999d, Table 44 (p. 184). Race, Native American, 1985: Indian Health Service, 1998, Table 3.7 (p. 46). Race, Native American, 1997: Indian Health Service, 1999.

Table 3.2

1. NCHS, 1999d, Table 37 (pp. 164–166), Table 38 (pp. 167–169), Table 39 (pp. 170–173), Table 42 (pp. 179–181).
2. 1985: NCHS, 1986, Tables 57, 58, 59 (pp. 82–87). 1996: NCHS, 1999b, Tables 57, 58, 59 (pp. 81–86).
3. 1985: NCHS, 1992b, Table 59 (p. 200). 1996: NCHS, 1999d, Table 59 (p. 210).
4. 1991–1992: McNeil, 1999a. 1994–1995: McNeil, 1999b.
5. 1985, ADLs: NCHS, 1989c, Table 28 (p. 38). 1985, IADLs: NCHS, 1999g. 1995, ADLs and IADLs: NCHS, 1999h.

Table 3.3

1. Centers for Disease Control and Prevention, 1998a, Table 2 (p. 311).
2. Centers for Disease Control and Prevention, 1999a, <13: Table 5 (p. 12, gender), and Table 15 (p. 22, race and ethnicity); 13+: Table 5 (p. 12, gender); and Tables 9 and 11 (pp. 16, 18, race and ethnicity).
3. Centers for Disease Control and Prevention, 1999a, Table 19 (p. 28).
4. NCHS, 1999d, Table 43 (pp. 182–183).

Table 3.4

1. 1997: Substance Abuse and Mental Health Services Administration, 1999c, Table 13.5 (p. 189).

Table 3.5

1. Rouse, 1998 (pp. 104, 106, 108, 110).

Table 3.6

1. NCHS, 1999g. NCHS, 1999h.

Table 3.7

1. 1985 (adjusted), past month use of any illicit drug, marijuana, cocaine, alcohol, cigarettes: Substance Abuse and Mental Health Services Administration, 1998c, Table 11 (p. 73), Table 12 (p. 74), Table 13 (p. 75), Table 14 (p. 76), Table 17 (p. 79). 1985 (adjusted), past year use of any illicit drug, marijuana, cocaine, alcohol, cigarettes: Substance Abuse and Mental Health Services Administration, 1997, Table 2.2 (p. 2–17). 1998, any illicit drug, marijuana and hashish, alcohol, cigarettes (past year), crack, hallucinogens (past year and past month by sex and race): Substance Abuse and Mental Health Services Administration, 1999d, Tables 2A–2D (pp. 19–21), Tables 3A–3D (pp. 25–27), Tables 4A–4D (pp. 31–33), Tables 5A–5D (pp. 37–39), Tables 7A–7D (pp. 49–51), Tables 13A–13D (pp. 85–87), Tables 14A–14D (pp. 91–93). 1998, any illicit drug, marijuana and hashish, cocaine, alcohol, cigarettes (past month by adult education): Substance Abuse and Mental Health Services Administration, 1999e, Tables 19–22, 25 (pp. 82–85, 88).
2. 1985, 1998: Johnston, O'Malley, & Bachman, 1999, Table 4–6 (pp. 79–81), Table 4–7 (pp. 82–84), Table 4–9 (pp. 86–88), Table D-2 (p. 371), Table D-6 (p. 375), Table D-8 (p. 377), Table D-10 (p. 379), Table D-14 (p. 383), Table D-16 (p. 385), Table D-28 (p. 397), Table D-34 (p. 403), Table D-36 (p. 405).
3. Indian Health Service, 1998, Table 4.29 (p. 96), Table 4.30 (p. 98).
4. Substance Abuse and Mental Health Services Administration, 1999f, Table 18 (p. 74), Table 22 (p. 78).

Table 3.8

1. 1997: NCHS, 1999d, Tables 46 and 47 (pp. 189–194).

Table 3.9

1. Administration for Children, Youth and Families, Children's Bureau, 1999 (pp. D14-D17).
2. Sedlak, Hantman, & Schultz, 1997: Harm standard: sex, Tables A-3A, A-3B (pp. A-4–A-8); age, Tables A-4A, A-4B (pp. A-9–A-21); race, Tables A-5A, A-5B (pp. A-22–A-28); income, Tables A-6A, A-6B (pp. A-29–A-35); family structure, Tables A-11A, A-11B (pp. A-56–A-66); endangerment standard: sex, Tables B-3A, B-3B (pp. B-4–B-8); age, Tables B-4A, B-4B (pp. B-9–B-21); race, Tables B-5A, B-5B (pp. B-22–B-28); income, Tables B-6A, B-6B (pp. B-29–B-35); family structure, Tables B-11A, B-11B (pp. B-56–B-66).

3. Tatara & Kuzmeskus, 1997, Table 9 (p. 22), Table 10 (p. 23), Table 11 (p. 24).
4. Greenfeld et al., 1998 (p. 43).

Table 3.10

1. Burt et al., 1999, Table 2.1 (p. 14).

Table 3.11

1. 1961–1970, 1971–1980: U.S. Bureau of the Census, 1991, Tables 7 and 10 (pp. 10–11).
1981–1990, 1991–1996: U.S. Bureau of the Census, 1999e, Tables 8 and 9 (pp. 11–12).

REFERENCES

Abbott, J. (1997). Injuries and illnesses of domestic violence. *Annals of Emergency Medicine, 29*(6), 781–785.

Achté, K. (1988). Suicidal tendencies in the elderly. *Suicide and Life-Threatening Behavior, 18,* 55–65.

Ackerman, L. K. (1997). Health problems of refugees. *Journal of the American Board of Family Practice, 10*(5), 337–348.

Adamek, M. E., & Kaplan, M. S. (1996). Managing elder suicide: A profile of American and Canadian crisis prevention centers. *Suicide and Life-Threatening Behavior, 26*(2), 122–131.

Aday, L. A. (1997). Vulnerable populations: A community-oriented perspective. *Family and Community Health, 19*(4), 1–18.

Aday, L. A., Aitken, M. J., & Wegener, D. H. (1988). *Pediatric home care: Results of a national evaluation of programs for ventilator assisted children.* Chicago: Pluribus Press.

Aday, L. A., Begley, C. E., Lairson, D. R., & Slater, C. H. (1998). *Evaluating the healthcare system: Effectiveness, efficiency, and equity* (2nd ed.). Chicago: Health Administration Press.

Aday, L. A., Begley, C. E., Lairson, D. R., Slater, C. H., Richard, A. J., & Montoya, I. D. (1999). A framework for assessing the effectiveness, efficiency, and equity of behavioral healthcare [Special issue]. *American Journal of Managed Care, 5,* SP25–44.

Administration for Children, Youth and Families. Children's Bureau. (1999). *Child maltreatment, 1997: Reports from the states to the National Child Abuse and Neglect Data System.* Washington, DC: National Clearinghouse on Child Abuse and Neglect Information.

Administration for Children, Youth and Families. National Center on Child Abuse and Neglect. (1999). *National Child Abuse and Neglect Data System: Summary data component tables 1990–1996, 1997* [diskette]. Washington, DC: National Clearinghouse on Child Abuse and Neglect Information.

Agency for Healthcare Research and Quality. (1990a). *AHCPR Conference Proceedings: Community-based Care of Persons with AIDS: Developing a Research Agenda* (DHHS Publication No. PHS 90–3456). Washington, DC: U.S. Government Printing Office.

Agency for Healthcare Research and Quality. (1990b). *AHCPR program note: Health services research on HIV/AIDS-related illnesses.* Rockville, MD: U.S. Department of Health and Human Services, Agency for Healthcare Research and Quality.

Agency for Healthcare Research and Quality. (1996). *Top five most expensive hospital diagnoses* [On-line]. Available: http://www.ahrq.gov/data/hcup/charts/5diag.htm [Accessed Mar. 20, 2000].

Agency for Healthcare Research and Quality. (1998). Low birthweight PORT publishes latest findings. *AHCPR Research Activities, 221,* 5–6.

Aguirre-Molina, M., & Gorman, D. M. (1996). Community-based approaches for the prevention of alcohol, tobacco, and other drug use. *Annual Review of Public Health, 17,* 337–358.

Ahearn, F. L., Jr., & Athey, J. L. (Eds.). (1991). *Refugee children: Theory, research, and services.* Baltimore, MD: Johns Hopkins University Press.

Alcohol, Drug Abuse, and Mental Health Administration. (1989a). *Report of the Secretary's Task Force on Youth Suicide: Vol. 1: Overview and recommendations* (DHHS Publication No. ADM 89–1621). Washington, DC: U.S. Government Printing Office.

Alcohol, Drug Abuse, and Mental Health Administration. (1989b). *Report of the Secretary's Task Force on Youth Suicide: Vol. 2: Risk factors for youth suicide* (DHHS Publication No. ADM 89–1622). (L. Davidson & M. Linnoila, Eds.). Washington, DC: U.S. Government Printing Office.

Alcohol, Drug Abuse, and Mental Health Administration. (1989c). *Report of the Secretary's Task Force on Youth Suicide: Vol. 3: Prevention and interventions in youth suicide* (DHHS Publication No. ADM 89–1623). (M. R. Feinleib, Ed.). Washington, DC: U.S. Government Printing Office.

Alcohol, Drug Abuse, and Mental Health Administration. (1989d). *Report of the Secretary's Task Force on Youth Suicide: Vol. 4: Strategies for the prevention of youth suicide* (DHHS Publication No. ADM 89–1624). (M. L. Rosenberg & K. Baer, Eds.). Washington, DC: U.S. Government Printing Office.

Alexander, G. R., & Korenbrot, C. C. (1995). The role of prenatal care in preventing low birth weight. *Future of Children, 5*(1), 103–120.

Allden, K., Poole, C., Chantavanich, S., Ohmar, K., Aung, N. N., & Mollica, R. F. (1996). Burmese political dissidents in Thailand: Trauma and survival among young adults in exile. *American Journal of Public Health, 86*(11), 1561–1569.

Allen, J. R., & Curran, J. W. (1988). Prevention of AIDS and HIV infection: Needs and priorities for epidemiologic research. *American Journal of Public Health, 78,* 381–386.

Allen, S. M. (1998). People and systems: Assessing the fit. In S. M. Allen & V. Mor (Eds.), *Living in the community with disability: Service needs, use, and systems* (pp. 372–387). New York: Springer.

Allen, S. M., & Mor V. (Eds.). (1998). *Living in the community with disability: Service needs, use, and systems.* New York: Springer.

Altamore, R., Mitchell, M., & Weber, C. M. (1990). Assuring good-quality care. In P. W. Brickner, L. K. Scharer, B. A. Conanan, M. Savarese, & B. C. Scanlan (Eds.), *Under the safety net: Health and social welfare of the homeless in the United States* (pp. 371–383). New York: Norton.

Amaro, H. (1999). An expensive policy: The impact of inadequate funding for substance abuse treatment. *American Journal of Public Health, 89*(5), 657–659.

American Association of Retired Persons. (1991). *The role of the Older Americans Act in providing long-term care* (FS1–1/91). Public Policy Institute Fact Sheet. Washington, DC: American Association of Retired Persons, Public Policy Institute.

American Association of Retired Persons. (1997). *Out-of-pocket health spending by Medicare beneficiaries age 65 and older: 1997 projections: Executive summary* [On-line]. Available:

http://www.research.aarp.org/health/9705_pocket_1.html [Accessed Oct. 25, 1999. Last updated Dec. 1997].

American Humane Association. (1989). *Highlights of official aggregate child neglect and abuse reporting, 1987*. Denver, CO: Author.

American Public Health Association. (1989). Senate passes landmark rights bill. *Nation's Health, 19*(10, 11), 4.

American Public Health Association. (1991). CDC announces expanded definition of AIDS. *Nation's Health, 21*(12), 4.

Anderson, K. H., & Mitchell, J. M. (1997). Expenditures on services for persons with acquired immunodeficiency syndrome under a Medicaid home and community-based waiver program. Are selection effects important? *Medical Care, 35*(5), 425–439.

Anderson, P. (1994). Overview: Public health, health promotion and addictive substances. *Addiction, 89*(11), 1523–1527.

Anderson, S. C., Boe, T., & Smith, S. (1988). Homeless women. *Affilia, 3*(2), 62–70.

Archambault, D. (1989). Adolescence: A physiological, cultural, and psychological no man's land. In G. W. Lawson & A. W. Lawson (Eds.), *Alcoholism and substance abuse in special populations* (pp. 223–245). Gaithersburg, MD: Aspen.

Arno, P. S., Bonuck, K. A., Green, J., Fleishman, J., Bennett, C. L., Fahs, M. C., Maffeo, C., & Drucker, E. (1996). The impact of housing status on health care utilization among persons with HIV disease. *Journal of Health Care for the Poor and Underserved, 7*(1), 36–49.

Arnstein, S. (1969). A ladder of citizen participation. *Journal of the American Institute of Planners, 35*, 216–224.

Aruffo, J. F., Coverdale, J. H., & Vallbona, C. (1991). AIDS knowledge in low-income and minority populations. *Public Health Reports, 106*, 115–119.

Auerbach, J. D., Wypijewska, C., & Brodie, H. K. H. (Eds.). (1994). *AIDS and behavior: An integrated approach*. Washington, DC: National Academy Press.

Bach, P. B., & Lantos, J. (1999). Methadone dosing, heroin affordability, and the severity of addiction. *American Journal of Public Health, 89*(5), 662–665.

Bailey, S. L., & Hubbard, R. L. (1990). Developmental variation in the context of marijuana initiation among adolescents. *Journal of Health and Social Behavior, 31*, 58–70.

Baker, F. M. (1987). The Afro-American life cycle: Success, failure, and mental health. *Journal of the National Medical Association, 79*, 625–633.

Baldwin, L. M., Larson, E. H., Connell, F. A., Nordlund, D., Cain, K. C., Cawthon, M. L., Byrns, P., & Rosenblatt, R. A. (1998). The effect of expanding Medicaid prenatal services on birth outcomes. *American Journal of Public Health, 88*(11), 1623–1629.

Bangert-Drowns, R. L. (1988). The effects of school-based substance abuse education: A meta-analysis. *Journal of Drug Education, 18*, 243–264.

Barber-Madden, R., & Kotch, J. B. (1990). Maternity care financing: Universal access or universal care? *Journal of Health Politics, Policy and Law, 15*, 797–814.

Barer, B. M., & Johnson, C. L. (1990). A critique of the caregiving literature. *Gerontologist, 30*, 26–29.

Barrows, D. C. (1998). The community orientation of social model and medical model recovery programs. *Journal of Substance Abuse Treatment, 15*(1), 55–64.

Bartels, S. J., & Colenda, C. C. (1998). Mental health services for Alzheimer's disease. Current trends in reimbursement and public policy, and the future under managed care. *American Journal of Geriatric Psychiatry, 6*(2 Suppl. 1), S85–100.

Baruffi, G., Strobino, D. M., & Paine, L. L. (1990). Investigation of institutional differences in primary cesarean birth rates. *Journal of Nurse Midwifery, 35*, 274–281.

Bassuk, E. L. (1993). Social and economic hardships of homeless and other poor women. *American Journal of Orthopsychiatry, 63*(3), 340–347.

Bassuk, E. L., Browne, A., & Buckner, J. C. (1996). Single mothers and welfare. *Scientific American, 275*(4), 60–63, 66–67.

Bassuk, E. L., Buckner, J. C., Weinreb, L. F., Browne, A., Bassuk, S. S., Dawson, R., & Perloff, J. N. (1997). Homelessness in female-headed families: Childhood and adult risk and protective factors. *American Journal of Public Health, 87*(2), 241–248.

Bassuk, E. L., Melnick, S., & Browne, A. (1998). Responding to the needs of low-income and homeless women who are survivors of family violence. *Journal of the American Medical Women's Association, 53*(2), 57–64.

Bassuk, E. L., & Weinreb, L. (1993). Homeless pregnant women: Two generations at risk. *American Journal of Orthopsychiatry, 63*(3), 348–357.

Bassuk, E. L., Weinreb, L. F., Dawson, R., Perloff, J. N., & Buckner, J. C. (1997). Determinants of behavior in homeless and low-income housed preschool children. *Pediatrics, 100*(1), 92–100.

Bayer, R. (1991). AIDS: The politics of prevention and neglect. *Health Affairs, 10*(1), 87–97.

Beachler, M. (1990). The mental health services program for youth. *Journal of Mental Health Administration, 17*, 115–121.

Bean, F. D., Edmonston, B., & Passel, J. S. (Eds.). (1990). *Undocumented migration to the United States: IRCA and the experience of the 1980s.* Santa Monica, CA: RAND Corporation.

Bean, F. D., Vernez, G., & Keely, C. B. (1989). *Opening and closing the doors: Evaluating immigration reform and control.* Santa Monica, CA: RAND Corporation.

Beauchamp, D. E. (1988). *The health of the republic: Epidemics, medicine, and moralism as challenges to democracy.* Philadelphia: Temple University Press.

Beauvais, F., Oetting, E. R., Wolf, W., & Edwards, R. W. (1989). American Indian youth and drugs, 1976–87: A continuing problem. *American Journal of Public Health, 79*, 634–636.

Bebbington, P. E. (1990). Population surveys of psychiatric disorder and the need for treatment. *Social Psychiatry and Psychiatric Epidemiology, 25*, 33–40.

Beck, A. J., & Mumola, C. J. (1999). *Prisoners in 1998* (Publication No. NCJ 175687). Washington, DC: U.S. Department of Justice, Bureau of Justice Statistics.

Becker, G. S., Grossman, M., & Murphy, K. M. (1994). An empirical analysis of cigarette addiction. *American Economic Review, 84* (3), 396–418.

Becker, M. H., & Joseph, J. G. (1988). AIDS and behavioral change to reduce risk: A review. *American Journal of Public Health, 78*, 394–410.

Beers, M. H., Fink, A., & Beck, J. C. (1991). Screening recommendations for the elderly. *American Journal of Public Health, 81*, 1131–1140.

Begley, C. E., Crane, M. M., & Perdue, G. (1990). Estimating the mortality cost of AIDS: Do estimates of earnings differ? *American Journal of Public Health, 80*, 1268–1270.

Bekemeier, B. (1995). Public health nurses and the prevention of and intervention in family violence. *Public Health Nursing, 12* (4), 222–227.

Bell, C. S., & Battjes, R. J. (Eds.). (1990). *Prevention research: Deterring drug abuse among children and adolescents* (DHHS Publication No. ADM 90–1334). Washington, DC: U.S. Government Printing Office.

Bellah, R. N., Madsen, R., Sullivan, W. M., Swidler, A., & Tipton, S. M. (1985). *Habits of the heart: Individualism and commitment in American life.* Berkeley: University of California Press.

Benjamin, A. E. (1989). Perspectives on a continuum of care for persons with HIV illnesses. In W. N. LeVee (Ed.), *Conference Proceedings: New Perspectives on HIV-related Illnesses: Progress in Health Services Research* (DHHS Publication No. PHS 89–3449) (pp. 145–158). Washington, DC: U.S. Government Printing Office.

Bennett, C. L. (1990). Quality of medical care for patients with AIDS and cancer. *Dissertation Abstracts International B, 50.* 5566. (University Microfilms No. AAD90–12735).

Bergner, M. (1989). Quality of life, health status, and clinical research. *Medical Care, 2*(Suppl.), S148-S156.

Berlin, I. N. (1987). Suicide among American Indian adolescents: An overview. *Suicide and Life-Threatening Behavior, 17*, 218–232.

Berne, A. S., Dato, C., Mason, D. J., & Rafferty, M. (1990). A nursing model for addressing the health needs of homeless families. *Image: Journal of Nursing Scholarship, 22*, 8–13.

Berry, D. E. (1993). The emerging epidemiology of rural AIDS. *Journal of Rural Health, 9*(4), 293–304.

Bevilacqua, J. J., Morris, J. A., & Pumariega, A. J. (1996). State services research capacity: Building a state infrastructure for mental health services research. *Community Mental Health Journal, 32*(6), 519–533.

Bickman, L., & Salzer, M. S. (1997). Measuring quality in mental health services. *Evaluation Review, 21*(3), 285–291.

Bienstock, J. L., Blakemore, K. J., Wang, E., Presser, D., Misra, D., & Pressman, E. K. (1997). Managed care does not lower costs but may result in poorer outcomes for patients with gestational diabetes. *American Journal of Obstetrics and Gynecology, 177*(5), 1035–1037.

Bilheimer, L. (1989). AIDS cost modeling in the U.S.: A pragmatic approach. *Health Policy, 11*, 147–168.

Bindman, A. B., Grumbach, K., Osmond, D., Komaromy, M., Vranizan, K., Lurie, N., Billings, J., & Stewart, A. (1995). Preventable hospitalizations and access to health care. *Journal of the American Medical Association, 274*(4), 305–311.

Bird, S. T., & Bauman, K. E. (1998). State-level infant, neonatal, and postneonatal mortality: The contribution of selected structural socioeconomic variables. *International Journal of Health Services, 28*(1), 13–27.

Björkman, T., Hansson, L., Svensson, B., & Berglund, I. (1995). What is important in psychiatric outpatient care? Quality of care from the patient's perspective. *International Journal for Quality in Health Care, 7*(4), 355–362.

Blank, N., & Diderichsen, F. (1996). The prediction of different experiences of longterm illness: A longitudinal approach in Sweden. *Journal of Epidemiology and Community Health, 50*(2), 156–161.

Blendon, R. J., Knox, R. A., Brodie, M., Benson, J. M., & Chervinsky, G. (1994). Americans compare managed care, Medicare, and fee-for-service. *Journal of American Health Policy. 4*(3), 42–47.

Blumstein, A., Cohen, J., Roth, J. A., & Visher, C. A. (Eds.). (1986a). *Criminal careers and "career criminals"* (Vol. 1). Washington, DC: National Academy Press.

Blumstein, A., Cohen, J., Roth, J. A., & Visher, C. A. (Eds.). (1986b). *Criminal careers and "career criminals"* (Vol. 2). Washington, DC: National Academy Press.

Bogard, C. J., McConnell, J. J., Gerstel, N., & Schwartz, M. (1999). Homeless mothers and depression: Misdirected policy. *Journal of Health and Social Behavior, 40*(1), 46–62.

Bonnie, R. J., Fulco, C. E., & Liverman, C. T. (1999). *Reducing the burden of injury: Advancing prevention and treatment.* Washington, DC: National Academy Press.

Borduin, C. M., Mann, B. J., Cone, L. T., Henggeler, S. W., Fucci, B. R., Blaske, D. M., & Williams, R. A. (1995). Multisystemic treatment of serious juvenile offenders: Long-term prevention of criminality and violence. *Journal of Consulting and Clinical Psychology, 63*(4), 569–578.

Bowering, J., Clancy, K. L., & Poppendieck, J. (1991). Characteristics of a random sample of emergency food program users in New York: II. Soup kitchens. *American Journal of Public Health, 81*, 914–917.

Bowlyow, J. E. (1990). Acute and long-term care linkages: A literature review. *Medical Care Review, 47*, 75–103.

Bozzette, S. A., & Asch, S. (1995). Developing quality review criteria from standards of care for HIV disease: A framework. *JAIDS: Journal of Acquired Immune Deficiency Syndromes, 8*(Suppl. 1), S45–52.

Bozzette, S. A., Berry, S. H., Duan, N., Frankel, M. R., Leibowitz, A. A., Lefkowitz, D., Emmons, C. A., Senterfitt, J. W., Berk, M. L., Morton, S. C., & Shapiro, M. F. (1998). The care of HIV-infected adults in the United States: HIV Cost and Services Utilization Study Consortium. *New England Journal of Medicine, 339*(26), 1897–1904.

Brach, C., Falik, M., Law, C., Robinson, G., Trent-Adams, S., Ulmer, C., & Wright, A. (1995). Mental health services: Critical component of integrated primary care and substance abuse treatment. *Journal of Health Care for the Poor and Underserved, 6*(3), 322–341.

Braun, D. (1991). *The rich get richer: The rise of income inequality in the United States and the world.* Chicago: Nelson-Hall.

Braveman, P., Bennett, T., Lewis, C., Egerter, S., & Showstack, J. (1993). Access to prenatal care following major Medicaid eligibility expansions. *Journal of the American Medical Association, 269*(10), 1285–1289.

Brent, D. A. (1989). The psychological autopsy: Methodological considerations for the study of adolescent suicide. *Suicide and Life-Threatening Behavior, 19*, 43–57.

Brickner, P. W., McAdam, J. M., Torres, R. A., Vicic, W. J., Conanan, B. A., Detrano, T., Piantieri, O., Scanlan, B., & Scharer, L. K. (1993). Providing health services for the homeless: A stitch in time. *Bulletin of the New York Academy of Medicine, 70*(3), 146–170.

Brickner, P. W., Scharer, L. K., Conanan, B. A., & Scanlan, B. C. (Eds.). (1990). *Under the safety net: Health and social welfare of the homeless in the United States.* New York: Norton.

Britt, C. L., Kleck, G., & Bordua, D. J. (1996). A reassessment of the D.C. gun law: Some cautionary notes on the use of interrupted time series designs for policy impact assessment. *Law and Society Review, 30*(2), 361–380.

Brody, B. E. (1988). Employee assistance programs: An historical and literature review. *American Journal of Health Promotion, 2*(3), 13–19.

Broer, J., & Garretsen, H. F. (1995). Simultaneous strategies to reduce demand for and problematic use of hard drugs. *Medicine and Law, 14*(3–4), 171–179.

Brook, R. H., Ware, J. E., Jr., Rogers, W. H., Keeler, E. B., Davies, A. R., Donald, C. A., Goldberg, G. A., Lohr, K. N., Masthay, P. C., & Newhouse, J. P. (1983). Does free care improve adults' health? Results from a randomized controlled trial. *New England Journal of Medicine, 309*, 1426–1434.

Brookoff, D., Campbell, E. A., & Shaw, L. M. (1993). The underreporting of cocaine-related trauma: Drug abuse warning network reports vs hospital toxicology tests. *American Journal of Public Health, 83*(3), 369–371.

Broughton, C. (1989, Sept.-Oct.). Serving refugee children and families in Head Start. *Children Today*, 6–10.

Brown, E. R., Wyn, R., & Ojeda, V. D. (1999). *Noncitizen children's rising uninsured rates threaten access to health care.* Los Angeles: UCLA Center for Health Policy Research.

Brown, F., & Tooley, J. (1989). Alcoholism in the black community. In G. W. Lawson, & A. W. Lawson (Eds.), *Alcoholism and substance abuse in special populations* (pp. 115–130). Gaithersburg, MD: Aspen.

Brown, M. A. (1997). Knowledge generation for the HIV-affected family. *Image—the Journal of Nursing Scholarship, 29*(3), 269–274.

Browne, G., Roberts, J., Gafni, A., Weir, R., Watt, S., & Byrne, C. (1995). More effective and less expensive: Lessons from five studies examining community approaches to care. *Health Policy, 34*(2), 95–112.

Browne, K., Davies, C., & Stratton, P. (Eds.). (1988). *Early prediction and prevention of child abuse.* New York: Wiley.

Bruneau, J., Lamothe, F., Franco, E., Lachance, N., Desy, M., Soto, J., & Vincelette, J. (1997). High rates of HIV infection among injection drug users participating in needle exchange programs in Montreal: Results of a cohort study. *American Journal of Epidemiology, 146*(12), 994–1002.

Brunskill, A. J. (1990). Some sources of error in the coding of birth weight. *American Journal of Public Health, 80*, 72–73.

Buchanan, R. J. (1996). Medicaid eligibility policies for people with AIDS. *Social Work in Health Care, 23*(2), 15–41.

Buchanan, R. J., & Smith, S. R. (1994a). Medicaid policies for HIV-related drug therapies: Perspectives of the state affiliates of the American Pharmaceutical Association. *Annals of Pharmacotherapy, 28*(4), 528–535.

Buchanan, R. J., & Smith, S. R. (1994b). Medicaid policies for HIV-related prescription drugs. *Health Care Financing Review, 15*(3), 43–61.

Buchanan, R. J., & Smith, S. R. (1998). State implementation of the AIDS drug assistance programs. *Health Care Financing Review, 19*(3), 39–62.

Buck, J. A., Teich, J. L., Umland, B., & Stein, M. (1999). Behavioral health benefits in employer-sponsored health plans, 1997. *Health Affairs, 18*(2), 67–78.

Buck, J. A., & Umland, B. (1997). Covering mental health and substance abuse services. *Health Affairs, 16*(4), 120–126.

Burke, D. S., Brundage, J. F., Redfield, R. R., Damato, J. J., Schable, C. A., Putman, P., Visintine, R., & Kim, H. I. (1988). Measurement of the false rate in a screening program for human immunodeficiency virus infections. *New England Journal of Medicine, 319*, 961–964.

Burkhauser, R. V., & Duncan, G. J. (1988). Life events, public policy, and the economic vulnerability of children and the elderly. In J. L. Palmer, T. Smeeding, & B. B. Torrey (Eds.), *The vulnerable* (pp. 55–88). Washington, DC: Urban Institute Press.

Burns, B. J., Wagner, H. R., Taube, J. E., Magaziner, J., Permutt, T., & Landerman, L. R. (1993). Mental health service use by the elderly in nursing homes. *American Journal of Public Health, 83*(3), 331–337.

Burt, M. R. (1986). Estimating the public costs of teenage childbearing. *Family Planning Perspectives, 18*, 221–226.

Burt, M. R. (1992). *Over the edge: The growth of homelessness in the 1980s.* New York: Russell Sage Foundation.

Burt, M. R., & Aron, L. Y. (2000). *America's homeless II: Populations and services* [On-line]. Available: http://www.urban.org/housing/homeless/numbers/index.htm [Accessed Feb. 29, 2000. Last updated Feb. 1, 2000].

Burt, M. R., Aron, L. Y., Douglas, T., Valente, J., Lee, E., & Iwen, B. (1999). *Homelessness: Programs and the people they serve: Findings of the National Survey of Homeless Assistance Providers and Clients.* Washington, DC: Urban Institute Press.

Burt, M. R., & Cohen, B. E. (1989). *America's homeless: Numbers, characteristics, and programs that serve them* (Urban Institute Report No. 89–3). Washington, DC: Urban Institute Press.

Busch, S. (1997). Carving-out mental health benefits to Medicaid beneficiaries: A shift toward managed care. *Administration and Policy in Mental Health, 24*(4), 301–321.

Calavita, K. (1996). The new politics of immigration: "Balanced-budget conservatism" and the symbolism of Proposition 187. *Social Problems, 43*(3), 284–305.

Canetto, S. S., & Lester, D. (1995). Gender and the primary prevention of suicide mortality. *Suicide and Life-Threatening Behavior, 25*(1), 58–69.

Canetto, S. S., & Sakinofsky, I. (1998). The gender paradox in suicide. *Suicide and Life-Threatening Behavior, 28*(1), 1–23.

Cano, C., Hennessy, K. D., Warren, J. L., & Lubitz, J. (1997). Medicare Part A utilization and expenditures for psychiatric services: 1995. *Health Care Financing Review, 18*(3), 177–193.

Capitman, J. A. (1988). Case management for long-term and acute medical care. *Health Care Financing Review, Annual Supplement*, 53–55.

Carcagno, G. J., & Kemper, P. (1988). The evaluation of the national long term care demonstration. *Health Services Research, 23*, 1–22.

Carney, T. (1989). A fresh approach to child protection practice and legislation in Australia. *Child Abuse and Neglect, 13,* 29–39.

Carpenter, L. (1988). Special report: Medicaid eligibility for persons in nursing homes. *Health Care Financing Review, 10*(2), 67–77.

Cartwright, W. S., & Ingster, L. M. (1993). A patient-based analysis of drug disorder diagnoses in the Medicare population. *Health Care Financing Review, 15*(2), 89–101.

Casarett, D. J., & Lantos, J. D. (1998). Have we treated AIDS too well? Rationing and the future of AIDS exceptionalism. *Annals of Internal Medicine, 128*(9), 756–759.

Caspi, Y., Poole, C., Mollica, R. F., & Frankel, M. (1998). Relationship of child loss to psychiatric and functional impairment in resettled Cambodian refugees. *Journal of Nervous and Mental Disease, 186*(8), 484–491.

Caulkins, J. P., & Reuter, P. (1997). Setting goals for drug policy: Harm reduction or use reduction? *Addiction, 92*(9), 1143–1150.

Caulkins, J. P., Rydell, C. P., Schwabe, W., & Chiesa, J. (1998). Are mandatory minimum drug sentences cost-effective? *Corrections Management Quarterly, 2*(1), 62–73.

Center for Mental Health Services. Substance Abuse and Mental Health Services Administration. (1998). *Managed behavioral health services: An annotated bibliography.* Washington, DC: U.S. Government Printing Office.

Center for Vulnerable Populations. (1992). *Familiar faces: The status of America's vulnerable populations: A chartbook.* Portland, ME: Center for Health Policy Development.

Centers for Disease Control and Prevention. (1985). Revision of the case definition of acquired immunodeficiency syndrome for national reporting—United States. *Morbidity and Mortality Weekly Report, 34,* 373–375.

Centers for Disease Control and Prevention. (1987). Revision of the CDC surveillance case definition for acquired immunodeficiency syndrome. *Morbidity and Mortality Weekly Report, 36* (Suppl. 1S), 3S-15S.

Centers for Disease Control and Prevention. (1990a). *National HIV seroprevalence surveys: Summary of results: Data from serosurveillance activities through 1989* (Publication No. HIV/CID/9–90/006). Atlanta, GA: Author.

Centers for Disease Control and Prevention. (1990b). State coalitions for prevention and control of tobacco use. *Morbidity and Mortality Weekly Report, 39*(28), 476–485.

Centers for Disease Control and Prevention. (1992). *National HIV serosurveillance summary: Results through 1990* (Publication No. HIV/NCID/11–91/011). Atlanta, GA: Author.

Centers for Disease Control and Prevention. (1993a). Assessment of street outreach for HIV prevention: Selected sites, 1991–1993. *Morbidity and Mortality Weekly Report, 42*(45), 873, 879–880.

Centers for Disease Control and Prevention. (1993b). Distribution of STD clinic patients along a stages-of-behavioral-change continuum: Selected sites 1993. *Morbidity and Mortality Weekly Report, 42*(45), 880–884.

Centers for Disease Control and Prevention. (1994a). HIV prevention practices of primary-care physicians: United States, 1992. *Morbidity and Mortality Weekly Report, 42*(51 & 52), 988–992.

Centers for Disease Control and Prevention. (1994b). *National HIV serosurveillance summary: Results through 1992* (Publication No. HIV/NCID/11–93–036). Atlanta, GA: Author.

Centers for Disease Control and Prevention. (1995). *National HIV serosurveillance summary: Results through 1993* (Publication No. HIV/DHAP/6–95–051). Atlanta, GA: Author.

Centers for Disease Control and Prevention. (1996). Community-level prevention of human immunodeficiency virus infection among high-risk populations: The AIDS community demonstration projects. *Morbidity and Mortality Weekly Report, 45*(RR-6), 1–16.

Centers for Disease Control and Prevention. (1997). Resources and priorities for chronic disease prevention and control, 1994. *Morbidity and Mortality Weekly Report, 46*(13), 286–287.

Centers for Disease Control and Prevention. (1998a). Diagnosis and reporting of HIV and AIDS in states with integrated HIV and AIDS surveillance: United States, January 1994–June 1997. *Morbidity and Mortality Weekly Report, 47*(15), 309–314.

Centers for Disease Control and Prevention. (1998b). *HIV/AIDS national prevalence surveys: 1997 summary*. Atlanta, GA: Author.

Centers for Disease Control and Prevention. (1998c). *HIV/AIDS surveillance report: U.S. HIV and AIDS cases reported through December 1997*. Atlanta, GA: Author.

Centers for Disease Control and Prevention. (1998d). *National HIV prevalence surveys: 1997 summary*. Atlanta, GA: Author.

Centers for Disease Control and Prevention. (1998e). Self-reported frequent mental distress among adults: United States, 1993–1996. *Morbidity and Mortality Weekly Report, 47*(16), 325–331.

Centers for Disease Control and Prevention. (1999a). *HIV/AIDS surveillance report: U.S. HIV and AIDS cases reported through June 1999*. Atlanta, GA: Author.

Centers for Disease Control and Prevention. (1999b). *HIV/AIDS surveillance report: U.S. HIV and AIDS cases reported through December 1998*. Atlanta, GA: Author.

Centers for Disease Control and Prevention. (1999c). Neighborhood safety and the prevalence of physical inactivity: Selected states, 1996. *Morbidity and Mortality Weekly Report, 48*(7), 143–146.

Centers for Disease Control and Prevention. (1999d). Prevalence of selected maternal and infant characteristics, Pregnancy Risk Assessment Monitoring System (PRAMS), 1997. *Morbidity and Mortality Weekly Report, 48*(SS-5).

Centers for Disease Control and Prevention AIDS Community Demonstration Projects Research Group. (1999). Community-level HIV intervention in five cities: Final outcome data from the CDC AIDS Community Demonstration Projects. *American Journal of Public Health, 89*(3), 336–345.

Chalk, R., & King, P. A. (Eds.). (1998). *Violence in families: Assessing prevention and treatment programs*. Washington, DC: National Academy Press.

Chaloupka, F. J., Grossman, M., & Saffer, H. (1998). The effects of price on the consequences of alcohol use and abuse. *Recent Developments in Alcoholism, 14*, 331–346.

Chaloupka, F. J., & Wechsler, H. (1997). Price, tobacco control policies and smoking among young adults. *Journal of Health Economics, 16*(3), 359–373.

Charles, C., & DeMaio, S. (1993). Lay participation in health care decision making: A conceptual framework. *Journal of Health Politics, Policy and Law, 18*(4), 881–904.

Chavkin, W. (Ed.). (1995). Women and HIV/AIDS. *Journal of the American Medical Women's Association, 50*(3 & 4).

Chavkin, W., Breitbart, V., Elman, D., & Wise, P. H. (1998). National survey of the states: Policies and practices regarding drug-using pregnant women. *American Journal of Public Health, 88*(1), 117–119.

Chavkin, W., Wise, P. H., & Elman, D. (1998). Policies towards pregnancy and addiction. Sticks without carrots. *Annals of the New York Academy of Sciences, 846*, 335–340.

Chen, M. S., Jr., Kuun, P., Guthrie, R., Li, W., & Zaharlick, A. (1991). Promoting heart health for Southeast Asians: A database for planning interventions. *Public Health Reports, 106*, 304–309.

Chenoweth, K., & Free, C. (1990). Homeless children come to school. *American Educator, 14*(3), 28–33.

Chilcoat, H. D., Breslau, N., & Anthony, J. C. (1996). Potential barriers to parent monitoring: Social disadvantage, marital status, and maternal psychiatric disorder. *Journal of the American Academy of Child and Adolescent Psychiatry, 35*(12), 1673–1682.

Children's Defense Fund. (1990). *S.O.S. America! A Children's Defense Fund budget*. Washington, DC: Author.

Children's Defense Fund. (1998). *The state of America's children: Yearbook, 1998*. Washington, DC: Author.

Children's Defense Fund. (1999). *Head Start FAQS (frequently asked questions)* [On-line]. Available: http://www.childrensdefense.org/headstart_faq.html [Accessed Oct. 25, 1999].

Chollet, D. J., Newman, J. F. Jr., & Sumner, A. T. (1996). The cost of poor birth outcomes in employer-sponsored health plans. *Medical Care, 34*(12), 1219–1234.

Christianson, J. B., & Osher, F. C. (1994). Health maintenance organizations, health care reform, and persons with serious mental illness. *Hospital and Community Psychiatry, 45*(9), 898–905.

Cicchetti, D., & Carlson, V. (1989). *Child maltreatment: Theory and research on the causes and consequences of child abuse and neglect.* New York: Cambridge University Press.

Clancy, K. L., Bowering, J., & Poppendieck, J. (1991). Characteristics of a random sample of emergency food program users in New York: I. Food pantries. *American Journal of Public Health, 81*, 911–914.

Clark, R. E., Teague, G. B., Ricketts, S. K., Bush, P. W., Xie, H., McGuire, T. G., Drake, R. E., McHugo, G. J., Keller, A. M., & Zubkoff, M. (1998). Cost-effectiveness of assertive community treatment versus standard case management for persons with co-occurring severe mental illness and substance use disorders. *Health Services Research, 33*(5 Pt. 1), 1285–1308.

Clark-Jones, F. (1997). Community violence, children and youth: Considerations for programs, policy, and nursing roles. *Pediatric Nursing, 23*(2), 131–137, 138–139.

Cleary, P. D. (1989). The need and demand for mental health services. In C. A. Taube, D. Mechanic, & A. A. Hohmann (Eds.), *The future of mental health services research* (DHHS Publication No. ADM 89–1600) (pp. 161–184). National Institute of Mental Health. Washington, DC: U.S. Government Printing Office.

Cleland, J. G., & van Ginneken, J. K. (1988). Maternal education and child survival in developing countries: The search for pathways of influence. *Social Science and Medicine, 27*, 1357–1368.

Cobas, J. A., Balcazar, H., Benin, M. B., Keith, V. M., & Chong, Y. (1996). Acculturation and low-birthweight infants among Latino women: A reanalysis of HHANES data with structural equation models. *American Journal of Public Health, 86*(3), 394–396.

Cohen, D. A., Farley, T. A., Bedimo-Etame, J. R., Scribner, R., Ward, W., Kendall, C., & Rice, J. (1999). Implementation of condom social marketing in Louisiana, 1993 to 1996. *American Journal of Public Health, 89*(2), 204–208.

Cohen, S., De Vos, E., & Newberger, E. (1997). Barriers to physician identification and treatment of family violence: Lessons from five communities. *Academic Medicine, 72*(1 Suppl.), S19–25.

Cohn, A. H., & Daro, D. (1987). Is treatment too late: What ten years of evaluative research tell us. *Child Abuse and Neglect, 11*, 433–442.

Cohn, A. H., & Lee, R. A. (1988). Child abuse and neglect. In H. M. Wallace, G. Ryan, Jr., & A. C. Oglesby (Eds.), *Maternal and child health practices* (3rd ed.) (pp. 497–503). Oakland, CA: Third Party Publishing Company.

Coleman, J. S. (1988). Social capital in the creation of human capital. *American Journal of Sociology, 94*(Suppl.), S95-120.

Coleman, J. S. (1990). *Foundations of social theory.* Cambridge, MA: Harvard University Press.

Coleman, J. S. (1993). The rational reconstruction of society. *American Sociological Review, 58*(1), 1–15.

Colenda, C. C., Banazak, D., & Mickus, M. (1998). Mental health services in managed care: Quality questions remain. *Geriatrics, 53*(8), 49–52, 59–60, 63–64.

Collins, A., Baumgartner, D., & Henry, K. (1995). U.S. prisoners' access to experimental HIV therapies. *Minnesota Medicine, 78*(11), 45–48.

Collins, J. J., & Zawitz, M. W. (1990). *Federal drug data for national policy*. Office of Justice Programs, Bureau of Justice Statistics, Drugs and Crime Data. Washington, DC: U.S. Department of Justice.

Collins, J. W. Jr., & Hawkes, E. K. (1997). Racial differences in post-neonatal mortality in Chicago: What risk factors explain the black infant's disadvantage? *Ethnicity and Health, 2*(1–2), 117–125.

Collins, R. L. (1996). The role of ethnic versus nonethnic sociocultural factors in substance use and misuse. *Substance Use and Misuse, 31*(1), 95–101.

Comerci, G. D. (1996). Efforts by the American Academy of Pediatrics to prevent and reduce violence and its effects on children and adolescents. *Bulletin of the New York Academy of Medicine, 73*(2), 398–410.

Committee to Identify Strategies to Raise the Profile of Substance Abuse and Alcoholism Research. Institute of Medicine. (1997). *Dispelling myths about addiction: Strategies to increase understanding and strengthen research*. Washington, DC: National Academy Press.

Committee on Law and Justice, National Research Council and JFK School of Government. Harvard University. (1994). *Violence in urban America: Mobilizing a response*. Washington, DC: National Academy Press.

Commonwealth Fund Commission on Elderly People Living Alone. (1987). *Old, alone and poor: A plan for reducing poverty among elderly people living alone*. Baltimore, MD: Author.

Commonwealth Fund Commission on Elderly People Living Alone. (1988). *Aging alone: Profiles and projections*. Baltimore, MD: Author.

Commonwealth Fund Commission on Elderly People Living Alone. (1989). *Help at home: Long-term care assistance for impaired elderly people*. Baltimore, MD: Author.

Conti, C. T. Sr. (1998). Emergency departments and abuse: policy issues, practice barriers, and recommendations. *Journal of the Association for Academic Minority Physicians, 9*(2), 35–39.

Conviser, R., Gamliel, S., & Honberg, L. (1998). Health-based payment for HIV/AIDS in Medicaid managed care programs. *Health Care Financing Review, 19*(3), 63–82.

Cook, P. J., Lawrence, B. A., Ludwig, J., & Miller, T. R. (1999). The medical costs of gunshot injuries in the United States. *Journal of the American Medical Association, 282*(5), 447–454.

Cooke, M., & Sande, M. A. (1989). The HIV epidemic and training in internal medicine: Challenges and recommendations. *New England Journal of Medicine, 321*, 1334–1337.

Coyle, S. L. (1998). Women's drug use and HIV risk: Findings from NIDA's Cooperative Agreement for Community-Based Outreach/Intervention Research Program. *Women and Health, 27*(1–2), 1–18.

Coyle, S. L., Boruch, R. F., & Turner, C. F. (Eds.). (1991). *Evaluating AIDS prevention programs*. Washington, DC: National Academy Press.

Craig, R. T. (1988a). Community care for persons with serious mental illness: Removing barriers and building supports. *National Conference of State Legislatures: State Legislative Report, 13*(35), 1–8.

Craig, R. T. (1988b). Mental health services for children and youth: Strengthening the promise of the future. *National Conference of State Legislatures: State Legislative Report, 13*(25), 1–10.

Crits-Christoph, P., Siqueland, L., Blaine, J., Frank, A., Luborsky, L., Onken, L. S., Muenz, L. R., Thase, M. E., Weiss, R. D., Gastfriend, D. R., Woody, G. E., Barber, J. P., Butler, S. F., Daley, D., Salloum, I., Bishop, S., Najavits, L. M., Lis, J., Mercer, D., Griffin, M. L., Moras, K., & Beck, A. T. (1999). Psychosocial treatments for cocaine dependence: National Institute on Drug Abuse Collaborative Cocaine Treatment Study. *Archives of General Psychiatry, 56*(6), 493–502.

Crocker, A. C. (1990). Medical care in the community for adults with mental retardation. *American Journal of Public Health, 80*, 1037–1038.

Croghan, T. W., Obenchain, R. L., & Crown, W. E. (1998). What does treatment of depression really cost? *Health Affairs, 17*(4), 198–208.

Cromwell, J., Bartosch, W. J., Fiore, M. C., Hasselblad, V., & Baker, T. (1997). Cost-effectiveness of the clinical practice recommendations in the AHCPR guideline for smoking cessation. Agency for Health Care Policy and Research. *Journal of the American Medical Association, 278*(21), 1759–1766.

Crowell, N. A., & Burgess, A. W. (Eds.). (1996). *Understanding violence against women.* Washington, DC: National Academy Press.

Culhane, D. P., Averyt, J. M., & Hadley, T. R. (1997). The rate of public shelter admission among Medicaid-reimbursed users of behavioral health services. *Psychiatric Services, 48*(3), 390–392.

Culhane, D. P., & Kuhn, R. (1998). Patterns and determinants of public shelter utilization among homeless adults in New York City and Philadelphia. *Journal of Policy Analysis and Management, 17*(1), 23–43.

Culhane, D. P., Lee, C. M., & Watcher, S. M. (1996). Where the homeless come from: A study of the prior address distribution of families admitted to public shelters in New York City and Philadelphia. *Housing Policy Debate, 7*(2), 327–365.

Culyer, A. J. (1992). The morality of efficiency in health care: Some uncomfortable implications. *Health Economics, 1*(1), 7–18.

Cummings, P., Koepsell, T. D., Grossman, D. C., Savarino, J., & Thompson, R. S. (1997). The association between the purchase of a handgun and homicide or suicide. *American Journal of Public Health, 87*(6), 974–978.

Cunningham, P. J., & Monheit, A. C. (1990). Insuring the children: A decade of change. *Health Affairs, 9*(4), 76–90.

Cunningham, W. E., Hays, R. D., Ettl, M. K., Dixon, W. J., Liu, R. C., Beck, C. K., & Shapiro, M. F. (1998). The prospective effect of access to medical care on health-related quality-of-life outcomes in patients with symptomatic HIV disease. *Medical Care, 36*(3), 295–306.

Curbow, B., Khoury, A. J., & Weisman, C. S. (1998). Provision of mental health services in women's health centers. *Women's Health, 4*(1), 71–91.

Curtis, J. R., Paauw, D. S., Wenrich, M. D., Carline, J. D., & Ramsey, P. G. (1995). Physicians' ability to provide initial primary care to an HIV-infected patient. *Archives of Internal Medicine, 155*(15), 1613–1618.

Damron-Rodriguez, J. (1993). Case management in two long-term-care populations: A synthesis of research. *Journal of Case Management, 2*(4), 125–129.

Dana, R. H., Conner, M. G., & Allen, J. (1996). Quality of care and cost-containment in managed mental health: Policy, education, research, advocacy. *Psychological Reports, 79*(3 Pt. 2), 1395–1422.

Dane, A. V., & Schneider, B. H. (1998). Program integrity in primary and early secondary prevention: Are implementation effects out of control? *Clinical Psychology Review, 18*(1), 23–45.

Daniels, N. (1990). Insurability and the HIV epidemic: Ethical issues in underwriting. *Milbank Quarterly, 68*, 497–524.

Daniels, N. (1991). Duty to treat or right to refuse? *Hastings Center Report, 21*(2), 36–46.

Daniels, N. (1996). Justice, fair procedures, and the goals of medicine. *Hastings Center Report, 26*(6), 10–12.

Daro, D. (1988). *Confronting child abuse: Research for effective program design.* New York: Free Press.

Davidson, A. J., Bertram, S. L., Lezotte, D. C., Marine, W. M., Rietmeijer, C. A., Hagglund, B. B., & Cohn, D. L. (1998). Comparison of health status, socioeconomic characteristics, and knowledge and use of HIV-related resources between HIV-infected women and men. *Medical Care, 36*(12), 1676–1684.

Davis, D. (1991). "Understanding AIDS": The national AIDS mailer. *Public Health Reports, 106*(6), 656–662.

Dean, A., & Ensel, W. M. (1983). Socially structured depression in men and women. *Research in Community and Mental Health, 3,* 113–139.

Dengelegi, L., Weber, J., & Torquato, S. (1990). Drug users' AIDS-related knowledge, attitudes, and behaviors before and after AIDS education sessions. *Public Health Reports, 105,* 504–510.

Densen, P. M. (1991). *Tracing the elderly through the health care system: An update.* Rockville, MD: U.S. Department of Health and Human Services, Agency for Health Care Policy and Research.

Dial, T. H., Kantor, A., Buck, J. A., & Chalk, M. E. (1996). Behavioral health care in HMOs. In R. W. Manderscheid & M. A. Sonnenschein (Eds.), *Mental health, United States, 1996* (pp. 27–58) (DHHS Publication No. SMA 96–3098). Washington, DC: U.S. Government Printing Office.

Diaz, T., Chu, S. Y., Conti, L., Nahlen, B. L., Whyte, B., Mokotoff, E., Shields, A., Checko, P. J., Herr, M., Mukhtar, Q., et al. (1994). Health insurance coverage among persons with AIDS: Results from a multistate surveillance project. *American Journal of Public Health, 84*(6), 1015–1018.

Dickey, B., & Azeni, H. (1996). Persons with dual diagnoses of substance abuse and major mental illness: Their excess costs of psychiatric care. *American Journal of Public Health, 86*(7), 973–977.

Dickey, B., & Wagenaar, H. (1994). Evaluating mental health care reform: Including the clinician, client, and family perspective. *Journal of Mental Health Administration, 21*(3), 313–319.

DiClemente, R. J., Lanier, M. M., Horan, P. F., & Lodico, M. (1991). Comparison of AIDS knowledge, attitudes, and behaviors among incarcerated adolescents and a public school sample in San Francisco. *American Journal of Public Health, 81,* 628–630.

Diez-Roux, A. V., Northridge, M. E., Morabia, A., Bassett, M. T., & Shea, S. (1999). Prevalence and social correlates of cardiovascular disease risk factors in Harlem. *American Journal of Public Health, 89*(3), 302–307.

DiFranceisco, W., Kelly, J. A., Sikkema, K. J., Somlai, A. M., Murphy, D. A., & Stevenson, L. Y. (1998). Differences between completers and early dropouts from two HIV intervention trials: A health belief approach to understanding prevention program attrition. *American Journal of Public Health, 88*(7), 1068–1073.

Dingemans, P. M. (1990). ICD-9-CM classification coding in psychiatry. *Journal of Clinical Psychology, 46,* 161–168.

Dixon, P. S., Flanigan, T. P., DeBuono, B. A., Laurie, J. J., De Ciantis, M. L., Hoy, J., Stein, M., Scott, H. D., & Carpenter, C. C. (1993). Infection with the human immunodeficiency virus in prisoners: Meeting the health care challenge. *American Journal of Medicine, 95*(6), 629–635.

Dohrenwend, B. P. (1990). Socioeconomic status (SES) and psychiatric disorders: Are the issues still compelling? *Social Psychiatry and Psychiatric Epidemiology, 25,* 41–47.

Dooley, D., Catalano, R., Rook, K., & Serxner, S. (1989a). Economic stress and suicide: Multilevel analyses: Part 1: Aggregate time-series analyses of economic stress and suicide. *Suicide and Life-Threatening Behavior, 19,* 321–336.

Dooley, D., Catalano, R., Rook, K., & Serxner, S. (1989b). Economic stress and suicide: Multilevel analyses: Part 2: Cross-level analyses of economic stress and suicidal ideation. *Suicide and Life-Threatening Behavior, 19,* 337–351.

Dowell, D. A., & Ciarlo, J. A. (1989). An evaluative overview of the community mental health centers program. In D. A. Rochefort (Ed.), *Handbook on mental health policy in the United States* (pp. 195–236). Westport, CT: Greenwood Press.

Downs, K., Bernstein, J., & Marchese, T. (1997). Providing culturally competent primary care for immigrant and refugee women: A Cambodian case study. *Journal of Nurse-Midwifery, 42*(6), 499–508.

Drake, R. D., Wallach, M. A., & Hoffman, J. S. (1989). Housing instability and homelessness among aftercare patients of an urban state hospital. *Hospital and Community Psychiatry, 40,* 46–51.

Dryfoos, J. G. (1990). *Adolescents-at-risk: Prevalence and prevention.* New York: Oxford University Press.

Dubay, L. C., Kenney, G. M., Norton, S. A., & Cohen, B. C. (1995). Local responses to expanded Medicaid coverage for pregnant women. *Milbank Quarterly, 73*(4), 535–563.

Dubowitz, H. (1990). Costs and effectiveness of interventions in child maltreatment. *Child Abuse and Neglect, 14,* 177–186.

Dunn, S. M. (1997). Medicaid AIDS waivers: Seeking cost-effective financing of AIDS care. *Journal of Health and Human Services Administration, 19*(3), 270–282.

DuPlessis, H. M., Inkelas, M., & Halfon, N. (1998). Assessing the performance of community systems for children. *Health Services Research, 33*(4 Pt 2), 1111–1142.

Durant, R. H., Pendergrast, R. A., & Cadenhead, C. (1994). Exposure to violence and victimization and fighting behavior by urban black adolescents. *Journal of Adolescent Health, 15*(4), 311–318.

Durlak, J. A., & Wells, A. M. (1997). Primary prevention mental health programs for children and adolescents: A meta-analytic review. *American Journal of Community Psychology, 25*(2), 115–152.

EchoHawk, M. (1997). Suicide: The scourge of Native American people. *Suicide and Life-Threatening Behavior, 27*(1), 60–67.

Eddy, D. M., Wolpert, R. L., & Rosenberg, M. L. (1989). Estimating the effectiveness of interventions to prevent youth suicides: A report to the Secretary's Task Force on Youth Suicide. In M. L. Rosenberg & K. Baer (Eds.), *Report of the Secretary's Task Force on Youth Suicide: Vol. 4: Strategies for the prevention of youth suicide* (DHHS Publication No. ADM 89–1624) (pp. 37–81). Alcohol, Drug Abuse, and Mental Health Administration. Washington, DC: U.S. Government Printing Office.

Eden, S. L., & Aguilar, R. J. (1989). The Hispanic chemically dependent client: Considerations for diagnosis and treatment. In G. W. Lawson & A. W. Lawson (Eds.), *Alcoholism and substance abuse in special populations* (pp. 205–222). Gaithersburg, MD: Aspen.

Edmonston, B. (Ed.). (1996). *Statistics on U.S. immigration: An assessment of data needs for future research.* Washington, DC: National Academy Press.

Edmunds, M., Frank, R., Hogan, M., McCarty, D., Robinson-Beale, R., & Weisner, C. (1997). *Managing managed care: Quality improvement in behavioral health.* Washington, DC: National Academy Press.

Edwards, P. W., & Donaldson, M. A. (1989). Assessment of symptoms in adult survivors of incest: A factor analytic study of the responses to childhood incest questionnaire. *Child Abuse and Neglect, 13,* 101–110.

Eggert, G. M., & Friedman, B. (1988). The need for special interventions for multiple hospital admission patients. *Health Care Financing Review, Annual Supplement,* 57–67.

el-Guebaly, N., Armstrong, S. J., & Hodgins, D. C. (1998). Substance abuse and the emergency room: Programmatic implications. *Journal of Addictive Diseases, 17*(2), 21–40.

Elias, C. J., Alexander, B. H., & Sokly, T. (1990). Infectious disease control in a long-term refugee camp: The role of epidemiologic surveillance and investigation. *American Journal of Public Health, 80,* 824–828.

Ellickson, P. L., & Bell, R. M. (1990a). Drug prevention in junior high: A multi-site longitudinal test. *Science, 247*(4948), 1299–1305.

Ellickson, P. L., & Bell, R. M. (1990b). *Prospects for preventing drug use among young adolescents* (R-3896-CHF). Santa Monica, CA: RAND Corporation.

Ellickson, P. L., Collins, R. L., & Bell, R. M. (1999). Adolescent use of illicit drugs other than marijuana: How important is social bonding and for which ethnic groups? *Substance Use and Misuse, 34*(3), 317–346.

Elliott, B. A. (1993). Community responses to violence. *Primary Care: Clinics in Office Practice, 20*(2), 495–502.

Elliott, R. L. (1997). Evaluating the quality of correctional mental health services: An approach to surveying a correctional mental health system. *Behavioral Sciences and the Law, 15*(4), 427–38.

Ellwood, M. R., & Burwell, B. (1990). Access to Medicaid and Medicare by the low-income disabled. *Health Care Financing Review, Annual Supplement,* 133–148.

Ellwood, M. R., & Kenney, G. (1995). Medicaid and pregnant women: Who is being enrolled and when. *Health Care Financing Review, 17*(2), 7–28.

Ellwood, M. R., & Ku, L. (1998). Welfare and immigration reforms: Unintended side effects for Medicaid. *Health Affairs, 17*(3), 137–151.

Enkin, M. W., Keirse, M. J., Renfrew, M. J., & Neilson, J. P. (1995). Effective care in pregnancy and childbirth: A synopsis. *Birth, 22*(2), 101–110.

Ennett, S. T., Bailey, S. L., & Federman, E. B. (1999). Social network characteristics associated with risky behaviors among runaway and homeless youth. *Journal of Health & Social Behavior, 40*(1), 63–78.

Ensign, J., & Santelli, J. (1997). Shelter-based homeless youth. Health and access to care. *Archives of Pediatrics and Adolescent Medicine, 151*(8), 817–823.

Ensign, J., & Santelli, J. (1998). Health status and service use: Comparison of adolescents at a school-based health clinic with homeless adolescents. *Archives of Pediatrics and Adolescent Medicine, 152*(1), 20–24.

Epstein, J., & Gfroerer, J. (1998). Changes affecting NHSDA estimates of treatment need for 1994–1996. In Substance Abuse and Mental Health Services Administration, *Analyses of substance abuse and treatment need issues* (pp. 127–133) (DHHS Publication No. SMA 98–3227). Washington, DC: U.S. Government Printing Office.

Epstein, M. R. (1990). Networking in a rural community focuses on at-risk children. *Public Health Reports, 105,* 428–430.

Epstein, S. (1996). *Impure science: AIDS, activism, and the politics of knowledge.* Berkeley: University of California Press.

Ernst, A. A., Nick, T. G., Weiss, S. J., Houry, D., & Mills, T. (1997). Domestic violence in an inner-city ED. *Annals of Emergency Medicine, 30*(2), 190–197.

Ershoff, D., Radcliffe, A., & Gregory, M. (1996). The Southern California Kaiser-Permanente Chemical Dependency Recovery Program evaluation: Results of a treatment outcome study in an HMO setting. *Journal of Addictive Diseases, 15*(3), 1–25.

Escobedo, L. G., Anda, R. F., Smith, P. F., Remington, P. L., & Mast, E. E. (1990). Sociodemographic characteristics of cigarette smoking initiation in the United States: Implications for smoking prevention policy. *Journal of the American Medical Association, 264,* 1550–1555.

Eskander, G. S., Jahan, M. S., & Carter, R. A. (1990). AIDS: Knowledge and attitudes among different ethnic groups. *Journal of the National Medical Association, 82,* 281–286.

Estes, C. L., & Close, L. (1998). Organization of health and social services for the frail elderly. In S. M. Allen & V. Mor (Eds.), *Living in the community with disability: Service needs, use, and systems* (pp. 73–91). New York: Springer.

Evans, R. G., Barer, M. L., & Marmor, T. R. (Eds.). (1994). *Why are some people healthy and others not? The determinants of health of populations.* New York: A. de Gruyter.

Evers, S. M., Van Wijk, A. S., & Ament, A. J. (1997). Economic evaluation of mental health care interventions. A review. *Health Economics, 6*(2), 161–177.

Fallek, S. B. (1997). Health care for illegal aliens: Why it is a necessity. *Houston Journal of International Law, 19*(3), 951–981.

Fama, T., Fox, P. D., & White, L. A. (1995). Do HMOs care for the chronically ill? *Health Affairs, 14*(1), 234–243.

Farkas, M. D., & Anthony, W. A. (1989). *Psychiatric rehabilitation programs: Putting theory into practice.* Baltimore, MD: Johns Hopkins University Press.

Farmer, P., Connors, M., & Simmons, J. (Eds.). (1996). *Women, poverty and AIDS: Sex, drugs, and structural violence.* Monroe, ME: Common Courage Press.

Fasciano, N. J., Cherlow, A. L., Turner, B. J., & Thornton, C. V. (1998). Profile of Medicare beneficiaries with AIDS: Application of an AIDS casefinding algorithm. *Health Care Financing Review, 19*(3), 19–38.

Feder, J. (1990). Health care of the disadvantaged: The elderly. *Journal of Health Politics, Policy and Law, 15,* 259–269.

Feinstein, A. R. (1989). Evaluation of prognosis and transitions: General strategic principles and applications to AIDS. In L. Sechrest, H. Freeman, & A. Mulley (Eds.), *Conference Proceedings: Health Services Research Methodology: A Focus on AIDS* (DHHS Publication No. PHS 89–3439) (pp. 189–195). Washington, DC: U.S. Government Printing Office.

Feldhaus, K. M., Koziol-McLain, J., Amsbury, H. L., Norton, I. M., Lowenstein, S. R., & Abbott, J. T. (1997). Accuracy of three brief screening questions for detecting partner violence in the emergency department. *Journal of the American Medical Association, 277*(17), 1357–1361.

Feldman, S. (1998). Behavioral health services: Carved out and managed. *American Journal of Managed Care, 4* (Suppl.), SP59–67.

Feldman, S., Baler, S., & Penner, S. (1997). The role of private-for-profit managed behavioral health in the public sector. *Administration and Policy in Mental Health, 24*(5), 379–389.

Fenton, J. J., Catalano, R., & Hargreaves, W. A. (1996). Effect of Proposition 187 on mental health service use in California: A case study. *Health Affairs, 15*(1), 182–190.

Fergusson, D. M., Horwood, L. J., & Beautrais, A. L. (1999). Is sexual orientation related to mental health problems and suicidality in young people? *Archives of General Psychiatry, 56*(10), 876–880.

Ferreira-Pinto, J. B., & Ramos, R. (1995). HIV/AIDS prevention among female sexual partners of injection drug users in Ciudad Juarez, Mexico. *AIDS Care, 7*(4), 477–488.

Ferrie, J. E., Shipley, M. J., Marmot, M. G., Stansfeld, S. A., & Smith, G. D. (1998). An uncertain future: The health effects of threats to employment security in white-collar men and women. *American Journal of Public Health, 88*(7), 1030–1036.

Filinson, R., & Ingman, S. R. (Eds.). (1989). *Elder abuse: Practice and policy.* New York: Human Sciences Press.

Fillmore, K. M. (1988). *Alcohol use across the life course: A critical review of seventy years of international longitudinal research.* Toronto: Addiction Research Foundation.

Fingerhut, L. A., & Kleinman, J. C. (1989). *Firearm mortality among children and youth* (DHHS Publication No. PHS 90–1250). National Center for Health Statistics, Advance Data No. 178. Washington, DC: U.S. Government Printing Office.

Fink, A., & McCloskey, L. (1990). Moving child abuse and neglect prevention programs forward: Improving program evaluations. *Child Abuse and Neglect, 14,* 187–206.

Finkelhor, D., Hotaling, G. T., & Yllo, K. (1988). *Stopping family violence: Research priorities for the coming decade.* Thousand Oaks, CA: Sage.

Finn, P., & Colson, S. (1990). *Civil protection orders: Legislation, current court practice, and enforcement.* Office of Justice Programs, National Institute of Justice. Washington, DC: U.S. Department of Justice.

Fiorentine, R., & Anglin, M. D. (1997). Does increasing the opportunity for counseling increase the effectiveness of outpatient drug treatment? *American Journal of Drug and Alcohol Abuse, 23*(3), 369–382.

Fisher, E. B., Auslander, W. F., Munro, J. F., Arfken, C. L., Brownson, R. C., & Owens, N. W. (1998). Neighbors for a Smoke Free North Side: Evaluation of a community organization approach to promoting smoking cessation among African Americans. *American Journal of Public Health, 88*(11), 1658–1663.

Fishman, P., Von Korff, M., Lozano, P., & Hecht, J. (1997). Chronic care costs in managed care. *Health Affairs, 16*(3), 239–247.

Fitzpatrick, K. M. (1997). Aggression and environmental risk among low-income African-American youth. *Journal of Adolescent Health, 21*(3), 172–178.

Flanagan, T. J., & Maguire, K. (Eds.). (1990). *Sourcebook of criminal justice statistics 1989* (NCJ-124224). Office of Justice Programs, Bureau of Justice Statistics. Washington, DC: U.S. Department of Justice.

Fleishman, J. A. (1998). Transitions in insurance and employment among people with HIV infection. *Inquiry, 35*(1), 36–48.

Fleishman, J. A., Hsia, D. C., & Hellinger, F. J. (1994). Correlates of medical service utilization among people with HIV infection. *Health Services Research, 29*(5), 527–548.

Fleishman, J. A., & Mor, V. (1993). Insurance status among people with AIDS: Relationships with sociodemographic characteristics and service use. *Inquiry, 30*(2), 180–188.

Fleishman, J. A., Mor, V., & Laliberte, L. L. (1995). Longitudinal patterns of medical service use and costs among people with AIDS. *Health Services Research, 30*(3), 403–424.

Flitcraft, A. (1997). Learning from the paradoxes of domestic violence. *Journal of the American Medical Association, 277*(17), 1400–1401.

Folland, S., Goodman, A. C., & Stano, M. (1997). *The economics of health and health care* (2nd ed.). Englewood Cliffs, NJ: Prentice Hall.

Fosset, J. W., Perloff, J. D., Peterson, J. A., & Kletke, P. R. (1990). Medicaid in the inner city: The case of maternity care in Chicago. *Milbank Quarterly, 68,* 111–141.

Fox, D. M., & Thomas, E. H. (Eds.). (1989). *Financing care for persons with AIDS: The first studies, 1985–1988.* Frederick, MD: University Publishing Group.

Fox, H. B., & Newacheck, P. W. (1990). Private health insurance of chronically ill children. *Pediatrics, 85,* 50–57.

Fox, H. B., Wicks, L. B., & Newacheck, P. W. (1993). Health maintenance organizations and children with special health needs. A suitable match? *American Journal of Diseases of Children, 147*(5), 546–552.

Fox, J., Merwin, E., & Blank, M. (1995). De facto mental health services in the rural south. *Journal of Health Care for the Poor and Underserved, 6*(4), 434–468.

Fox, K., Merrill, J. C., Chang, H. H., & Califano, J. A. Jr. (1995). Estimating the costs of substance abuse to the Medicaid hospital care program. *American Journal of Public Health, 85*(1), 48–54.

Fox, P. D., Etheredge, L., & Jones, S. B. (1998). Addressing the needs of chronically ill persons under Medicare. *Health Affairs, 17*(2), 144–151.

Frank, R. G. (1989). The medically indigent mentally ill: Approaches to financing. *Hospital and Community Psychiatry, 40,* 9–12.

Frank, R. G., & Kamlet, M. S. (1985). Direct costs and expenditures for mental health care in the United States in 1980. *Hospital and Community Psychiatry, 36,* 165–168.

Frank, R. G., Koyanagi, C., & McGuire, T. G. (1997). The politics and economics of mental health "parity" laws. *Health Affairs, 16*(4), 108–119.

Frank, R. G., McGuire, T. G., & Newhouse, J. P. (1995). Risk contracts in managed mental health care. *Health Affairs, 14*(3), 50–64.

Frank, R. G., McGuire, T. G., Notman, E. H., & Woodward, R. M. (1996). Developments in Medicaid managed behavioral health care. In R. W. Manderscheid, & M. A. Sonnenschein (Eds.), *Mental health, United States, 1996* (pp. 138–153) (DHHS Publication No. SMA 96–3098). Center for Mental Health Services. Substance Abuse and Mental Health Services Administration. Washington, DC: U.S. Government Printing Office.

Freeman, K. R., & Estrada-Mullaney, T. (1988). *Using dolls to interview child victims: Legal concerns and interview procedures.* Office of Justice Programs, National Institute of Justice. Washington, DC: U.S. Department of Justice.

Freeman, R. B., & Hall, B. (1986). *Permanent homelessness in America?* Working Paper No. 2013. Cambridge, MA: National Bureau of Economic Research.

Freire, P. (1970). *Pedagogy of the oppressed* (M. B. Ramos, Trans.). New York: Seabury Press.

French, M. T., Dunlap, L. J., Zarkin, G. A., McGeary, K. A., & McLellan, A. T. (1997). A structured instrument for estimating the economic cost of drug abuse treatment. The Drug Abuse Treatment Cost Analysis Program (DATCAP). *Journal of Substance Abuse Treatment, 14*(5), 445–455.

French, M. T., & Martin, R. F. (1996). The costs of drug abuse consequences: A summary of research findings. *Journal of Substance Abuse Treatment, 13*(6), 453–466.

French, M. T., Mauskopf, J. A., Teague, J. L., & Roland, E. J. (1996). Estimating the dollar value of health outcomes from drug-abuse interventions. *Medical Care, 34*(9), 890–910.

French, M. T., & McGeary, K. A. (1997). Estimating the economic cost of substance abuse treatment. *Health Economics, 6*(5), 539–544.

Freudenberg, N., Wilets, I., Greene, M. B., & Richie, B. E. (1998). Linking women in jail to community services: Factors associated with rearrest and retention of drug-using women following release from jail. *Journal of the American Medical Women's Association, 53*(2), 89–93.

Friday, J. C. (1995). The psychological impact of violence in underserved communities. *Journal of Health Care for the Poor & Underserved, 6*(4), 403–409.

Friedland, R. B., & Pankaj, V. (1997). *Welfare and elderly legal immigrants* (Prepared for the Henry J. Kaiser Family Foundation). Washington, DC: National Academy on Aging.

Friedman, R. M., Katz-Leavy, J. W., Manderscheid, R. W., & Sondheimer, D. L. (1998). Prevalence of serious emotional disturbance: An update. In R. W. Manderscheid & M. J. Henderson (Eds.), *Mental health, United States, 1998* (pp. 110–112) (DHHS Publication No. SMA 99–3285). Center for Mental Health Services. Substance Abuse and Mental Health Services Administration. Washington, DC: U.S. Government Printing Office.

Friedman, S. R., Neaigus, A., Jose, B., Curtis, R., Goldstein, M., Ildefonso, G., Rothenberg, R. B., & Des Jarlais, D. C. (1997). Sociometric risk networks and risk for HIV infection. *American Journal of Public Health, 87*(8), 1289–1296.

Fries, J. F. (1989). The compression of morbidity: Near or far? *Milbank Quarterly, 67*, 208–232.

Frisman, L. K., & McGuire, T. G. (1989). The economics of long-term care for the mentally ill. *Journal of Social Issues, 45*, 119–130.

Fritz, M. E. (1989). Full circle or forward. *Child Abuse and Neglect, 13*, 313–318.

Frye, B. A., & D'Avanzo, C. D. (1994). Cultural themes in family stress and violence among Cambodian refugee women in the inner city. *Advances in Nursing Science, 16*(3), 64–77.

Fryer, G. E. Jr., & Miyoshi, T. J. (1995). A cluster analysis of detected and substantiated child maltreatment incidents in rural Colorado. *Child Abuse and Neglect, 19*(3), 363–369.

Fulco, C. E., Liverman, C. T., & Bonnie, R. J. (Eds.). (1996). *Pathways of addiction: Opportunities in drug abuse research.* Washington, DC: National Academy Press.

Fuller, M. G. (1994). A new day: Strategies for managing psychiatric and substance abuse benefits. *Health Care Management Review, 19*(4), 20–24.

Fullilove, M. T. (1996). Psychiatric implications of displacement: Contributions from the psychology of place. *American Journal of Psychiatry, 153*(12), 1516–1523.

Fullilove, M. T., Green, L., & Fullilove, R. E. III. (1999). Building momentum: An ethnographic study of inner-city redevelopment. *American Journal of Public Health, 89*(6), 840–844.

Fullilove, M. T., Héon, V., Jimenez, W., Parsons, C., Green, L. L., & Fullilove, R. E. (1998). Injury and anomie: Effects of violence on an inner-city community. *American Journal of Public Health, 88*(6), 924–927.

Gallagher, T. C., Andersen, R. M., Koegel, P., & Gelberg, L. (1997). Determinants of regular source of care among homeless adults in Los Angeles. *Medical Care, 35*(8), 814–830.

Garbarino, J. (1986). Can we measure success in preventing child abuse? Issues in policy, programming and research. *Child Abuse and Neglect, 10*, 143–156.

Gardner, J. F., Nudler, S., & Chapman, M. S. (1997). Personal outcomes as measures of quality. *Mental Retardation, 35*(4), 295–305.

Garnick, D. W., Horgan, C. M., Hendricks, A. M., & Constock, C. (1996). Using health insurance claims data to analyze substance abuse charges and utilization. *Medical Care Research and Review, 53*(3), 350–368.

Gelberg, L., Doblin, B. H., & Leake, B. D. (1996). Ambulatory health services provided to low-income and homeless adult patients in a major community health center. *Journal of General Internal Medicine, 11*(3), 156–162.

Gelberg, L., Gallagher, T. C., Andersen, R. M., & Koegel, P. (1997). Competing priorities as a barrier to medical care among homeless adults in Los Angeles. *American Journal of Public Health, 87*(2), 217–220.

Gelberg, L., Panarites, C. J., Morgenstern, H., Leake, B., Andersen, R. M., & Koegel, P. (1997). Tuberculosis skin testing among homeless adults. *Journal of General Internal Medicine, 12*(1), 25–33.

Gelberg, L., Stein, J. A., & Neumann, C. G. (1995). Determinants of undernutrition among homeless adults. *Public Health Reports, 110*(4), 448–454.

Gelles, R. J., & Cornell, C. P. (1990). *Intimate violence in families* (2nd ed.). Thousand Oaks, CA: Sage.

Gelles, R. J., & Straus, M. A. (1988). *Intimate violence: Causes and consequences of abuse in the American family.* New York: Simon & Schuster.

General Accounting Office. (1985). *Homelessness: A complex problem and the federal response* (GAO-HRD-85–40). Washington, DC: U.S. Government Printing Office.

General Accounting Office. (1987). *Prenatal care: Medicaid recipients and uninsured women obtain insufficient care* (GAO-HRD-87–137). Washington, DC: U.S. Government Printing Office.

General Accounting Office. (1988a). *Homeless mentally ill: Problems and options in estimating numbers and trends* (GAO-PEMD-88–24). Washington, DC: U.S. Government Printing Office.

General Accounting Office. (1988b). *Long-term care for the elderly: Issues of need, access, and cost* (GAO-HRD-89–4). Washington, DC: U.S. Government Printing Office.

General Accounting Office. (1989a). *Board and care: Insufficient assurances that residents' needs are identified and met* (GAO-HRD-89–50). Washington, DC: U.S. Government Printing Office.

General Accounting Office. (1989b). *Children and youths: About 68,000 homeless and 186,000 in shared housing at any given time* (GAO-PEMD-89–14). Washington, DC: U.S. Government Printing Office.

General Accounting Office. (1989c). *Health care: Home care experiences of families with chronically ill children* (GAO-HRD-89–73). Washington, DC: U.S. Government Printing Office.

General Accounting Office. (1989d). *Mental health: Prevention of mental disorders and research on stress-related disorders* (GAO-HRD-89–97). Washington, DC: U.S. Government Printing Office.

General Accounting Office. (1990a). *Drug abuse: Research on treatment may not address current needs* (GAO-HRD-90–114). Washington, DC: U.S. Government Printing Office.

General Accounting Office. (1990b). *Homelessness: Access to McKinney Act programs improved but better oversight needed* (GAO-RCED-91–29). Washington, DC: U.S. Government Printing Office.

General Accounting Office. (1990c). *Home visiting: A promising early intervention strategy for at-risk families* (GAO-HRD-90–83). Washington, DC: U.S. Government Printing Office.

General Accounting Office. (1991). *Trauma care: Lifesaving system threatened by unreimbursed costs and other factors* (GAO-HRD-91–57). Washington, DC: U.S. Government Printing Office.

General Accounting Office. (1999). *Homelessness: Coordination and evaluation of programs are essential* (GAO-RCED-99–49). Washington, DC: U. S. Government Printing Office.

Gerbert, B., Macguire, B. T., & Coates, T. J. (1990). Are patients talking to their physicians about AIDS? *American Journal of Public Health, 80*, 467–469.

Gerstein, D. R., & Green, L. W. (Eds.). (1993). *Preventing drug abuse: What do we know?* Washington, DC: National Academy Press.

Gerstein, D. R., & Harwood, H. J. (Eds.). (1990). *Treating drug problems* (Vol. 1). Washington, DC: National Academy Press.

Gibbs, J. T. (1988). Conceptual, methodological, and sociocultural issues in black youth suicide: Implications for assessment and early intervention. *Suicide and Life-Threatening Behavior, 18*, 73–89.

Gielen, A. C., O'Campo, P., Faden, R. R., & Eke, A. (1997). Women's disclosure of HIV status: Experiences of mistreatment and violence in an urban setting. *Women and Health, 25*(3), 19–31.

Glied, S. (1998). Too little time? The recognition and treatment of mental health problems in primary care. *Health Services Research, 33*(4 Pt. 1), 891–910.

Glied, S., Hoven, C. W., Moore, R. E., Garrett, A. B., & Regier, D. A. (1997). Children's access to mental health care: Does insurance matter? *Health Affairs, 16*(1), 167–174.

Golding, J. M., & Lipton, R. I. (1990). Depressed mood and major depressive disorder in two ethnic groups. *Journal of Psychiatric Research, 24*, 65–82.

Goldsmith, H. F., Lin, E., Bell, R. A., & Jackson, D. J. (Eds.). (1988). *Needs assessment: Its future* (DHHS Publication No. ADM 88–1550). Washington, DC: U.S. Government Printing Office.

Goldstrom, I., Henderson, M., Male, A., & Manderscheid, R. W. (1998). Jail mental health services: A national survey. In R. W. Manderscheid & M. J. Henderson (Eds.), *Mental health, United States, 1998* (pp. 176–187) (DHHS Publication No. SMA 99–3285). Center for Mental Health Services. Substance Abuse and Mental Health Services Administration. Washington, DC: U.S. Government Printing Office.

Goodman, E., & Cohall, A. T. (1989). Acquired immunodeficiency syndrome and adolescents: Knowledge, attitudes, beliefs, and behaviors in a New York City adolescent minority population. *Pediatrics, 84*, 36–42.

Gorsky, R. D., & Colby, J. P., Jr. (1989). The cost effectiveness of prenatal care in reducing low birth weight in New Hampshire. *Health Services Research, 24*, 583–598.

Gortmaker, S. L., Clark, C. J. G., Graven, S. N., Sobol, A. M., & Geronimus, A. T. (1989). Reducing infant mortality in rural America: Evaluation of the rural infant care program. In G. H. DeFriese, T. C. Ricketts III, & J. S. Stein (Eds.), *Methodological advances in health services research* (pp. 91–116). Ann Arbor MI: Health Administration Press.

Gould, M. S., Wallenstein, S., & Davidson, L. (1989). Suicide clusters: A critical review. *Suicide and Life-Threatening Behavior, 19*, 17–29.

Grabbe, L., Demi, A., Camann, M. A., & Potter, L. (1997). The health status of elderly persons in the last year of life: A comparison of deaths by suicide, injury, and natural causes. *American Journal of Public Health, 87*(3), 434–437.

Graham, J. W., Johnson, C. A., Hansen, W. B., Flay, B. R., & Gee, M. (1990). Drug use prevention programs, gender, and ethnicity: Evaluation of three seventh-grade project SMART cohorts. *Preventive Medicine, 19*, 305–313.

Graham, R. P., Forrester, M. L., Wysong, J. A., Rosenthal, T. C., & James, P. A. (1995). HIV/AIDS in the rural United States: Epidemiology and health services delivery. *Medical Care Research & Review, 52*(4), 435–452.

Graitcer, P. L. (1989). Evaluating community interventions to reduce drunken driving. *American Journal of Public Health, 79*, 271.

Grazier, K. L. (1989). Long-term care services for the chronically mentally ill: Reimbursement system structure, effects, and alternatives. *Medical Care Review, 46*, 45–73.

Green, J., Oppenheimer, G. M., & Wintfeld, N. (1994). The $147,000 misunderstanding: Repercussions of overestimating the cost of AIDS. *Journal of Health Politics, Policy and Law, 19*(1), 69–90.

Greenberg, M., & Schneider, D. (1994). Violence in American cities: Young black males is the answer, but what was the question? *Social Science and Medicine, 39*(2), 179–187.

Greenfeld, L. A., Rand, M. R., Craven, D., Klaus, P. A., Perkins, C. A., Ringel, C., Warchol, G., Maston, C., & Fox, J. A. (1998). *Violence by intimates: Analysis of data on crimes by current or former spouses, boyfriends, and girlfriends* (Publication No. NCJ-167237). Washington, DC: U.S. Department of Justice, Bureau of Justice Statistics.

Greenwald, H. P., Polissar, N. L., Borgatta, E. F., McCorkle, R., & Goodman, G. (1998). Social factors, treatment, and survival in early-stage non–small cell lung cancer. *American Journal of Public Health, 88*(11), 1681–1684.

Grella, C. E. (1997). Services for perinatal women with substance abuse and mental health disorders: The unmet need. *Journal of Psychoactive Drugs, 29*(1), 67–78.

Griffin, J. F., Hogan, J. W., Buechner, J. S., & Leddy, T. M. (1999). The effect of a Medicaid managed care program on the adequacy of prenatal care utilization in Rhode Island. *American Journal of Public Health, 89*(4), 497–501.

Griss, B. (1988). Measuring the health insurance needs of persons with disabilities and persons with chronic illness. *Access to Health Care, 1*(1,2), 1–63.

Griss, B. (1989). Strategies for adapting the private and public health insurance systems to the health related needs of persons with disabilities or chronic illness. *Access to Health Care, 1*(3,4), 1–91.

Grob, G. N. (1991). *From asylum to community: Mental health policy in modern America.* Princeton, NJ: Princeton University Press.

Grossman, D. C., Milligan, B. C., & Deyo, R. A. (1991). Risk factors for suicide attempts among Navajo adolescents. *American Journal of Public Health, 81*, 870–874.

Grossman, M., & Chaloupka, F. J. (1998). The demand for cocaine by young adults: A rational addiction approach. *Journal of Health Economics, 17*(4), 427–474.

Guinan, M. E., Farnham, P. G., & Holtgrave, D. R. (1994). Estimating the value of preventing a human immunodeficiency virus infection. *American Journal of Preventive Medicine, 10*(1), 1–4.

Gurr, T. R. (Ed.). (1989). *Violence in America: The history of crime* (Vol. 1). Thousand Oaks, CA: Sage.

Gust, S. W., & Walsh, J. M. (Eds.). (1989). *Drugs in the workplace: Research and evaluation data* (DHHS Publication No. ADM 89–1612). Washington, DC: U.S. Government Printing Office.

Gustafson, J. S., & Darby, M. (Eds.). (1999). *Connection: A newsletter linking the users and producers of drug abuse services research* (February 1999 issue). Washington, DC: Association for Health Services Research.

Haack, M. R. (1997). *Drug-dependent mothers and their children: Issues in public policy and public health.* New York: Springer.

Haaga, J., & Reuter, P. (Eds.). (1991). *Improving data for federal drug policy decisions: A RAND note.* Santa Monica, CA: RAND, Drug Policy Research Center.

Habermas, J. (1995). *Moral consciousness and communicative action* (C. Lenhardt & S. W. Nicholsen, Trans.). Cambridge, MA: MIT Press.

Habermas, J. (1996). *Between facts and norms: Contributions to a discourse theory of law and democracy* (W. Rehg, Trans.). Cambridge, MA: MIT Press.

Habib, J., Manton, K., Danon, D., Dowd, J. E., Galinsky, D., Kovar, M. G., Olshansky, S. J., & Suzman, R. (1988). Workshop: Forecasting the care needs of the elderly: Methodology and limitations. *Public Health Reports, 103*, 541–543.

Haines, D. W. (Ed.). (1989). *Refugees as immigrants: Cambodians, Laotians, and Vietnamese in America.* Lanham, MD: Rowman and Littlefield.

Halfon, N., Schuster, M., Valentine, W., & McGlynn, E. (1998). Improving the quality of healthcare for children: Implementing the results of the AHSR research agenda conference. *Health Services Research, 33*(4 Pt. 2), 955–976.

Halfon, N., Wood, D. L., Valdez, R. B., Pereyra, M., & Duan, N. (1997). Medicaid enrollment and health services access by Latino children in inner-city Los Angeles. *Journal of the American Medical Association, 277*(8), 636–641.

Hamilton, V. L., Broman, C. L., Hoffman, W. S., & Renner, D. S. (1990). Hard times and vulnerable people: Initial effects of plant closing on autoworkers' mental health. *Journal of Health and Social Behavior, 31*, 123–140.

Hanke, P. J., & Gundlach, J. H. (1995). Damned on arrival: A preliminary study of the relationship between homicide, emergency medical care, and race. *Journal of Criminal Justice, 23*(4), 313–323.

Hannan, E. L., van Ryn, M., Burke, J., Stone, D., Kumar, D., Arani, D., Pierce, W., Rafii, S., Sanborn, T. A., Sharma, S., Slater, J., & DeBuono, B. A. (1999). Access to coronary artery bypass surgery by race/ethnicity and gender among patients who are appropriate for surgery. *Medical Care, 37*(1), 68–77.

Hardwick, P. J., & Rowton-Lee, M. A. (1996). Adolescent homicide: Towards assessment of risk. *Journal of Adolescence, 19*(3), 263–276.

Hardy, A. M. (1990). National Health Interview Survey data on adult knowledge of AIDS in the United States. *Public Health Reports, 105*, 629–634.

Hargraves, M. A. (1996). Immigrants needing health care in Texas. *Texas Medicine, 92*(10), 64–77.

Hargreaves, W. A., & Shumway, M. (1989). Effectiveness of mental health services for the severely mentally ill. In C. A. Taube, D. Mechanic, & A. A. Hohmann (Eds.), *The future of mental health services research* (DHHS Publication No. ADM 89–1600) (pp. 253–286). National Institute of Mental Health. Washington, DC: U.S. Government Printing Office.

Harrington, C., & Newcomer, R. J. (1991). Social health maintenance organizations' service use and costs, 1985–89. *Health Care Financing Review, 12*(3), 37–52.

Hart, K. D., Kunitz, S. J., Sell, R. R., & Mukamel, D. B. (1998). Metropolitan governance, residential segregation, and mortality among African Americans. *American Journal of Public Health, 88*(3), 434–438.

Harwood, H., Fountain, D., Livermore, G., & the Lewin Group. (1998). *The economic costs of alcohol and drug abuse in the United States 1992* (NIH Publication No. 98–4327). National Institute on Drug Abuse. Washington, DC: U.S. Government Printing Office.

Haugaard, J. J., & Emery, R. E. (1989). Methodological issues in child sexual abuse research. *Child Abuse and Neglect, 13*, 89–100.

Haugaard, J. J., & Reppucci, N. D. (1989). *The sexual abuse of children: A comprehensive guide to current knowledge and intervention strategies.* San Francisco: Jossey-Bass.

Havens, P. L., Cuene, B. E., & Holtgrave, D. R. (1997). Lifetime cost of care for children with human immunodeficiency virus infection. *Pediatric Infectious Disease Journal, 16*(6), 607–610.

Hay Group. (1999). *Health care plan design and cost trends: 1988 through 1998.* Arlington, VA: Author.

Hayden, S. R., Barton, E. D., & Hayden, M. (1997). Domestic violence in the emergency department: How do women prefer to disclose and discuss the issues? *Journal of Emergency Medicine, 15*(4), 447–451.

Hayes, C. D. (Ed.). (1987). *Risking the future: Adolescent sexuality, pregnancy, and childbearing.* Washington, DC: National Academy Press.

Health Care Financing Administration. (1998a). *Medicaid and Acquired Immune Deficiency Syndrome (AIDS) and Human Immunodeficiency Virus (HIV) infection* [On-line]. Available:

http://www.hcfa.gov/medicaid/obs11.htm [Accessed Sept. 13, 1999. Last updated Mar. 10, 1998].

Health Care Financing Administration. (1998b). *National summary of Medicaid managed care programs and enrollment* [On-line]. Available: http://www.hcfa.gov/medicaid/trends98.htm [Accessed Sept, 13, 1999. Last updated Apr. 8, 1999].

Health Care Financing Administration. (1998c). *Program of all-inclusive care for the elderly (PACE)* [On-line]. Available: http://www.hcfa.gov/medicaid/pace/pacegen.htm [Accessed Sept. 14, 1999. Last updated Nov. 2, 1998].

Health Care Financing Administration. (1999). *Medicaid waivers and demonstrations* [On-line]. Available: http://www.hcfa.gov/medicaid/hpg1.htm [Accessed Apr. 20, 2000. Last updated Dec. 2, 1999].

Healton, C., Messeri, P., Abramson, D., Howard, J., Sorin, M. D., & Bayer, R. (1996). A balancing act: The tension between case-finding and primary prevention strategies in New York State's voluntary HIV counseling and testing program in women's health care settings. *American Journal of Preventive Medicine, 12*(4 Suppl.), 53–60.

Heath, K., Hogg, R. S., Singer, J., Schechter, M. T., O'Shaughnessy, M. V., & Montaner, J. S. (1997). Physician concurrence with primary care guidelines for persons with HIV disease. *International Journal of STD & AIDS, 8*(10), 609–613.

Hedrick, S. C., Koepsell, T. D., & Inui, T. (1989). Meta-analysis of home-care effects on mortality and nursing-home placement. *Medical Care, 27*, 1015–1026.

Hedrick, S. C., Rothman, M. L., Chapko, M., Inui, T. S., Kelly, J. R., Ehreth, J., & the Adult Day Health Care Evaluation Development Group. (1991). Adult day health care evaluation study: Methodology and implementation. *Health Services Research, 25*, 935–960.

Helfer, R. E., & Kempe, R. S. (Eds.). (1987). *The battered child* (4th ed., rev. and exp.). Chicago: University of Chicago Press.

Hellinger, F. J. (1988a). Forecasting the personal medical care costs of AIDS from 1988 through 1991. *Public Health Reports, 103*, 309–319.

Hellinger, F. J. (1988b). National forecasts of the medical care costs of AIDS: 1988–1992. *Inquiry, 25*, 469–484.

Hellinger, F. J. (1990). Updated forecasts of the costs of medical care for persons with AIDS, 1989–1993. *Public Health Reports, 105*, 1–12.

Hellinger, F. J. (1991). Forecasting the medical care costs of the HIV epidemic: 1991–1994. *Inquiry, 28*, 213–224.

Hellinger, F. J. (1993a). The lifetime cost of treating a person with HIV. *Journal of the American Medical Association, 270*(4), 474–478.

Hellinger, F. J. (1993b). The use of health services by women with HIV infection. *Health Services Research, 28*(5), 543–561.

Hellinger, F. J. (1998). Cost and financing of care for persons with HIV disease: An overview. *Health Care Financing Review, 19*(3), 5–18.

Hellinger, F. J., Fleishman, J. A., & Hsia, D. C. (1994). AIDS treatment costs during the last months of life: Evidence from the ACSUS. *Health Services Research, 29*(5), 569–581.

Helzer, J. E., Spitznagel, E. L., & McEvoy, L. (1987). The predictive validity of lay diagnostic interview schedule diagnoses in the general population. *Archives of General Psychiatry, 44*, 1069–1077.

Henderson, D. C., & Anderson, S. C. (1989). Adolescents and chemical dependency. *Social Work in Health Care, 14*, 87–105.

Henry, K. (1988). Setting AIDS priorities: The need for a closer alliance of public health and clinical approaches toward the control of AIDS. *American Journal of Public Health, 78*, 1210–1212.

Hermann, R. C., Ettner, S. L., & Dorwart, R. A. (1998). The influence of psychiatric disorders on patients' ratings of satisfaction with health care. *Medical Care, 36*(5), 720–727.

Hernandez, D., & Charney, E. (Eds.). (1998). *From generation to generation: The health and well-being of children in immigrant families.* Washington, DC: National Academy Press.

Herz, E. J., Chawla, A. J., & Gavin, N. I. (1998). Preventive services for children under Medicaid, 1989 and 1992. *Health Care Financing Review, 19*(4), 25–44.

Hessol, N. A., Fuentes-Afflick, E., & Bacchetti, P. (1998). Risk of low birth weight infants among black and white parents. *Obstetrics and Gynecology, 92*(5), 814–822.

Hexter, A. C., Harris, J. A., Roeper, P., Croen, L. A., Krueger, P., & Gant, D. (1990). Evaluation of the hospital discharge diagnoses index and the birth certificate as sources of information on birth defects. *Public Health Reports, 105,* 296–307.

Heymann, S. J., & Earle, A. (1999). The impact of welfare reform on parents' ability to care for their children's health. *American Journal of Public Health, 89*(4), 502–505.

Hill, I. T. (1990). Improving state Medicaid programs for pregnant women and children. *Health Care Financing Review, Annual Supplement,* 75–87.

Hinton-Walker, P. (1993). Care of the chronically ill: Paradigm shifts and directions for the future. *Holistic Nursing Practice, 8*(1), 56–66.

Holden, C. (1988). Health problems of the homeless. *Science, 242*(4876), 188–189.

Holtgrave, D. R., & Pinkerton, S. D. (1997). Updates of cost of illness and quality of life estimates for use in economic evaluations of HIV prevention programs. *JAIDS: Journal of Acquired Immune Deficiency Syndromes, 16*(1), 54–62.

Hombs, M. E., & Snyder, M. (1982). *Homelessness in America: Forced march to nowhere* (1st ed.). Washington, DC: Community for Creative Non-Violence.

Hombs, M. E., & Snyder, M. (1983). *Homelessness in America: Forced march to nowhere* (2nd ed.). Washington, DC: Community for Creative Non-Violence.

Honigfeld, L. S., & Kaplan, D. W. (1987). Native American postneonatal mortality. *Pediatrics, 80,* 575–578.

Hoppe, S. K., & Martin, H. W. (1986). Patterns of suicide among Mexican Americans and anglos, 1960–1980. *Social Psychiatry, 21,* 83–88.

Horbar, J. D., & Lucey, J. F. (1995). Evaluation of neonatal intensive care technologies. *Future of Children, 5*(1), 139–161.

Hotaling, G. T., Finkelhor, D., Kirkpatrick, J. T., & Straus, M. A. (Eds.). (1988a). *Coping with family violence: Research and policy perspectives.* Thousand Oaks, CA: Sage.

Hotaling, G. T., Finkelhor, D., Kirkpatrick, J. T., & Straus, M. A. (Eds.). (1988b). *Family abuse and its consequences: New directions in research.* Thousand Oaks, CA: Sage.

Hough, R. L., Landsverk, J. A., Karno, M., Burnam, M. A., Timbers, D. M., Escobar, J. I., & Regier, D. A. (1987). Utilization of health and mental health services by Los Angeles Mexican Americans and non-Hispanic whites. *Archives of General Psychiatry, 44,* 702–709.

Hser, Y. I., Joshi, V., Anglin, M. D., & Fletcher, B. (1999). Predicting posttreatment cocaine abstinence for first-time admissions and treatment repeaters. *American Journal of Public Health, 89*(5), 666–671.

Huba, G., & Melchior, L. (1994). *Evaluation of the effects of Ryan White Title I funding on services for HIV-infected drug abusers: Baseline data: Year I: Summary report* (HRSA-RD-SP-94–8). Washington, DC: Health Resources & Services Administration.

Huby, G. (1997). Interpreting silence, documenting experience: An anthropological approach to the study of health service users' experience with HIV/AIDS care in Lothian, Scotland. *Social Science and Medicine, 44*(8), 1149–1160.

Hughes, S. L. (1985). Apples and oranges? A review of evaluations of community-based long-term care. *Health Services Research, 20,* 461–488.

Hunter, J. K., Crosby, F., Ventura, M. R., & Warkentin, L. (1997). Factors limiting evaluation of health care programs for the homeless. *Nursing Outlook, 45*(5), 224–228.

Hurley, S. F., Kaldor, J. M., Carlin, J. B., Gardiner, S., Evans, D. B., Chondros, P., Hoy, J., Spelman, D., Spicer, W. J., Wraight, H., et al. (1995). The usage and costs of health services for HIV infection in Australia. *AIDS, 9*(7), 777–785.

Immigration and Naturalization Service. (1999a). *Asylees, fiscal year 1997.* Washington, DC: U.S. Department of Justice.

Immigration and Naturalization Service. (1999b). *Legal immigration, fiscal year 1998.* Washington, DC: U.S. Department of Justice.

Immigration and Naturalization Service. (1999c). *Refugees, fiscal year 1997.* Washington, DC: U.S. Department of Justice.

Indian Health Service. (1998). *Trends in Indian health 1997.* Washington, DC: U.S. Government Printing Office.

Indian Health Service. (1999). [Selected vital statistics]. Unpublished data.

Infant Health and Development Program. (1990). Enhancing the outcomes of low-birth-weight, premature infants: A multisite, randomized trial. *Journal of the American Medical Association, 263,* 3035–3042.

Ingster, L. M., & Cartwright, W. S. (1995). Drug disorders and cardiovascular disease: The impact on annual hospital length of stay for the Medicare population. *American Journal of Drug and Alcohol Abuse, 21*(1), 93–110.

Institute of Medicine. (1985). *Preventing low birthweight.* Washington, DC: National Academy Press.

Institute of Medicine. (1986). *Confronting AIDS: Directions for public health, health care, and research.* Washington, DC: National Academy Press.

Institute of Medicine. (1987). *Causes and consequences of alcohol problems: An agenda for research.* Washington, DC: National Academy Press.

Institute of Medicine. (1988a). *Confronting AIDS: Update 1988.* Washington, DC: National Academy Press.

Institute of Medicine. (1988b). *The future of public health.* Washington, DC: National Academy Press.

Institute of Medicine. (1988c). *Homelessness, health, and human needs.* Washington, DC: National Academy Press.

Institute of Medicine. (1988d). *Prenatal care: Reaching mothers, reaching infants* (S. S. Brown, Ed.). Washington, DC: National Academy Press.

Institute of Medicine. (1989a). *Medical professional liability and the delivery of obstetrical care* (Vol. 1). Washington, DC: National Academy Press.

Institute of Medicine. (1989b). *Medical professional liability and the delivery of obstetrical care* (Vol. 2). Washington, DC: National Academy Press.

Institute of Medicine. (1989c). *Prevention and treatment of alcohol problems: Research opportunities* (Publication IOM-89–13). Washington, DC: National Academy Press.

Institute of Medicine. (1989d). *Research on children and adolescents with mental, behavioral, and developmental disorders: Mobilizing a national initiative.* Washington, DC: National Academy Press.

Institute of Medicine. (1990). *Broadening the base of treatment for alcohol problems.* Washington, DC: National Academy Press.

Institute of Medicine. (1991a). *The AIDS research program of the National Institutes of Health.* Washington, DC: National Academy Press.

Institute of Medicine. (1991b). *Disability in America: Toward a national agenda for prevention.* Washington, DC: National Academy Press.

Institute of Medicine. (1991c). *The second fifty years: Promoting health and preventing disability.* Washington, DC: National Academy Press.

Interagency Forum on Aging-Related Statistics. (1989). *Measuring the activities of daily living among the elderly: A guide to national surveys.* Federal Forum: A Final Report. Washington, DC: Brookings Institution.

International Center for the Disabled. (1986). *The ICD survey of disabled Americans: Bringing disabled Americans into the mainstream.* New York: Louis Harris and Associates.

Irazuzta, J. E., McJunkin, J. E., Danadian, K., Arnold, F., & Zhang, J. (1997). Outcome and cost of child abuse. *Child Abuse & Neglect, 21*(8), 751–757.

Ireys, H. T., Anderson, G. F., Shaffer, T. J., & Neff, J. M. (1997). Expenditures for care of children with chronic illnesses enrolled in the Washington State Medicaid program, fiscal year 1993. *Pediatrics, 100*(2 Pt. 1), 197–204.

Israel, B. A., Schulz, A. J., Parker, E. A., & Becker, A. B. (1998). Review of community-based research: Assessing partnership approaches to improve public health. *Annual Review of Public Health, 19*, 173–202.

Issel, L. M. (1996). Use of community resources by prenatal case managers. *Public Health Nursing, 13*(1), 3–12.

Ivey, S. L., & Kramer, E. J. (1998). Immigrant women and the emergency department: The juncture with welfare and immigration reform. *Journal of the American Medical Women's Association, 53*(2), 94–95, 107.

Ivey, S. L., Scheffler, R., & Zazzali, J. L. (1998). Supply dynamics of the mental health workforce: Implications for health policy. *Milbank Quarterly, 76*(1), 25–58.

Jacobs, P., & McDermott, S. (1989). Family caregiver costs of chronically ill and handicapped children: Method and literature review. *Public Health Reports, 104*, 158–163.

Jarvik, M. E. (1990). The drug dilemma: Manipulating the demand. *Science, 250*(4979), 387–392.

Jaskulski, T., & Robinson, G. K. (1990). *The community support program: A review of a federal-state partnership.* Washington, DC: Mental Health Policy Resource Center.

Jellinek, M. S., Murphy, J. M., Bishop, S., Poitrast, F., & Quinn, S. D. (1990). Protecting severely abused and neglected children: An unkept promise. *New England Journal of Medicine, 323*, 1628–1630.

Jencks, C., & Peterson, P. E. (Eds.). (1991). *The urban underclass.* Washington, DC: Brookings Institution.

Jenkins, C.N.H., McPhee, S. J., Bird, J. A., & Bonilla, N. H. (1990). Cancer risks and prevention practices among Vietnamese refugees. *Western Journal of Medicine, 153*, 34–39.

Jerrell, J. M., & Hu, T. W. (1996). Estimating the cost impact of three dual diagnosis treatment programs. *Evaluation Review, 20*(2), 160–180.

Jobes, D. A., Berman, A. L., & Josselson, A. R. (1987). Improving the validity and reliability of medical-legal certifications of suicide. *Suicide and Life-Threatening Behavior, 17*, 310–325.

Johnson, J. G., Cohen, P., Brown, J., Smailes, E. M., & Bernstein, D. P. (1999). Childhood maltreatment increases risk for personality disorders during early adulthood. *Archives of General Psychiatry, 56*(7), 600–606.

Johnson, J. G., Spitzer, R. L., Williams, J. B., Kroenke, K., Linzer, M., Brody, D., deGruy, F., & Hahn, S. (1995). Psychiatric comorbidity, health status, and functional impairment associated with alcohol abuse and dependence in primary care patients: Findings of the PRIME MD-1000 study. *Journal of Consulting and Clinical Psychology, 63*(1), 133–140.

Johnson, R. A., Gerstein, D. R., & Rasinski, K. A. (1998). Adjusting survey estimates for response bias: An application to trends in alcohol and marijuana use. *Public Opinion Quarterly, 62*, 354–377.

Johnston, L. D., O'Malley, P. M., & Bachman, J. G. (1999). *National survey results on drug use from the Monitoring the Future Study, 1975–1998: Vol. 1: Secondary school students* (NIH Publication No. 99–4660). Washington, DC: U.S. Government Printing Office.

Jones, C. L., & Battjes, R. J. (1990a). The context and caveats of prevention research on drug abuse. In C. L. Jones & R. J. Battjes (Eds.), *Etiology of drug abuse: Implications for prevention* (DHHS Publication No. ADM 90–1335) (pp. 1–12). Washington, DC: U.S. Government Printing Office.

Jones, C. L., & Battjes, R. J. (Eds.). (1990b). *Etiology of drug abuse: Implications for prevention* (DHHS Publication No. ADM 90–1335). Washington, DC: U.S. Government Printing Office.

Jones, E. W., Densen, P. M., & Brown, S. D. (1989). Posthospital needs of elderly people at home: Findings from an eight-month follow-up study. *Health Services Research, 24*, 643–664.

Joyce, T., Corman, H., & Grossman, M. (1988). A cost-effectiveness analysis of strategies to reduce infant mortality. *Medical Care, 26*, 348–360.

Justice, A. C., Feinstein, A. R., & Wells, C. K. (1989). A new prognostic staging system for the acquired immunodeficiency syndrome. *New England Journal of Medicine, 320*, 1388–1393.

Justice, B., & Justice, R. (1990). *The abusing family* (Rev. ed.). New York: Plenum Press.

Kaiser Family Foundation. (1997). *Medicaid facts: The Medicaid program at a glance.* Washington, DC: Author.

Kaiser Family Foundation. (1999). *Medicare and Medicaid for the elderly and disabled poor.* Washington, DC: Author.

Kane, C. F., & Ennis, J. M. (1996). Health care reform and rural mental health: Severe mental illness. *Community Mental Health Journal, 32*(5), 445–62.

Kane, R. A., & Kane, R. L. (1988). Long-term care: Variations on a quality assurance theme. *Inquiry, 25*, 132–146.

Kane, R. L. (1990). Promoting the art of the possible in long-term care. *American Journal of Public Health, 80*, 15–16.

Kanouse, D. E., Mathews, W. C., & Bennett, C. L. (1989). Quality-of-care issues for HIV illness: Clinical and health services research. In W. N. LeVee (Ed.), *Conference Proceedings: New Perspectives on HIV-related Illnesses: Progress in Health Services Research* (DHHS Publication No. PHS 89–3449) (pp. 159–169). Washington, DC: U.S. Government Printing Office.

Kaplan, M. S., Adamek, M. E., & Johnson, S. (1994). Trends in firearm suicide among older American males: 1979–1988. *Gerontologist, 34*(1), 59–65.

Kaplan, M. S., & Geling, O. (1998). Firearm suicides and homicides in the United States: Regional variations and patterns of gun ownership. *Social Science and Medicine, 46*(9), 1227–1233.

Kastner, T. A., Walsh, K. K., & Criscione, T. (1997). Overview and implications of Medicaid managed care for people with developmental disabilities. *Mental Retardation, 35*(4), 257–269.

Katz, M. B. (1989). *The undeserving poor.* New York: Pantheon Books.

Kawachi, I., & Kennedy, B. P. (1997). The relationship of income inequality to mortality: Does the choice of indicator matter? *Social Science & Medicine, 45*(7), 1121–1127.

Kegeles, S. M., Hays, R. B., & Coates, T. J. (1996). The Mpowerment Project: A community-level HIV prevention intervention for young gay men. *American Journal of Public Health, 86*(8 Pt 1), 1129–1136.

Kelly, J. A. (1997). Substance abuse and mental health care. Managed care, access, and clinical outcomes. *AAOHN Journal, 45*(9), 439–445.

Kennedy, B. P., Kawachi, I., Lochner, K., Jones, C., & Prothrow-Stith, D. (1997). (Dis)respect and black mortality. *Ethnicity & Disease, 7*(3), 207–214.

Kennedy, B. P., Kawachi, I., Prothrow-Stith, D., Lochner, K., & Gupta, V. (1998). Social capital, income inequality, and firearm violent crime. *Social Science and Medicine, 47*(1), 7–17.

Kennedy, R. D., & Deapen, R. E. (1991). Differences between Oklahoma Indian infant mortality and other races. *Public Health Reports, 106*, 97–99.

Kessler, R. C. (1994). Building on the ECA: The National Comorbidity Survey and the Children's ECA. *International Journal of Methods in Psychiatric Research, 4*(2), 81–94.

Kessler, R. C. (1995). The National Comorbidity Survey: Preliminary results and future directions. *International Journal of Methods in Psychiatric Research, 5*(2), 139–151.

Kessler, R. C., Berglund, P. A., Walters, E. E., Leaf, P. J., Kouzis, A. C., Bruce, M. L., Friedman, R. M., Grosser, R. C., Kennedy, C., Kuehnel, T. G., Laska, E. M., Manderscheid, R. W., Narrow, W. E., Rosenheck, R. A., & Schneir, M. (1998). A methodology for estimating the twelve-month prevalence of serious mental illness. In R. W. Manderscheid & M. J. Henderson (Eds.), *Mental health, United States, 1998* (pp. 99–109) (DHHS Publication

No. SMA 99–3285). Center for Mental Health Services. Substance Abuse and Mental Health Services Administration. Washington, DC: U.S. Government Printing Office.

Kessler, R. C., Borges, G., & Walters, E. E. (1999). Prevalence of and risk factors for lifetime suicide attempts in the National Comorbidity Survey. *Archives of General Psychiatry, 56*(7), 617–626.

Kessler, R. C., McGonagle, K. A., Zhao, S., Nelson, C. B., Hughes, M., Eshleman, S., Wittchen, H. U., & Kendler, K. S. (1994). Lifetime and twelve-month prevalence of DSM-III-R psychiatric disorders in the United States. Results from the National Comorbidity Survey. *Archives of General Psychiatry, 51*(1), 8–19.

Khabbaz, R. F., Hartley, T. M., Lairmore, M. D., & Kaplan, J. E. (1990). Epidemiologic assessment of screening tests for antibody to human T lymphotropic virus type 1 (HTLV-1). *American Journal of Public Health, 80,* 190–192.

Kim, S., Coletti, S. D., Crutchfield, C. C., Williams, C., & Hepler, N. (1995). Benefit-cost analysis of drug abuse prevention programs: A macroscopic approach. *Journal of Drug Education, 25*(2), 111–127.

Kim, Y., & Grant, D. (1997). Immigration patterns, social support, and adaptation among Korean immigrant women and Korean American women. *Cultural Diversity and Mental Health, 3*(4), 235–245.

Kindig, D. A. (1997). *Purchasing population health: Paying for results.* Ann Arbor: University of Michigan Press.

Kington, R. S., & Smith, J. P. (1997). Socioeconomic status and racial and ethnic differences in functional status associated with chronic diseases. *American Journal of Public Health, 87*(5), 805–810.

Kinney, E. D., & Steinmetz, S. K. (1994). Notes from the insurance underground: How the chronically ill cope. *Journal of Health Politics, Policy and Law, 19*(3), 633–642.

Kirby, R. S. (1997). The quality of vital perinatal statistics data, with special reference to prenatal care. *Paediatric and Perinatal Epidemiology, 11*(1), 122–128.

Kirp, D. L., Epstein, S., Franks, M. S., Simon, J., Conaway, D., & Lewis, J. (1989). *Learning by heart: AIDS and schoolchildren in America's communities.* New Brunswick, NJ: Rutgers University Press.

Kleinman, P. K., Blackbourne, B. D., Marks, S. C., Karellas, A., & Belanger, P. L. (1989). Radiologic contributions to the investigation and prosecution of cases of fatal infant abuse. *New England Journal of Medicine, 320,* 507–511.

Klerman, G. L. (1989). Psychiatric diagnostic categories: Issues of validity and measurement: An invited comment on Mirowsky and Ross. *Journal of Health and Social Behavior, 30,* 26–32.

Klinkman, M. S., Gorenflo, D. W., & Ritsema, T. S. (1997). The effects of insurance coverage on the quality of prenatal care. *Archives of Family Medicine, 6*(6), 557–566.

Knudsen, D. D. (1988). *Child protective services: Discretion, decisions, dilemmas.* Springfield, IL: Thomas.

Koegel, P., Melamid, E., & Burnam, M. A. (1995). Childhood risk factors for homelessness among homeless adults. *American Journal of Public Health, 85*(12), 1642–1649.

Koff, T. H. (1988). *New approaches to health care for an aging population: Developing a continuum of chronic care services.* San Francisco: Jossey-Bass.

Koob, G. F., & Le Moal, M. (1997). Drug abuse: Hedonic homeostatic dysregulation. *Science, 278*(5335), 52–58.

Kosberg, J. I., Cairl, R. E., & Keller, D. M. (1990). Components of burden: Interventive implications. *Gerontologist, 30,* 236–242.

Kotch, J. B. (1997). *Maternal and child health: Programs, problems and policy in public health.* Gaithersburg, MD: Aspen.

Kovess, V., & Fournier, L. (1990). The DISSA: An abridged self-administered version of the DIS: Approach by episode. *Social Psychiatry and Psychiatric Epidemiology, 25,* 179–186.

Kozol, J. (1991). *Savage inequalities: Children in America's schools.* New York: HarperCollins.

Kposowa, A. J., Breault, K., & Singh, G. K. (1995). White male suicide in the United States: A multivariate individual-level analysis. *Social Forces, 74*(1), 315–325.

Kramer, A. M., Shaughnessy, P. W., Bauman, M. K., & Crisler, K. S. (1990). Assessing and assuring the quality of home health care: A conceptual framework. *Milbank Quarterly, 68,* 413–443.

Kreider, B., & Nicholson, S. (1997). Health insurance and the homeless. *Health Economics, 6*(1), 31–41.

Kreitman, N. (1988). The two traditions in suicide research: Dublin Lecture. *Suicide and Life-Threatening Behavior, 18,* 66–72.

Krueger, P., & Patterson, C. (1997). Detecting and managing elder abuse: Challenges in primary care. The Research Subcommittee of the Elder Abuse and Self-Neglect Task Force of Hamilton-Wentworth. *Canadian Medical Association Journal, 157*(8), 1095–1100.

Krugman, R. D. (1989). The more we learn, the less we know "with reasonable medical certainty"? *Child Abuse and Neglect, 13,* 165–166.

Kuhlthau, K., Walker, D. K., Perrin, J. M., Bauman, L., Gortmaker, S. L., Newacheck, P. W., & Stein, R. E. (1998). Assessing managed care for children with chronic conditions. *Health Affairs, 17*(4), 42–52.

Kulig, J. C. (1990). A review of the health status of Southeast Asian refugee women. *Health Care for Women International, 11,* 49–63.

Kunnes, R., Niven, R., Gustafson, T., Brooks, N., Levin, S. M., Edmunds, M., Trumble, J. G., & Coye, M. J. (1993). Financing and payment reform for primary health care and substance abuse treatment. *Journal of Addictive Diseases, 12*(2), 23–42.

Kurland, D. (1995). A review of quality evaluation systems for mental health services. *American Journal of Medical Quality, 10*(3), 141–148.

Kyriacou, D. N., McCabe, F., Anglin, D., Lapesarde, K., & Winer, M. R. (1998). Emergency department–based study of risk factors for acute injury from domestic violence against women. *Annals of Emergency Medicine, 31*(4), 502–506.

Labonte, R. (1993). Community development and partnerships. *Canadian Journal of Public Health, 84*(4), 237–240.

Labonte, R. (1994). Health promotion and empowerment: Reflections on professional practice. *Health Education Quarterly, 21*(2), 253–268.

Laine, C., Markson, L. E., McKee, L. J., Hauck, W. W., Fanning, T. R., & Turner, B. J. (1998). The relationship of clinic experience with advanced HIV and survival of women with AIDS. *AIDS, 12*(4), 417–424.

Lairson, D. R., Schulmeier, G., Begley, C. E., Aday, L. A., Coyle, Y., & Slater, C. H. (1997). Managed care and community-oriented care: Conflict or complement? *Journal of Health Care for the Poor and Underserved, 8*(1), 36–55.

Lam, J. A., & Rosenheck, R. (1999). Social support and service use among homeless persons with serious mental illness. *International Journal of Social Psychiatry, 45*(1), 13–28.

Lamb, S., Greenlick, M. R., & McCarty, D. (Eds.). (1998). *Bridging the gap between practice and research: Forging partnerships with community-based drug and alcohol treatment.* Washington, DC: National Academy Press.

Lambert, D., & Agger, M. S. (1995). Access of rural AFDC Medicaid beneficiaries to mental health services. *Health Care Financing Review, 17*(1), 133–145.

Lang, E. L. (1998). Datasets for exploring aspects of disability. *American Sociological Association Footnotes, 26*(11), 7.

Langenbucher, J. (1994a). Offsets are not add-ons: The place of addictions treatment in American health care reform. *Journal of Substance Abuse, 6*(1), 117–122.

Langenbucher, J. (1994b). Rx for health care costs: Resolving addictions in the general medical setting. *Alcoholism: Clinical and Experimental Research, 18*(5), 1033–1036.

Last, J. M., et al. (Eds.). (1995). *A dictionary of epidemiology* (3rd ed.). New York: Oxford University Press.

Laudicina, S. S., & Burwell, B. (1988). A profile of Medicaid home and community-based care waivers, 1985: Findings of a national survey. *Journal of Health Politics, Policy and Law, 13,* 525–546.

Laumann, E. O., Gagnon, J. H., Michaels, S., Michael, R. T., & Coleman, J. S. (1989). Monitoring the AIDS epidemic in the United States: A network approach. *Science, 244*(4909), 1186–1189.

Lave, J. R., & Goldman, H. H. (1990). Medicare financing for mental health care. *Health Affairs, 9*(1), 19–30.

Lawrence, R. A. (1994). The anatomy of violence. *Medicine and Law, 13*(5–6), 407–416.

Lawson, A. W. (1989). Substance abuse problems of the elderly: Considerations for treatment and prevention. In G. W. Lawson & A. W. Lawson (Eds.), *Alcoholism and substance abuse in special populations* (pp. 95–113). Gaithersburg, MD: Aspen.

Lê, C. T., Winter, T. D., Boyd, K. J., Ackerson, L., & Hurley, L. B. (1998). Experience with a managed care approach to HIV infection: Effectiveness of an interdisciplinary team. *American Journal of Managed Care, 4*(5), 647–657.

LeClere, F. B., Rogers, R. G., & Peters, K. (1998). Neighborhood social context and racial differences in women's heart disease mortality. *Journal of Health and Social Behavior, 39*(2), 91–107.

Lee, E. (1988). Cultural factors in working with Southeast Asian refugee adolescents. *Journal of Adolescence, 11,* 167–179.

Leenaars, A. A. (1989). Are young adults' suicides psychologically different from those of other adults? Shneidman lecture. *Suicide and Life-Threatening Behavior, 19,* 249–263.

Leenaars, A. A., Yang, B., & Lester, D. (1993). The effect of domestic and economic stress on suicide rates in Canada and the United States. *Journal of Clinical Psychology, 49*(6), 918–921.

Leff, H. S., & Woocher, L. S. (1998). Trends in the evaluation of managed mental health care. *Harvard Review of Psychiatry, 5*(6), 344–347.

Lehrman, S. E., Gentry, D., & Fogarty, T. E. (1998). Predictors of California nursing facilities' acceptance of people with HIV/AIDS. *Health Services Research, 32*(6), 867–880.

Leukefeld, C. G., & Tims, F. R. (1993). Drug abuse treatment in prisons and jails. *Journal of Substance Abuse Treatment, 10*(1), 77–84.

Leutz, W. N., Greenlick, M. R., & Capitman, J. A. (1994). Integrating acute and long-term care. *Health Affairs, 13*(4), 58–74.

Levi, J. (1998). Can access to care for people living with HIV be expanded? *AIDS and Public Policy Journal, 13*(2), 56–74.

Levi, J., Sogocio, K., Gambrell, A. E., & Jones, P. M. (1999). *Can access to the private individual insurance market be increased for people living with HIV?* Washington, DC: George Washington University School of Public Health and Health Services, Center for Health Policy Research.

Levine, C. (1990). AIDS and changing concepts of family. *Milbank Quarterly, 68*(Suppl. 1), 33–57.

Levine, D. S., & Levine, D. R. (1975). *The cost of mental illness, 1971* (DHEW Publication No. ADM 76–265). National Institute of Mental Health. Washington, DC: U.S. Government Printing Office.

Levine, D. S., & Willner, S. G. (1976). *The cost of mental illness, 1974.* National Institute of Mental Health, Statistical Note No. 125. Washington, DC: U.S. Government Printing Office.

Levine, I. S., & Haggard, L. K. (1989). Homelessness as a public health problem. In D. A. Rochefort (Ed.), *Handbook on mental health policy in the United States* (pp. 293–310). Westport, CT: Greenwood Press.

Levinson, A., & Ullman, F. (1998). Medicaid managed care and infant health. *Journal of Health Economics, 17*(3), 351–368.

Levitan, S. A. (1990). *Programs in aid of the poor* (6th ed.). Baltimore: Johns Hopkins University Press.

Lewis, R. A., Haller, D. L., Branch, D., & Ingersoll, K. S. (1996). Retention issues involving drug-abusing women in treatment research. *NIDA Research Monograph, 166,* 110–122.

Lewit, E. M., Baker, L. S., Corman, H., & Shiono, P. H. (1995). The direct cost of low birth weight. *Future of Children, 5*(1), 35–56.

Lia-Hoagberg, B., Rode, P., Skovholt, C. J., Oberg, C. N., Berg, C., Mullet, S., & Choi, T. (1990). Barriers and motivators to prenatal care among low-income women. *Social Science and Medicine, 30,* 487–495.

Liao, Y., McGee, D. L., Kaufman, J. S., Cao, G., & Cooper, R. S. (1999). Socioeconomic status and morbidity in the last years of life. *American Journal of Public Health, 89*(4), 569–572.

Limata, C., Schoen, E. J., Cohen, D., Black, S. B., & Quesenberry, C. P. Jr. (1997). Compliance with voluntary prenatal HIV testing in a large health maintenance organization (HMO). *JAIDS: Journal of Acquired Immune Deficiency Syndromes, 15*(2), 126–130.

Lindan, C. P., Hearst, N., Singleton, J. A., Trachtenberg, A. I., Riordan, N. M., Tokagawa, D. A., & Chu, G. S. (1990). Underreporting of minority AIDS deaths in San Francisco Bay area, 1985–86. *Public Health Reports, 105,* 400–405.

Lin-Fu, J. S. (1988). Population characteristics and health care needs of Asian Pacific Americans. *Public Health Reports, 103,* 18–27.

Link, B. G., & Phelan, J. (1995). Social conditions as fundamental causes of disease. *Journal of Health and Social Behavior* (Spec. No), 80–94.

Link, B., Phelan, J., Bresnahan, M., Stueve, A., Moore, R., & Susser, E. (1995). Lifetime and five-year prevalence of homelessness in the United States: New evidence on an old debate. *American Journal of Orthopsychiatry, 65*(3), 347–354.

Link, B. G., Susser, E., Stueve, A., Phelan, J., Moore, R. E., & Struening, E. (1994). Lifetime and five-year prevalence of homelessness in the United States. *American Journal of Public Health, 84*(12), 1907–1912.

Lipsey, M. W., & Wilson, D. B. (1993). The efficacy of psychological, educational, and behavioral treatment. Confirmation from meta-analysis. *American Psychologist, 48*(12), 1181–1209.

Liu, K., Manton, K. G., & Liu, B. M. (1990). Morbidity, disability, and long-term care of the elderly: Implications for insurance financing. *Milbank Quarterly, 68,* 445–450.

Liu, Z., Shilkret, K. L., Tranotti, J., Freund, C. G., & Finelli, L. (1998). Distinct trends in tuberculosis morbidity among foreign-born and US-born persons in New Jersey, 1986 through 1995. *American Journal of Public Health, 88*(7), 1064–1067.

Loring, M. T., & Smith, R. W. (1994). Health care barriers and interventions for battered women. *Public Health Reports, 109*(3), 328–338.

Lorion, R. P., & Allen, L. (1989). Preventive services in mental health. In D. A. Rochefort (Ed.), *Handbook on mental health policy in the United States* (pp. 403–432). Westport, CT: Greenwood Press.

Loue, S. (Ed.). (1998). *Handbook of immigrant health.* New York: Plenum.

Lowe, B. F. (1988). Future directions for community-based long-term care research. *Milbank Quarterly, 66,* 552–571.

Lu, M. C., Lin, Y. G., Prietto, N. M., & Garite, T. J. (2000). Elimination of public funding of prenatal care for undocumented immigrants in California: A cost/benefit analysis. *American Journal of Obstetrics and Gynecology, 182*(1 Pt. 1), 233–239.

Luckey, J. W. (1987). Justifying alcohol treatment on the basis of cost savings: The "Offset" literature. *Alcohol Health and Research World, 12*(1), 8–15.

Lundgren, R. I., & Lang, R. (1989). "There is no sea, only fish": Effects of United States policy on the health of the displaced in El Salvador. *Social Science and Medicine, 28,* 697–706.

Lynch, J. W., Kaplan, G. A., & Shema, S. J. (1997). Cumulative impact of sustained economic hardship on physical, cognitive, psychological, and social functioning. *New England Journal of Medicine, 337*(26), 1889–1895.

Lynn, L. E., Jr., & McGeary, M.G.H. (Eds.). (1990). *Inner-city poverty in the United States.* Washington, DC: National Academy Press.

Lyons, J., Howard, K., O'Mahoney, M., & Lish, J. (1997). *The measurement and management of clinical outcomes in mental health.* New York: Wiley.

MacAdam, M., Capitman, J., Yee, D., Prottas, J., Leutz, W., & Westwater, D. (1989). Case management for frail elders: The Robert Wood Johnson Foundation's program for hospital initiatives in long-term care. *Gerontologist, 29,* 737–744.

Macher, A., Goosby, E., Barker, L., Volberding, P., Goldschmidt, R., Balano, K. B., Williams, A., Hoenig, L., Gould, B., & Daniels, E. (1994). Educating primary care providers about HIV disease: Multidisciplinary interactive mechanisms. *Public Health Reports, 109*(3), 305–310.

Macklin, E. D. (Ed.). (1989). *AIDS and families: Report of the AIDS Task Force: Groves Conference on Marriage and the Family.* New York: Haworth Press.

Magaziner, J., & Cadigan, D. A. (1988). Community care of older women living alone. *Women and Health, 14,* 121–138.

Maiuro, R. D., & Eberle, J. E. (1989). New developments in research on aggression: An international report. *Violence and Victims, 4,* 3–15.

Manderscheid, R. W., & Henderson, M. J. (1996). The growth and direction of managed care. In R. W. Manderscheid & M. A. Sonnenschein (Eds.), *Mental health, United States, 1996* (pp. 17–26) (DHHS Publication No. SMA 96–3098). Center for Mental Health Services. Substance Abuse and Mental Health Services Administration. Washington, DC: U.S. Government Printing Office.

Mane, P., Aggleton, P., Dowsett, G., Parker, R., Gupta, G. R., Anderson, S., Bertozzi, S., Chevallier, E., Clark, M., Kaleeba, N., Kingma, S., Manthey, G., Smedberg, M., & Timberlake, S. (1996). Summary of track D: social science: research, policy and action. *AIDS, 10*(Suppl. 3), S123–132.

Mansfield, C. J., Wilson, J. L., Kobrinski, E. J., & Mitchell, J. (1999). Premature mortality in the United States: The roles of geographic area, socioeconomic status, household type, and availability of medical care. *American Journal of Public Health, 89*(6), 893–898.

Manton, K. G. (1989). Epidemiological, demographic, and social correlates of disability among the elderly. *Milbank Quarterly, 67*(Suppl. 2), 13–58.

Manton, K. G., Stallard, E., & Corder, L. S. (1998). The dynamics of dimensions of age-related disability 1982 to 1994 in the U.S. elderly population. *Journals of Gerontology. Series A, Biological Sciences and Medical Sciences, 53*(1), B59–70.

Mark, T., McKusick, D., King, E., Harwood, H., & Genuardi, J. (1998). *National expenditures for mental health, alcohol and other drug abuse treatment, 1996* (DHHS Publication No. SMA 98–3255). Substance Abuse and Mental Health Services Administration. Washington, DC: U.S. Government Printing Office.

Mark, T., & Mueller, C. (1996). Access to care in HMOs and traditional insurance plans. *Health Affairs, 15*(4), 81–87.

Marlatt, G. A. (1996). Harm reduction: Come as you are. *Addictive Behaviors, 21*(6), 779–788.

Marlatt, G. A. (Ed.). (1998). *Harm reduction: Pragmatic strategies for managing high risk behaviors.* New York, NY: Guilford Press.

Martell, J. V., Seitz, R. S., Harada, J. K., Kobayashi, J., Sasaki, V. K., & Wong, C. (1992). Hospitalization in an urban homeless population: The Honolulu Urban Homeless Project. *Annals of Internal Medicine, 116*(4), 299–303.

Martinez, R. J., Jr. (1996). Latinos and lethal violence: The impact of poverty and inequality. *Social Problems, 43*(2), 131–146.

Massey, D. S., & Espinosa, K. E. (1997). What's driving Mexico-U.S. migration? A theoretical, empirical, and policy analysis. *American Journal of Sociology, 102*(4), 939–999.

Mayfield, J. A., Rosenblatt, R. A., Baldwin, L.-M., Chu, J., & Logerfo, J. P. (1990). The relation of obstetrical volume and nursery level to perinatal mortality. *American Journal of Public Health, 80*, 819–823.

McAdam, J. M., Brickner, P. W., Scharer, L. L., Crocco, J. A., & Duff, A. E. (1990). The spectrum of tuberculosis in a New York City men's shelter clinic (1982–1988). *Chest, 97*(4), 798–805.

McCann, K., Wadsworth, E., & Beck, E. J. (1993). Planning health care for people with HIV infection and AIDS. *Health Services Management Research, 6*(3), 167–177.

McCaslin, R. (1988). Reframing research on service use among the elderly: An analysis of recent findings. *Gerontologist, 28*, 592–599.

McCaughrin, W. C., & Howard, D. L. (1996). Variation in access to outpatient substance abuse treatment: Organizational factors and conceptual issues. *Journal of Substance Abuse, 8*(4), 403–415.

McCloskey, L. A., Figueredo, A. J., & Koss, M. P. (1995). The effects of systemic family violence on children's mental health. *Child Development, 66*(5), 1239–1261.

McCloskey, L. A., Southwick, K., Fernandez-Esquer, M. E., & Locke, C. (1995). The psychological effects of political and domestic violence on Central American and Mexican immigrant mothers and children. *Journal of Community Psychology, 23*(2), 95–116.

McCormick, M. C., & Richardson, D. K. (1995). Access to neonatal intensive care. *Future of Children, 5*(1), 162–175.

McCoy, H. V., McCoy, C. B., & Lai, S. (1998). Effectiveness of HIV interventions among women drug users. *Women and Health, 27*(1–2), 49–66.

McCrone, P., & Weich, S. (1996). Mental health care costs: Paucity of measurement. *Social Psychiatry and Psychiatric Epidemiology, 31*(2), 70–77.

McDermott, J., Drews, C., Green, D., & Berg, C. (1997). Evaluation of prenatal care information on birth certificates. *Paediatric and Perinatal Epidemiology, 11*(1), 105–121.

McDowell, I., & Newell, C. (1996). *Measuring health: A guide to rating scales and questionnaires* (2nd ed.). New York: Oxford University Press.

McFarland, B. H. (1994). Health maintenance organizations and persons with severe mental illness. *Community Mental Health Journal, 30*(3), 221–242.

McGlynn, E. A. (1996). Choosing chronic disease measures for HEDIS: Conceptual framework and review of seven clinical areas. *Managed Care Quarterly, 4*(3), 54–77.

McKinlay, J. B., & Marceau, L. D. (1999). A tale of three tails. *American Journal of Public Health, 89*(3), 295–298.

McKusick, D., Mark, T. L., King, E., Harwood, R., Buck, J. A., Dilonardo, J., & Genuardi, J. S. (1998). Spending for mental health and substance abuse treatment, 1996. *Health Affairs, 17*(5), 147–157.

McLeod, J. D., & Kessler, R. C. (1990). Socioeconomic status differences in vulnerability to undesirable life events. *Journal of Health and Social Behavior, 31*, 162–172.

McMurchie, M. (1993). The role of the primary care physician. *Journal of Acquired Immune Deficiency Syndromes, 6*(Suppl. 1), S77–83.

McMurray-Avila, M. (1997). *Organizing health services for homeless people: A practical guide.* Nashville, TN: National Health Care for the Homeless Council.

McNeil, J. M. (1997). *Americans with disabilities, 1994–95.* Current Population Reports, No. P70–61. Washington, DC: U.S. Government Printing Office.

McNeil, J. M. (1999a). [Selected 1991–1992 data on disability status from the Survey of Income and Program Participation]. Unpublished data.

McNeil, J. M. (1999b). [Selected 1994–1995 data on disability status from the Survey of Income and Program Participation]. Unpublished data.

McNellis, D. (1988). Specific federal programs for improving reproductive health care: What have we learned? In H. M. Wallace, G. Ryan, Jr., & A. C. Oglesby (Eds.), *Maternal and child health practices* (3rd ed.) (pp. 401–407). Oakland, CA: Third Party Publishing Company.

McShane, D. (1988). An analysis of mental health research with American Indian youth. *Journal of Adolescence, 11*, 87–116.

Mechanic, D. (1990). Treating mental illness: Generalist versus specialist. *Health Affairs, 9*(4), 61–75.

Mechanic, D. (1996a). Changing medical organization and the erosion of trust. *Milbank Quarterly, 74*(2), 171–189.

Mechanic, D. (1996b). Emerging issues in international mental health services research. *Psychiatric Services, 47*(4), 371–375.

Mechanic, D. (1996c). Key policy considerations for mental health in the managed care era. In R. W. Manderscheid & M. A. Sonnenschein (Eds.), *Mental health, United States, 1996* (pp. 1–16) (DHHS Publication No. SMA 96–3098). Center for Mental Health Services. Substance Abuse and Mental Health Services Administration. Washington, DC: U.S. Government Printing Office.

Mechanic, D. (1998). Emerging trends in mental health policy and practice. *Health Affairs, 17*(6), 82–98.

Mechanic, D., & Aiken, L. H. (1989). Lessons from the past: Responding to the AIDS crisis. *Health Affairs, 9*(3), 16–32.

Medicine/Public Health Initiative. (1999). Available: http://www.sph.uth.tmc.edu/mph/ [Accessed Oct. 22, 1999. Last updated Oct. 20, 1999].

Merlis, M. (1999). *Financing long-term care in the twenty-first century: The public and private roles*. New York: Commonwealth Fund.

Meropol, S. B. (1995). Health status of pediatric refugees in Buffalo, NY. *Archives of Pediatrics and Adolescent Medicine, 149*(8), 887–892.

Metha, A., Weber, B., & Webb, L. D. (1998). Youth suicide prevention: A survey and analysis of policies and efforts in the fifty states. *Suicide and Life-Threatening Behavior, 28*(2), 150–164.

Mhatre, S. L., & Deber, R. B. (1992). From equal access to health care to equitable access to health: A review of Canadian provincial health commissions and reports. *International Journal of Health Services, 22*(4), 645–668.

Michael, S., & Gany, F. (1996). Welfare and immigration reform: Immigrant access to health services. *Current Issues in Public Health, 2*, 199–204.

Miller, H. G., Turner, C. F., & Moses, L. E. (Eds.). (1990). *AIDS: The second decade*. Washington, DC: National Academy Press.

Miller, N. A. (1997). Patient centered long-term care. *Health Care Financing Review, 19*(2), 1–10.

Miller, R. H., & Luft, H. S. (1994). Managed care plan performance since 1980. A literature analysis. *Journal of the American Medical Association, 271*(19), 1512–1519.

Minkoff, H., Bauer, T., & Joyce, T. (1997). Welfare reform and the obstetrical care of immigrants and their newborns. *New England Journal of Medicine, 337*(10), 705–707.

Mirowsky, J., & Ross, C. E. (1989a). Psychiatric diagnosis as reified measurement. *Journal of Health and Social Behavior, 30*, 11–25.

Mirowsky, J., & Ross, C. E. (1989b). Rejoinder—Assessing the type and severity of psychological problems: An alternative to diagnosis. *Journal of Health and Social Behavior, 30*, 38–40.

Mitchell, J. B. (1991). Physician participation in Medicaid revisited. *Medical Care, 29*, 645–653

Mitchell, M. K. (1997). Domestic violence: Teaming communities with providers for effective intervention. *Advanced Practice Nursing Quarterly, 2*(4), 51–58.

Moffitt, R., & Wolfe, B. L. (1993). Medicaid, welfare dependency, and work: Is there a causal link? *Health Care Financing Review, 15*(1), 123–133.

Mollica, R. F., McInnes, K., Pham, T., Smith Fawzi, M. C., Murphy, E., & Lin, L. (1998). The dose-effect relationships between torture and psychiatric symptoms in Vietnamese ex-political detainees and a comparison group. *Journal of Nervous and Mental Disease, 186*(9), 543–553.

Moncher, M. S., Holden, G. W., & Trimble, J. E. (1990). Substance abuse among Native-American youth. *Journal of Consulting and Clinical Psychology, 58,* 408–415.

Montgomery, R.J.V. (1988). Respite care: Lessons from a controlled design study. *Health Care Financing Review, Annual Supplement,* 133–138.

Montoya, I. D., Richard, A. J., Bell, D. C., & Atkinson, J. S. (1997). An analysis of unmet need for HIV services: The Houston Study. *Journal of Health Care for the Poor and Underserved, 8*(4), 446–460.

Moon, M., Gaberlavage, G., & Newman, S. J. (Eds.). (1989). *Preserving independence, supporting needs: The role of board and care homes.* Washington, DC: American Association of Retired Persons, Public Policy Institute.

Moore, P., & Hepworth, J. T. (1994). Use of perinatal and infant health services by Mexican-American Medicaid enrollees. *Journal of the American Medical Association, 272*(4), 297–304.

Mor, V., Fleishman, J. A., Allen, S. M., & Piette, J. D. (1994). *Networking AIDS services.* Ann Arbor, MI: Health Administration Press.

Mor, V., Fleishman, J. A., Dresser, M., & Piette, J. (1992). Variation in health service use among HIV-infected patients. *Medical Care, 30,* 17–29.

Mor, V., Fleishman, J. A., Piette, J. D., & Allen, S. M. (1993). Developing AIDS community service consortia. *Health Affairs, 12*(1), 186–199.

Moran, J. S., Janes, H. R., Peterman, T. A., & Stone, K. M. (1990). Increase in condom sales following AIDS education and publicity, United States. *American Journal of Public Health, 80,* 607–608.

Morenoff, J. D., & Sampson, R. J. (1997). Violent crime and the spatial dynamics of neighborhood transition: Chicago, 1970–1990. *Social Forces, 76*(1), 31–64.

Morrissey, J. P. (1989). The changing role of the public health hospital. In D. A. Rochefort (Ed.), *Handbook on mental health policy in the United States* (pp. 311–338). Westport, CT: Greenwood Press.

Morrissey, J. P., & Levine, I. S. (1987). Researchers discuss latest findings, examine needs of homeless mentally ill persons. *Hospital and Community Psychiatry, 38,* 811–812.

Moscicki, E. K. (1989). Epidemiologic surveys as tools for studying suicidal behavior: A review. *Suicide and Life-Threatening Behavior, 19,* 131–146.

Moss, N., Baumeister, L., & Biewener, J. (1996). Perspectives of Latina immigrant women on Proposition 187. *Journal of the American Medical Women's Association, 51*(4), 161–165.

Mrazek, P. J., & Haggerty, R. J. (Eds.). (1994). *Reducing risks for mental disorders: Frontiers for preventive intervention research.* Washington, DC: National Academy Press.

Mullahy, J., & Sindelar, J. (1989). Life-cycle effects of alcoholism on education, earnings, and occupation. *Inquiry, 26,* 272–282.

Muller, C., Fahs, M. C., Mulak, G., Walther, V., Blumenfield, S., & Fulop, G. (1996). Pediatric AIDS at Mount Sinai Medical Center 1988–89: A study of costs and social severity. *Social Work in Health Care, 22*(4), 1–20.

Murphy, T. F. (1991). No time for an AIDS backlash. *Hastings Center Report, 21*(2), 7–11.

Mushinski, M. (1994). Violence in America's public schools. *Statistical Bulletin—Metropolitan Insurance Companies, 75*(2), 2–9.

Nadelson, C. C. (1998). Gender and health policy. *Harvard Review of Psychiatry, 5*(6), 340–343.

National Alliance to End Homelessness. (1988). *Housing and homelessness.* Washington, DC: Author.

National Center on Child Abuse and Neglect. (1988). *Study findings: Study of national incidence and prevalence of child abuse and neglect: 1988.* Washington, DC: U.S. Government Printing Office.

National Center for Health Statistics. (1979). *Vital statistics of the United States, 1975: Vol. 2, Mortality Part A* (DHHS Publication No. PHS 79–1114). Washington, DC: U.S. Government Printing Office.

National Center for Health Statistics. (1980). *Health, United States, 1980, with prevention profile* (DHHS Publication No. PHS 81–1232). Washington, DC: U.S. Government Printing Office.

National Center for Health Statistics. (1982). *Health, United States, 1982* (DHHS Publication No. PHS 83–1232). Washington, DC: U.S. Government Printing Office.

National Center for Health Statistics. (1983). *Health, United States, 1983* (DHHS Publication No. PHS 84–1232). Washington, DC: U.S. Government Printing Office.

National Center for Health Statistics. (1986). *Current estimates from the National Health Interview Survey: United States, 1985* (DHHS Publication No. PHS 86–1588). Washington, DC: U.S. Government Printing Office.

National Center for Health Statistics. (1987). *Current estimates from the National Health Interview Survey: United States, 1986* (DHHS Publication No. PHS 87–1592). Washington, DC: U.S. Government Printing Office.

National Center for Health Statistics. (1988a). *Current estimates from the National Health Interview Survey: United States, 1987* (DHHS Publication No. PHS 88–1594). Washington, DC: U.S. Government Printing Office.

National Center for Health Statistics. (1988b). *Health of an aging America: Issues on data for policy analysis* (DHHS Publication No. PHS 89–1488). Washington, DC: U.S. Government Printing Office.

National Center for Health Statistics. (1988c). *Vital statistics of the United States, 1985: Vol. 1, Natality* (DHHS Publication No. PHS 88–1113). Washington, DC: U.S. Government Printing Office.

National Center for Health Statistics. (1989a). *Current estimates from the National Health Interview Survey: United States, 1988* (DHHS Publication No. PHS 89–1501). Washington, DC: U.S. Government Printing Office.

National Center for Health Statistics. (1989b). *Health characteristics by occupation and industry of longest employment* (DHHS Publication No. PHS 89–1596). Washington, DC: U.S. Government Printing Office.

National Center for Health Statistics. (1989c). *The National Nursing Home Survey: 1985 summary for the United States* (DHHS Publication No. PHS 89–1758). Washington, DC: U.S. Government Printing Office.

National Center for Health Statistics. (1990a). *Current estimates from the National Health Interview Survey: United States, 1989* (DHHS Publication No. PHS 90–1504). Washington, DC: U.S. Government Printing Office.

National Center for Health Statistics. (1990b). *Health, United States, 1989* (DHHS Publication No. PHS 90–1232). Washington, DC: U.S. Government Printing Office.

National Center for Health Statistics. (1990c). *Long-term care for the functionally dependent elderly* (DHHS Publication No. PHS 90–1765). Washington, DC: U.S. Government Printing Office.

National Center for Health Statistics. (1991a). *Current estimates from the National Health Interview Survey: United States, 1990* (DHHS Publication No. PHS 92–1509). Washington, DC: U.S. Government Printing Office.

National Center for Health Statistics. (1991b). *Health, United States, 1990* (DHHS Publication No. PHS 91–1232). Washington, DC: U.S. Government Printing Office.

National Center for Health Statistics. (1992a). *Current estimates from the National Health Interview Survey: United States, 1991* (DHHS Publication No. PHS 93–1512). Washington, DC: U.S. Government Printing Office.

National Center for Health Statistics. (1992b). *Health, United States, 1991, and prevention profile* (DHHS Publication No. PHS 92–1232). Washington, DC: U.S. Government Printing Office.

National Center for Health Statistics. (1993). *Health, United States, 1992, and healthy people 2000 review* (DHHS Publication No. PHS 93–1232). Washington, DC: U.S. Government Printing Office.

National Center for Health Statistics. (1994a). *Current estimates from the National Health Interview Survey: United States, 1992* (DHHS Publication No. PHS 94–1517). Washington, DC: U.S. Government Printing Office.

National Center for Health Statistics. (1994b). *Current estimates from the National Health Interview Survey: United States, 1993* (DHHS Publication No. PHS 95–1518). Washington, DC: U.S. Government Printing Office.

National Center for Health Statistics. (1994c). *Health, United States, 1993* (DHHS Publication No. PHS 94–1232). Washington, DC: U.S. Government Printing Office.

National Center for Health Statistics. (1995a). *Health, United States, 1994* (DHHS Publication No. PHS 95–1232). Washington, DC: U.S. Government Printing Office.

National Center for Health Statistics. (1995b). *Trends in the health of older Americans: United States, 1994* (DHHS Publication No. PHS 95–1414). Washington, DC: U.S. Government Printing Office.

National Center for Health Statistics. (1996a). *Current estimates from the National Health Interview Survey: United States, 1994* (DHHS Publication No. PHS 96–1521). Washington, DC: U.S. Government Printing Office.

National Center for Health Statistics. (1996b). *Health, United States, 1995* (DHHS Publication No. PHS 96–1232). Washington, DC: U.S. Government Printing Office.

National Center for Health Statistics. (1997). *Health, United States, 1996–97, and injury chartbook* (DHHS Publication No. PHS 97–1232). Washington, DC: U.S. Government Printing Office.

National Center for Health Statistics. (1998a). *Current estimates from the National Health Interview Survey: United States, 1995* (DHHS Publication No. PHS 98–1527). Washington, DC: U.S. Government Printing Office.

National Center for Health Statistics. (1998b). *Deaths: Final data for 1996.* National Vital Statistics Report Vol. 47, No. 9. Washington, DC: U.S. Government Printing Office.

National Center for Health Statistics. (1998c). *Health, United States, 1998, with socioeconomic status and health chartbook* (DHHS Publication No. PHS 98–1232). Washington, DC: U.S. Government Printing Office.

National Center for Health Statistics. (1999a). *Births: Final data for 1997.* National Vital Statistics Report Vol. 47, No. 18. Washington, DC: U.S. Government Printing Office.

National Center for Health Statistics. (1999b). *Current estimates from the National Health Interview Survey: United States, 1996* (DHHS Publication No. PHS 99–1528). Washington, DC: U.S. Government Printing Office.

National Center for Health Statistics. (1999c). *Deaths: Final data for 1997.* National Vital Statistics Report Vol. 47, No. 19. Washington, DC: U.S. Government Printing Office.

National Center for Health Statistics. (1999d). *Health, United States, 1999, with health and aging chartbook* (DHHS Publication No. PHS 99–1232). Washington, DC: U.S. Government Printing Office.

National Center for Health Statistics. (1999e). *Infant mortality statistics from the 1997 period linked birth / infant death data set.* National Vital Statistics Reports Vol. 47, No. 23. Washington, DC: U.S. Government Printing Office.

National Center for Health Statistics. (1999f). *National health interview survey on disability (NHIS-D)* [On-line]. Available: http://www.cdc.gov/nchswww/about/major/nhis_dis/nhis_dis.htm [Accessed Sept. 16, 1999. Last updated Sept. 9, 1998].

National Center for Health Statistics. (1999g). [Selected data from the 1985 National Nursing Home Survey]. Unpublished data.

National Center for Health Statistics. (1999h). [Selected data from the 1995 National Nursing Home Survey]. Unpublished data.

National Commission on Children. (1991). *Beyond rhetoric: A new American agenda for children and families.* Washington, DC: National Commission on Children.

National Commission to Prevent Infant Mortality. (1988a). *Death before life: The tragedy of infant mortality.* Washington, DC: Author.

National Commission to Prevent Infant Mortality. (1988b). *Malpractice and liability: An obstetrical crisis.* Washington, DC: Author.

National Commission to Prevent Infant Mortality. (1989). *Home visiting: Opening doors for America's pregnant women and children.* Washington, DC: Author.

National Institute on Aging. (1989). *Dimensions of long-term care research at the National Institute on Aging: A report to the National Advisory Council on Aging.* Washington, DC: U.S. Government Printing Office.

National Institute on Drug Abuse. (1990). *National Drug and Alcoholism Treatment Unit Survey (NDATUS): 1989 main findings report* (DHHS Publication No. ADM 91–1729). Washington, DC: U.S. Government Printing Office.

National Institute on Drug Abuse. (1991). *Drug abuse and drug abuse research: Third triennial report to Congress from the Secretary, Department of Health and Human Services* (DHHS Publication No. ADM 91–1704). Washington, DC: U.S. Government Printing Office.

National Research Council. (1985). *Injury in America: A continuing public health problem.* Washington, DC: National Academy Press.

National Research Council. (1988). *Injury control: A review of the status and progress of the Injury Control Program at the Centers for Disease Control.* Washington, DC: National Academy Press.

National Research Council. (1993). *The social impact of AIDS in the United States.* Washington, DC: National Academy Press.

National Research Council Panel on Research and Child Abuse and Neglect. (1993). *Understanding child abuse and neglect.* Washington, DC: National Academy Press.

Neal, L. J. (1998). Functional assessment of the home health client. *Home Healthcare Nurse, 16*(10), 670–677.

Needleman, H. L. (1991). Childhood lead poisoning: A disease for the history texts. *American Journal of Public Health, 81*, 685–687.

Neergaard, J. A. (1990). A proposal for a foster grandmother intervention program to prevent child abuse. *Public Health Reports, 105*, 89–93.

Neff, J. M., & Anderson, G. (1995). Protecting children with chronic illness in a competitive marketplace. *Journal of the American Medical Association, 274*(23), 1866–1869.

Neighbors, H. W., Jackson, J. S., Campbell, L., & Williams, D. (1989). The influence of racial factors on psychiatrtic diagnosis: A review and suggestions for research. *Community Mental Health Journal, 25*, 301–311.

Nelson, C. R., & Stussman, B. J. (1994). *Alcohol- and drug-related visits to hospital emergency departments: 1992 National Hospital Ambulatory Medical Care Survey* (DHHS Publication No. PHS 94–1250). Washington, DC: U.S. Government Printing Office.

Newacheck, P. W. (1994). Poverty and childhood chronic illness. *Archives of Pediatrics and Adolescent Medicine, 148*(11), 1143–1149.

Newacheck, P. W., Stoddard, J. J., & McManus, M. (1993). Ethnocultural variations in the prevalence and impact of childhood chronic conditions. *Pediatrics, 91*(5 Pt. 2), 1031–1039.

Newcomer, R., Harrington, C., & Friedlob, A. (1990). Social health maintenance organizations: Assessing their initial experience. *Health Services Research, 25*, 425–454.

Newschaffer, C. J., Cocroft, J., Hauck, W. W., Fanning, T., & Turner, B. J. (1998). Improved birth outcomes associated with enhanced Medicaid prenatal care in drug-using women infected with the human immunodeficiency virus. *Obstetrics and Gynecology, 91*(6), 885–891.

Nicaragua Health Study Collaborative at Harvard, Centro para Investigaciones y Estudios de Salud Publica, and Universidad Nacional Autonoma de Nicaragua. (1989). Health effects of the war in two rural communities in Nicaragua. *American Journal of Public Health, 79*, 424–429.

NIMH Multisite HIV Prevention Trial Group. (1998). The NIMH Multisite HIV Prevention Trial: Reducing HIV sexual risk behavior. The National Institute of Mental Health (NIMH) Multisite HIV Prevention Trial Group. *Science, 280*(5371), 1889–1894.

Noland, M. P., Kryscio, R. J., Riggs, R. S., Linville, L. H., Ford, V. Y., & Tucker, T. C. (1998). The effectiveness of a tobacco prevention program with adolescents living in a tobacco-producing region. *American Journal of Public Health, 88*(12), 1862–1865.

Normand, J., Vlahov, D., & Moses, L. E. (Eds.). (1995). *Preventing HIV transmission: The role of sterile needles and bleach.* Washington, DC: National Academy Press.

Norquist, G. S., & Magruder, K. M. (1998). Views from funding agencies. National Institute of Mental Health. *Medical Care, 36*(9), 1306–1308.

Norton, S. A., Kenney, G. M., & Ellwood, M. R. (1996). Medicaid coverage of maternity care for aliens in California. *Family Planning Perspectives, 28*(3), 108–112.

Nyamathi, A., Stein, J. A., & Brecht, M. L. (1995). Psychosocial predictors of AIDS risk behavior and drug use behavior in homeless and drug addicted women of color. *Health Psychology, 14*(3), 265–273.

Nyman, J. A., Cyphert, S. T., Russell, D. W., & Wallace, R. B. (1989). The ratio of impaired elderly in the community to those in nursing homes in two rural Iowa counties. *Medical Care, 27,* 920–927.

Oberg, C. N., Lia-Hoagberg, B., Hodkinson, E., Skovholt, C. J., & Vanman, R. (1990). Prenatal care comparisons among privately insured, uninsured, and Medicaid-enrolled women. *Public Health Reports, 105,* 533–535.

O'Brien, E., Rowland, D., & Keenan, P. (1999). *Medicare and Medicaid for the elderly and disabled poor.* Washington, DC: Kaiser Family Foundation.

O'Campo, P., Gielen, A. C., Faden, R. R., Xue, X., Kass, N., & Wang, M. C. (1995). Violence by male partners against women during the childbearing year: A contextual analysis. *American Journal of Public Health, 85*(8 Pt. 1), 1092–1097.

O'Campo, P., Xue, X., Wang, M. C., & Caughy, M. (1997). Neighborhood risk factors for low birthweight in Baltimore: A multilevel analysis. *American Journal of Public Health, 87*(7), 1113–1118.

O'Carroll, P. W. (1989). A consideration of the validity and reliability of suicide mortality data. *Suicide and Life-Threatening Behavior, 19,* 1–16.

O'Carroll, P. W., Loftin, C., Waller, J. B., Jr., McDowall, D., Bukoff, A., Scott, R. O., Mercy, J. A., & Wiersema, B. (1991). Preventing homicide: An evaluation of the efficacy of a Detroit gun ordinance. *American Journal of Public Health, 81,* 576–581.

O'Donnell, L., Stueve, A., San Doval, A., Duran, R., Haber, D., Atnafou, R., Johnson, N., Grant, U., Murray, H., Juhn, G., Tang, J., & Piessens, P. (1999). The effectiveness of the Reach for Health Community Youth Service learning program in reducing early and unprotected sex among urban middle school students. *American Journal of Public Health, 89*(2), 176–181.

Oddone, E. Z., Cowper, P., Hamilton, J. D., Matchar, D. B., Hartigan, P., Samsa, G., Simberkoff, M., & Feussner, J. R. (1993). Cost effectiveness analysis of early zidovudine treatment of HIV infected patients. *British Medical Journal, 307*(6915), 1322–1325.

Office of Assistant Secretary for Planning and Evaluation. (1995). *Conditions and impairments among the working-age population with disabilities* [On-line]. Available: http://aspe.hhs.gov/daltcp/reports/conimpwa.htm [Accessed Sept. 16, 1999. Last updated 1995].

Office of Assistant Secretary for Planning and Evaluation. (1996). *Encyclopedia of financial gerontology: Federal disability programs section* [On-line]. Available: http://aspe.hhs.gov/daltcp/reports/encyclo.htm [Accessed Sept. 16, 1999. Last updated 1996].

Office of Technology Assessment. (1986). *Children's mental health: Problems and services— A background paper* (OTA-BP-H-33). Washington, DC: U.S. Government Printing Office.

Office of Technology Assessment. (1987a). *Neonatal intensive care for low birthweight infants: Costs and effectiveness* (OTA-HCS-38). Washington, DC: U.S. Government Printing Office.

Office of Technology Assessment. (1987b). *Technology-dependent children: Hospital v. home care- A technical memorandum* (OTA-TM-H-38). Washington, DC: U.S. Government Printing Office.

Office of Technology Assessment. (1988). *Healthy children: Investing in the future* (OTA-H-345). Washington, DC: U.S. Government Printing Office.

Office of Technology Assessment. (1989). *The use of preventive services by the elderly* (Staff Paper 2). Washington, DC: U.S. Government Printing Office.

Office of Technology Assessment. (1990). *Indian adolescent mental health* (OTA-H-446). Washington, DC: U.S. Government Printing Office.

Oktay, J. S., & Volland, P. J. (1990). Post-hospital support program for the frail elderly and their caregivers: A quasi-experimental evaluation. *American Journal of Public Health, 80,* 39–46.

Oldenettel, D., Dye, T. D., & Artal, R. (1997). Prenatal HIV screening in pregnant women: A medical-legal review. *Birth, 24*(3), 165–172.

Oleske, D. M., Branca, M. L., Schmidt, J. B., Ferguson, R., & Linn, E. S. (1998). A comparison of capitated and fee-for-service Medicaid reimbursement methods on pregnancy outcomes. *Health Services Research, 33*(1), 55–73.

Olfson, M., Sing, M., & Schlesinger, H. J. (1999). Mental health/medical care cost offsets: Opportunities for managed care. *Health Affairs, 18*(2), 79–90.

Olshansky, S. J., & Ault, A. B. (1986). The fourth stage of the epidemiologic transition: The age of delayed degenerative diseases. *Milbank Quarterly, 64,* 355–391.

Oppenheimer, G. M., & Padgug, R. A. (1986). AIDS: The risks to insurers, the threat to equity. *Hastings Center Report, 16*(5), 18–22.

Osborne, C. M. (1996). HIV/AIDS in resource-poor settings: Comprehensive care across a continuum. *AIDS, 10*(Suppl. 3), S61–67.

Osgood, N. J., & McIntosh, J. L. (Eds.). (1986). *Suicide and the elderly: An annotated bibliography and review.* Westport, CT: Greenwood Press.

Osofsky, J. D., Wewers, S., Hann, D. M., & Fick, A. C. (1993). Chronic community violence: What is happening to our children? *Psychiatry, 56*(1), 36–45.

Padgett, D. K., Patrick, C., Burns, B. J., & Schlesinger, H. J. (1994). Ethnicity and the use of outpatient mental health services in a national insured population. *American Journal of Public Health, 84*(2), 222–226.

Padgett, D. K., Struening, E. L., Andrews, H., & Pittman, J. (1995). Predictors of emergency room use by homeless adults in New York City: The influence of predisposing, enabling and need factors. *Social Science & Medicine, 41*(4), 547–56.

Pallak, M. S., Cummings, N. A., Dorken, H., & Henke, C. J. (1993). Managed mental health, Medicaid, and medical cost offset. *New Directions for Mental Health Services, 59,* 27–40.

Palmer, R. F., Graham, J. W., White, E. L., & Hansen, W. B. (1998). Applying multilevel analytic strategies in adolescent substance use prevention research. *Preventive Medicine, 27*(3), 328–336.

Paneth, N. (1990). Technology at birth. *American Journal of Public Health, 80,* 791–792.

Parikh, S. V., Lin, E., & Lesage, A. D. (1997). Mental health treatment in Ontario: Selected comparisons between the primary care and specialty sectors. *Canadian Journal of Psychiatry, 42*(9), 929–934.

Partnership for the Homeless. (1987). *National growth in homelessness: Winter 1987: "Broken promises-broken lives."* New York: Author.

Partnership for the Homeless. (1989). *Moving forward: A national agenda to address homelessness in 1990 and beyond and a status report on homelessness in America.* New York: Author.

Patrick, D. L., & Peach, H. (Eds.). (1989). *Disablement in the community.* New York: Oxford University Press.

Payne, S. F., Rutherford, G. W., Lemp, G. F., & Clevenger, A. C. (1990). Effect of the revised AIDS case definition on AIDS reporting in San Francisco: Evidence of increased reporting in intravenous drug users. *AIDS, 4,* 335–339.

Pennbridge, J. N., Yates, G. L., David, T. G., & Mackenzie, R. G. (1990). Runaway and homeless youth in Los Angeles County, California. *Journal of Adolescent Health Care, 11,* 159–165.

Pepper Commission: U.S. Bipartisan Commission on Comprehensive Health Care. (1990). *A call for action: Final report* (S. Prt. 101–114). Washington, DC: U.S. Government Printing Office.

Perloff, J. D., Kletke, P. R., Fossett, J. W., & Banks, S. (1997). Medicaid participation among urban primary care physicians. *Medical Care, 35*(2), 142–157.

Perrin, E. B., & Koshel, J. J. (Eds.). (1997). *Assessment of performance measures for public health, substance abuse, and mental health*. Washington, DC: National Academy Press.

Perrin, J. M. (1998). Services for children with chronic physical disorders and their families. In S. M. Allen & V. Mor (Eds.), *Living in the community with disability: Service needs, use, and systems* (pp. 329–349). New York: Springer.

Peterson, R. D., & Krivo, L. J. (1993). Racial segregation and black urban homicide. *Social Forces, 71*(4), 1001–1026.

Pettit, G. S. (1997). The developmental course of violence and aggression. Mechanisms of family and peer influence. *Psychiatric Clinics of North America, 20*(2), 283–299.

Pfeffer, C. R. (Ed.). (1989). *Suicide among youth: Perspectives on risk and prevention*. Washington, DC: American Psychiatric Press.

Phillips, C. D., Zimmerman, D., Bernabei, R., & Jonsson, P. V. (1997). Using the Resident Assessment Instrument for quality enhancement in nursing homes. *Age and Ageing, 26*(Suppl. 2), 77–81.

Phillips, J. A. (1997). Variation in African-American homicide rates: An assessment of potential explanations. *Criminology, 35*(4), 527–556.

Phillips, K. (1990). *The politics of rich and poor: Wealth and the American electorate in the Reagan aftermath*. New York: Random House.

Phillips, K. (1993). *Boiling point: Democrats, Republicans, and the decline of middle-class prosperity*. New York: HarperCollins.

Phillips, K. A., Morrison, K. R., Sonnad, S. S., & Bleecker, T. (1997). HIV counseling and testing of pregnant women and women of childbearing age by primary care providers: Self-reported beliefs and practices. *JAIDS: Journal of Acquired Immune Deficiency Syndromes, 14*(2), 174–178.

Pich, E. M., Pagliusi, S. R., Tessari, M., Talabot-Ayer, D., Hooft van Huijsduijnen, R., & Chiamulera, C. (1997). Common neural substrates for the addictive properties of nicotine and cocaine. *Science, 275*(5296), 83–86.

Pickens, R. W., & Svikis, D. S. (Eds.). (1988). *Biological vulnerability to drug abuse* (DHHS Publication No. ADM 88–1590). Washington, DC: U.S. Government Printing Office.

Piette, J. D., Fleishman, J. A., Stein, M. D., Mor, V., & Mayer, K. (1993). Perceived needs and unmet needs for formal services among people with HIV disease. *Journal of Community Health, 18*(1), 11–23.

Pine, P. L. (1998). Changing environments of AIDS/HIV service delivery and financing: An overview. *Health Care Financing Review, 19*(3), 1–3.

Pinkerton, S. D., Holtgrave, D. R., DiFranceisco, W. J., Stevenson, L. Y., & Kelly, J. A. (1998). Cost-effectiveness of a community-level HIV risk reduction intervention. *American Journal of Public Health, 88*(8), 1239–1242.

Piper, J. M., Mitchel, E. F. Jr., & Ray, W. A. (1994). Presumptive eligibility for pregnant Medicaid enrollees: Its effects on prenatal care and perinatal outcome. *American Journal of Public Health, 84*(10), 1626–1630.

Piper, J. M., Ray, W. A., & Griffin, M. R. (1990). Effects of Medicaid eligibility expansion on prenatal care and pregnancy outcome in Tennessee. *Journal of the American Medical Association, 264*, 2219–2223.

Plant, M. A., Orford, J., & Grant, M. (1989). The effects on children and adolescents of parents' excessive drinking: An international review. *Public Health Reports, 104*, 433–442.

Pless, I. B. (1998). Service needs of children with chronic physical disorders and their families. In S. M. Allen & V. Mor (Eds.), *Living in the community with disability: Service needs, use, and systems* (pp. 311–328). New York: Springer.

Popkin, B. M., & Udry, J. R. (1998). Adolescent obesity increases significantly in second and third generation U.S. immigrants: The National Longitudinal Study of Adolescent Health. *Journal of Nutrition, 128* (4), 701–706.

Popkin, M. K., Lurie, N., Manning, W., Harman, J., Callies, A., Gray, D., & Christianson, J. (1998). Changes in the process of care for Medicaid patients with schizophrenia in Utah's Prepaid Mental Health Plan. *Psychiatric Services, 49*(4), 518–523.

Portes, A. (1998). Social capital: Its origins and applications in modern sociology. *Annual Review of Sociology, 24,* 1–24.

President's Commission on Mental Health. (1978a). *Report to the President* (Vol. 1). Washington, DC: U.S. Government Printing Office.

President's Commission on Mental Health. (1978b). *Appendix: Task panel reports* (Vol. 2). Washington DC: U.S. Government Printing Office.

President's Commission on Mental Health. (1978c). *Appendix: Task panel reports* (Vol. 3). Washington, DC: U.S. Government Printing Office.

Presidential Commission on the Human Immunodeficiency Virus Epidemic. (1988). *The report on human immunodeficiency virus epidemic.* Washington, DC: U.S. Government Printing Office.

Prothrow-Stith, D. B. (1995). The epidemic of youth violence in America: Using public health prevention strategies to prevent violence. *Journal of Health Care for the Poor and Underserved, 6*(2), 95–101.

Public Health Service. (1989). *Caring for our future: The content of prenatal care.* Washington, DC: U.S. Government Printing Office.

Public Health Service. (1990). *Healthy people 2000: National health promotion and disease prevention objectives: Full report, with commentary* (DHHS Publication No. PHS 91–50212). Washington, DC: U.S. Government Printing Office.

Public Health Service Task Force on Drug Abuse Data. (1990). *Report of the Public Health Service Task Force on Drug Abuse Data: Improving drug abuse statistics.* Washington, DC: Office of the Assistant Secretary for Planning and Evaluation.

Putnam, R. D. (1993). *Making democracy work: Civic traditions in modern Italy.* Princeton, NJ: Princeton University Press.

Putnam, R. D. (1995). Bowling alone: America's declining social capital. *Journal of Democracy, 6*(1), 65–78.

Quinn, M. J., & Tomita, S. K. (1986). *Elder abuse and neglect: Causes, diagnosis, and intervention strategies.* New York: Springer.

Quirk, G. J., & Casco, L. (1994). Stress disorders of families of the disappeared: A controlled study in Honduras. *Social Science and Medicine, 39*(12), 1675–1679.

Rahkonen, O., Lahelma, E., & Huuhka, M. (1997). Past or present? Childhood living conditions and current socioeconomic status as determinants of adult health. *Social Science and Medicine, 44*(3), 327–336.

Raine, A., Brennan, P., Mednick, B., & Mednick, S. A. (1996). High rates of violence, crime, academic problems, and behavioral problems in males with both early neuromotor deficits and unstable family environments. *Archives of General Psychiatry, 53*(6), 544–549.

Ramirez-Valles, J., Zimmerman, M. A., & Newcomb, M. D. (1998). Sexual risk behavior among youth: Modeling the influence of prosocial activities and socioeconomic factors. *Journal of Health and Social Behavior, 39*(3), 237–253.

RAND. (1998a). *Helping adolescents resist drugs: Project ALERT* (RAND Document No. RB-4518). Santa Monica, CA: Author.

RAND. (1998b). *How does managed care affect the cost of mental health services* (RAND Document No. RB-4515). Santa Monica, CA: Author.

RAND. (1998c). *Improving the quality and cost-effectiveness of treatment of depression* (RAND Document No. RB-4500–1). Santa Monica, CA: Author.

RAND. (1999). *A portrait of the HIV+ population in America: Initial results from the HIV Cost and Services Utilization Study* (RAND Document No. RB-4523). Santa Monica, CA: Author.

RAND. Institute for Civil Justice. (1999). *Helping shape civil justice policy: 1998 annual report* (RAND Document No. AR-7006-ICJ). Santa Monica, CA: Author.

Randall, T. (1990). Domestic violence intervention calls for more than treating injuries. *Journal of the American Medical Association, 264*, 939–940.

Rauschenbach, B., Frongillo, E. A., Jr., Thompson, F. E., Anderson, E.J.Y., & Spicer, D. A. (1990). Dependency on soup kitchens in urban areas of New York State. *American Journal of Public Health, 80*, 57–60.

Raube, K., & Merrell, K. (1999). Maternal minimum-stay legislation: Cost and policy implications. *American Journal of Public Health, 89*(6), 922–923.

Ray, W. A., Gigante, J., Mitchel, E. F. Jr., & Hickson, G. B. (1998). Perinatal outcomes following implementation of TennCare. *Journal of the American Medical Association, 279*(4), 314–316.

Ray, W. A., Mitchel, E. F. Jr., & Piper, J. M. (1997). Effect of Medicaid expansions on preterm birth. *American Journal of Preventive Medicine, 13*(4), 292–297.

Redfield, R. R., & Tramont, E. C. (1989). Toward a better classification system for HIV infection. *New England Journal of Medicine, 320*, 1414–1416.

Regier, D. A., Farmer, M. E., Rae, D. S., Locke, B. Z., Keith, S. J., Judd, L. L., & Goodwin, F. K. (1990). Comorbidity of mental disorders with alcohol and other drug abuse: Results from the epidemiologic catchment area (ECA) study. *Journal of the American Medical Association, 264*, 2511–2518.

Reich, T., Cloninger, C. R., Van Eerdewegh, P., Rice, J. P., & Mullaney, J. (1988). Secular trends in the familial transmission of alcoholism. *Alcoholism: Clinical and Experimental Research, 12*, 458–464.

Reiniger, A., Robison, E., & McHugh, M. (1995). Mandated training of professionals: A means for improving reporting of suspected child abuse. *Child Abuse and Neglect, 19*(1), 63–69.

Reiss, A. J., Jr., & Roth, J. A. (Eds.). (1993). *Understanding and preventing violence.* Washington, DC: National Academy Press.

Remafedi, G. (1999). Sexual orientation and youth suicide. *Journal of the American Medical Association, 282*(13), 1291–1292.

Renaud, M., & Kresse E. (1997). *Profiles of activities to reduce perinatal transmission of HIV: Assessing the response.* Washington, DC: U.S. Conference of Mayors.

Reuter, P. (1991). *On the consequences of toughness* (N-3447-DPRC). Santa Monica, CA: RAND.

Reuter, P., & Caulkins, J. P. (1995). Redefining the goals of national drug policy: recommendations from a working group. *American Journal of Public Health, 85*(8 Pt. 1), 1059–1063.

Rice, D. P., Kelman, S., Miller, L. S., & Dunmeyer, S. (1990). *The economic costs of alcohol and drug abuse and mental illness: 1985.* San Francisco: Institute for Health and Aging, University of California.

Ridgely, M. S., & Goldman, H. H. (1989). Mental health insurance. In D. A. Rochefort (Ed.), *Handbook on mental health policy in the United States* (pp. 341–361). Westport, CT: Greenwood Press.

Riemer, J. G., Van Cleve, L., & Galbraith, M. (1995). Barriers to well child care for homeless children under age 13. *Public Health Nursing, 12*(1), 61–66.

Rietmeijer, C. A., Kane, M. S., Simons, P. Z., Corby, N. H., Wolitski, R. J., Higgins, D. L., Judson, F. N., & Cohn, D. L. (1996). Increasing the use of bleach and condoms among injecting drug users in Denver: Outcomes of a targeted, community-level HIV prevention program. *AIDS, 10*(3), 291–298.

Riley, M. W., Ory, M. G., & Zablotsky, D. (Eds.). (1989). *AIDS in an aging society: What we need to know.* New York: Springer.

Ringwalt, C. L., Greene, J. M., Robertson, M., & McPheeters, M. (1998). The prevalence of homelessness among adolescents in the United States. *American Journal of Public Health, 88*(9), 1325–1329.

Rissel, C. (1994). Empowerment: The holy grail of health promotion? *Health Promotion International, 9*(1), 39–47.

Rivlin, A. M., Wiener, J. M., Hanley, R., & Spence, D. (1988). *Caring for the disabled elderly: Who will pay?* Washington, DC: Brookings Institution.

Rizzo, J. A., Marder, W. D., & Willke, R. J. (1990). Physician contact with and attitudes toward HIV-seropositive patients: Results from a national survey. *Medical Care, 28,* 251–260.

Robert Wood Johnson Foundation. (1985). *The perinatal program—what has been learned.* Princeton, NJ: Author.

Robert Wood Johnson Foundation. (1986). *The rural infant care program.* Princeton, NJ: Author.

Robert Wood Johnson Foundation. (1989). *Interfaith volunteer caregivers.* Special Report Number One. Princeton, NJ: Author.

Robert Wood Johnson Foundation. (1990). Day care center closes gap in services for disabled children. *Robert Wood Johnson Foundation-Advances, 4,* 10. Princeton, NJ: Author.

Robert Wood Johnson Foundation. (1994). *Making connections: AIDS and communities: Summary of selected Robert Wood Johnson Foundation Projects.* Princeton, NJ: Author.

Robertson, A., & Minkler, M. (1994). New health promotion movement: A critical examination. *Health Education Quarterly, 21*(3), 295–312.

Robins, L. N. (1989). Cross-cultural differences in psychiatric disorder. *American Journal of Public Health, 79,* 1479–1480.

Robins, L. N. (1990). Psychiatric epidemiology—a historic review. *Social Psychiatry and Psychiatric Epidemiology, 25,* 16–26.

Robins, L. N., & Regier, D. A. (Eds.). (1991). *Psychiatric disorders in America: The Epidemiologic Catchment Area Study.* New York: Free Press.

Robinson, G. K., Meisel, J., & Guthierrez, L. (1990). *Long-term care legislation and mental illness: An analysis of current proposals.* Washington, DC: Mental Health Policy Resource Center.

Robinson, G. K., & Toff-Bergman, G. (1990). *Choices in case management: Current knowledge and practice for mental health programs.* Washington, DC: Mental Health Policy Resource Center.

Roche, A. M., Evans, K. R., & Stanton, W. R. (1997). Harm reduction: Roads less travelled to the holy grail. *Addiction, 92*(9), 1207–1212.

Rochefort, D. A. (1997). *From poorhouses to homelessness: Policy analysis and mental health care* (2nd ed.). Westport, CT: Auburn House.

Rodriguez, M. A., & Brindis, C. D. (1995). Violence and Latino youth: Prevention and methodological issues. *Public Health Reports, 110*(3), 260–267.

Rogler, L. H. (1989). The meaning of culturally sensitive research in mental health. *American Journal of Psychiatry, 146,* 296–303.

Rogowski, J. (1998). Cost-effectiveness of care for very low birth weight infants. *Pediatrics, 102*(1 Pt. 1), 35–43.

Rogowski, J. A. (1993). *Private versus public sector insurance coverage for drug abuse* (RAND Document No. MR-166-DPRC). Santa Monica, CA: RAND.

Rokaw, W. M., Mercy, J. A., & Smith, J. C. (1990). Comparing death certificate data with FBI crime reporting statistics on U.S. homicides. *Public Health Reports, 105,* 447–455.

Rooks, J. P., Weatherby, N. L., Ernst, E.K.M., Stapleton, S., Rosen, D., & Rosenfield, A. (1989). Outcomes of care in birth centers: The national birth center study. *New England Journal of Medicine, 321,* 1804–1825.

Roos, N. P., & Havens, B. (1991). Predictors of successful aging: A twelve-year study of Manitoba elderly. *American Journal of Public Health, 81,* 63–68.

Rosenbach, M. L., & Ammering, C. J. (1997). Trends in Medicare Part B mental health utilization and expenditures: 1987–92. *Health Care Financing Review, 18*(3), 19–42.

Rosenbaum, S., Hughes, D. C., & Johnson, K. (1988). Maternal and child health services for medically indigent children and pregnant women. *Medical Care, 26,* 315–332.

Rosenberg, M. L., Gelles, R. J., Holinger, P. C., Zahn, M. A., Stark, E., Conn, J. M., Fajman, N. N., & Karlson, T. A. (1987). Violence: Homicide, assault, and suicide. In R. W. Amler & H. B. Dull (Eds.), *Closing the gap: The burden of unnecessary illness* (pp. 164–178). New York: Oxford University Press.

Rosenblatt, R. A. (1989). The perinatal paradox: Doing more and accomplishing less. *Health Affairs, 8*(3), 158–204.

Rosenfeld, A. A., Pilowsky, D. J., Fine, P., Thorpe, M., Fein, E., Simms, M. D., Halfon, N., Irwin, M., Alfaro, J., Saletsky, R., & Nickman, S. (1997). Foster care: An update. *Journal of the American Academy of Child and Adolescent Psychiatry, 36*(4), 448–457.

Rosenfield, S. (1989). Psychiatric epidemiology: An overview of methods and findings. In D. A. Rochefort (Ed.), *Handbook on mental health policy in the United States* (pp. 45–65). Westport, CT: Greenwood Press.

Rosenheck, R., Frisman, L., & Kasprow, W. (1999). Improving access to disability benefits among homeless persons with mental illness: An agency-specific approach to services integration. *American Journal of Public Health, 89*(4), 524–528.

Rosenheck, R., Gallup, P., Leda, C., Gorchov, L., & Errera, P. (1990, May). Help for the homeless: A progress report on the HCMI veterans program. *VA Practitioner,* 53–56.

Rosenheck, R., & Lam, J. A. (1997). Client and site characteristics as barriers to service use by homeless persons with serious mental illness. *Psychiatric Services, 48*(3), 387–390.

Rosenheck, R., Morrissey, J., Lam, J., Calloway, M., Johnsen, M., Goldman, H., Randolph, F., Blasinsky, M., Fontana, A., Calsyn, R., & Teague, G. (1998). Service system integration, access to services, and housing outcomes in a program for homeless persons with severe mental illness. *American Journal of Public Health, 88*(11), 1610–1615.

Rosenheck, R., & Seibyl, C. L. (1998). Homelessness: Health service use and related costs. *Medical Care, 36*(8), 1256–1264.

Rossi, P. H. (1989). *Down and out in America: The origins of homelessness.* Chicago: University of Chicago Press.

Rossi, P. H. (1990). The old homeless and the new homelessness in historical perspective. *American Psychologist, 45,* 954–959.

Rossi, P. H., Wright, J. D., Fisher, G. A., & Willis, G. (1987). The urban homeless: Estimating composition and size. *Science, 235*(4794), 1336–1341.

Rost, K., Zhang, M., Fortney, J., Smith, J., & Smith, G. R. Jr. (1998). Rural-urban differences in depression treatment and suicidality. *Medical Care, 36*(7), 1098–1107.

Rothenberg, K. H., & Paskey, S. J. (1995). The risk of domestic violence and women with HIV infection: Implications for partner notification, public policy, and the law. *American Journal of Public Health, 85* (11), 1569–1576.

Rothenberg, R. B., & Koplan, J. P. (1990). Chronic disease in the 1990s. *Annual Review of Public Health, 11,* 267–296.

Rouse, B. A. (1996). Epidemiology of illicit and abused drugs in the general population, emergency department drug-related episodes, and arrestees. *Clinical Chemistry, 42*(8 Pt. 2), 1330–1336.

Rouse, B. A. (1998). *Substance abuse and mental health statistics sourcebook–1998* (DHHS Publication No. SMA 98–3170). Washington, DC: U.S. Government Printing Office.

Rowe, M. J., & Keintz, R. (1989). National survey of state spending for AIDS. *Intergovernmental AIDS Reports, George Washington University, 2*(3), 1–12.

Roy, A. W., Ford, A. B., & Folmar, S. J. (1990). The elderly and risk factors for institutionalization: Evidence from the Cleveland General Accounting Office (GAO) study, 1975–1984. *Journal of Applied Social Sciences, 14,* 177–195.

Rudd, M. D. (1990). An integrative model of suicidal ideation. *Suicide and Life-Threatening Behavior, 20,* 16–30.

Rudzinski, K. A., Marconi, K. M., & McKinney, M. M. (1994). Federal funding for health services research on AIDS, 1986–1991. *Health Affairs, 13*(3), 261–266.

Ruiz, P. (1993). Access to health care for uninsured Hispanics: policy recommendations. *Hospital & Community Psychiatry, 44*(10), 958–962.

Rumbaut, R. G., Chavez, L. R., Moser, R. J., Pickwell, S. M., & Wishik, S. M. (1988). The politics of migrant health care: A comparative study of Mexican immigrants and Indochinese refugees. *Research in the Sociology of Health Care, 7,* 143–202.

Rydell, C. P., & Everingham, S. S. (1994). *Controlling cocaine: Supply versus demand programs* (RAND Document No. MR-331-ONDCP/A/DPRC). Santa Monica, CA: RAND.

Sable, M. R., Stockbauer, J. W., Schramm, W. F., & Land, G. H. (1990). Differentiating the barriers to adequate prenatal care in Missouri, 1987–88. *Public Health Reports, 105,* 549–555.

Sadowsky, D., & Kunzel, C. (1996). Predicting dentists' willingness to treat HIV-infected patients. *AIDS Care, 8*(5), 581–588.

Safren, S. A., & Heimberg, R. G. (1999). Depression, hopelessness, suicidality, and related factors in sexual minority and heterosexual adolescents. *Journal of Consulting and Clinical Psychology, 67*(6), 859–866.

St. Clair, P. A., Smeriglio, V. L., Alexander, C. S., & Celentano, D. D. (1989). Social network structure and prenatal care utilization. *Medical Care, 27,* 823–832.

St. Clair, P. A., Smeriglio, V. L., Alexander, C. S., Connell, F. A., & Niebyl, J. R. (1990). Situational and financial barriers to prenatal care in a sample of low-income, inner-city women. *Public Health Reports, 105,* 264–267.

Salit, S. A., Kuhn, E. M., Hartz, A. J., Vu, J. M., & Mosso, A. L. (1998). Hospitalization costs associated with homelessness in New York City. *New England Journal of Medicine, 338*(24), 1734–1740.

Salkever, D., Domino, M. E., Burns, B. J., Santos, A. B., Deci, P. A., Dias, J., Wagner, H. R., Faldowski, R. A., & Paolone, J. (1999). Assertive community treatment for people with severe mental illness: The effect on hospital use and costs. *Health Services Research, 34*(2), 577–601.

Samet, J. H., Libman, H., LaBelle, C., Steger, K., Lewis, R., Craven, D. E., & Freedberg, K. A. (1995). A model clinic for the initial evaluation and establishment of primary care for persons infected with human immunodeficiency virus. *Archives of Internal Medicine, 155*(15), 1629–1633.

Sanborn, C. J. (1990). Gender socialization and suicide: American Association of Suicidology Presidential Address, 1989. *Suicide and Life-Threatening Behavior, 20,* 148–155.

Sandrick, K. (1993). Learning from experience: In AIDS treatment, knowledge means quality. *Hospitals, 67*(7), 32–35.

Sardell, A. (1990). Child health policy in the U.S.: The paradox of consensus. *Journal of Health Politics, Policy and Law, 15,* 271–304.

Sargent, M. (1989). Update on programs for the homeless mentally ill. *Hospital and Community Psychiatry, 40,* 1015–1016.

Sawyer, S. M., Blair, S., & Bowes, G. (1997). Chronic illness in adolescents: Transfer or transition to adult services? *Journal of Paediatrics and Child Health, 33*(2), 88–90.

Scallet, L. J. (1990). Paying for public mental health care: Crucial questions. *Health Affairs, 9*(1), 117–124.

Scallet, L. J., Marvelle, K., & Davidson, L. (1990). *Protection and advocacy for mentally ill individuals: Legislative history and analysis of P.L. 99–319.* Washington, DC: Mental Health Policy Resource Center.

Scanlon, W. J. (1988). A perspective on long-term care for the elderly. *Health Care Financing Review, Annual Supplement,* 7–15.

Schene, P., & Bond, K. (Eds.). (1989). *Research issues in risk assessment for child protection.* Denver, CO: American Association for Protecting Children.

Schietinger, H., & Schechter, C. (1998). *Medical coverage for Medicare beneficiaries with HIV/AIDS: Issues and implications.* Washington, DC: Academy for Educational Development.

Schlesinger, M., & Kronebusch, K. (1990). The failure of prenatal care policy for the poor. *Health Affairs, 9*(4), 91–111.

Schmidt, L., Weisner, C., & Wiley, J. (1998). Substance abuse and the course of welfare dependency. *American Journal of Public Health, 88*(11), 1616–1622.

Schone, B. S., & Weinick, R. M. (1998). Health-related behaviors and the benefits of marriage for elderly persons. *Gerontologist, 38*(5), 618–627.

Schore, J., Harrington, M., & Crystal, S. (1998). *Serving a changing population: Home- and community-based services for people with AIDS.* Princeton, NJ: Mathematica Policy Research.

Schulberg, H. C., & Burns, B. J. (1988). Mental disorders in primary care: Epidemiologic, diagnostic, and treatment research directions. *General Hospital Psychiatry, 10*, 79–87.

Schurman, R. A., Kramer, P. D., & Mitchell, J. B. (1985). The hidden mental health network. *Archives of General Psychiatry, 42*, 89–94.

Schwartz, R. H. (1993). Syringe and needle exchange programs: Part I. *Southern Medical Journal, 86*(3), 318–322.

Scitovsky, A. A. (1988). The economic impact of AIDS in the United States. *Health Affairs, 7*(4), 32–45.

Scitovsky, A. A. (1989a). Past lessons and future directions: The economics of health services delivery for HIV-related illnesses. In W. N. LaVee (Ed.), *Conference Proceedings: New Perspectives on HIV-related Illness: Progress in Health Services Research* (DHHS Publication No. PHS 89–3449) (pp. 21–33). Washington, DC: U.S. Government Printing Office.

Scitovsky, A. A. (1989b). Studying the cost of HIV-related illnesses: Reflections on the moving target. *Milbank Quarterly, 67*, 318–344.

Scitovsky, A. A., & Rice, D. P. (1987). Estimates of the direct and indirect costs of acquired immunodeficiency syndrome in the United States, 1985, 1986, and 1991. *Public Health Reports, 102*, 5–17.

Scott, J., & Rantz, M. (1997). Managing chronically ill older people in the midst of the health care revolution. *Nursing Administration Quarterly, 21*(2), 55–64.

Scribner, R., & Dwyer, J. H. (1989). Acculturation and low birthweight among Latinos in the Hispanic HANES. *American Journal of Public Health, 79*, 1263–1267.

Sechrest, L., Freeman, H., & Mulley, A. (Eds.). (1989). *Conference Proceedings: Health Services Research Methodology: A Focus on AIDS* (DHHS Publication No. PHS 89–3439). Washington, DC: U.S. Government Printing Office.

Sedlak, A. J. (1991). *National incidence and prevalence of child abuse and neglect: 1988, Revised report.* Rockville, MD: Westat.

Sedlak, A. J., & Broadhurst, D. D. (1996). *Third National Incidence Study of Child Abuse and Neglect: Final report.* Washington, DC: Administration on Children, Youth and Families, National Center on Child Abuse and Neglect.

Sedlak, A. J., Hantman, I., & Schultz, D. (1997). *Third National Incidence Study of Child Abuse and Neglect: Final report appendices.* Washington, DC: Administration on Children, Youth and Families, National Center on Child Abuse and Neglect.

Segal, S. P., & Kotler, P. (1989). Community residential care. In D. A. Rochefort (Ed.), *Handbook on mental health policy in the United States* (pp. 237–265). Westport, CT: Greenwood Press.

Selden, T. M., Banthin, J. S., & Cohen, J. W. (1999). Waiting in the wings: Eligibility and enrollment in the State Children's Health Insurance Program. *Health Affairs, 18*(2), 126–133.

Selik, R. M., Buehler, J. W., Karon, J. M., Chamberland, M. E., & Berkelman, R. L. (1990). Impact of the 1987 revision of the case definition of acquired immune deficiency syndrome in the United States. *Journal of Acquired Immune Deficiency Syndromes, 3*, 73–82.

Seltzer, G. B., & Essex, E. L. (1998). Service needs of persons with mental retardation and other developmental disabilities. In S. A. Mor & V. Mor, *Living in the community with disability: Service needs, use, and systems* (pp. 197–218). New York: Springer.

Seltzer, M. M. (1998). Service use and delivery for persons with mental retardation and other developmental disabilities. In S. A. Mor & V. Mor, *Living in the community with disability: Service needs, use, and systems* (pp. 219–242). New York: Springer.

Shadish, W. R., Jr. (1989). Critical multiplism: A research strategy and its attendant tactics. In L. Sechrest, H. Freeman, & A. Mulley (Eds.), *Conference Proceedings: Health Services Research Methodology: A Focus on AIDS* (DHHS Publication No. PHS 89–3439) (pp. 5–28). Washington, DC: U.S. Government Printing Office.

Shadish, W. R., Jr., & Reis, J. (1984). A review of studies of the effectiveness of programs to improve pregnancy outcome. *Evaluation Review, 8,* 747–775.

Shapiro, E., & Tate, R. (1988). Who is really at risk of institutionalization? *Gerontologist, 28,* 237–245.

Shapiro, M. F., Morton, S. C., McCaffrey, D. F., Senterfitt, J. W., Fleishman, J. A., Perlman, J. F., Athey, L. A., Keesey, J. W., Goldman, D. P., Berry, S. H., & Bozzette, S. A. (1999). Variations in the care of HIV-infected adults in the United States: Results from the HIV Cost and Services Utilization Study. *Journal of the American Medical Association, 281*(24), 2305–2315.

Shaughnessy, P. W. (1985). Long-term care research and public policy. *Health Services Research, 20,* 490–499.

Shaughnessy, P. W., Crisler, K. S., Schlenker, R. E., & Arnold, A. G. (1997). Outcomes across the care continuum: Home health care. *Medical Care, 35*(11 Suppl.), NS115–123.

Shaughnessy, P. W., & Kramer, A. (1990). The increased needs of patients in nursing homes and patients receiving home health care. *New England Journal of Medicine, 322,* 21–27.

Shelp, E. E., DuBose, E. R., & Sunderland, R. H. (1990). The infrastructure of religious communities: A neglected resource for care of people with AIDS. *American Journal of Public Health, 80,* 970–972.

Shelton, T. L., Jeppson, E. S., & Johnson, B. H. (1989). *Family-centered care for children with special health care needs* (2nd ed.). Washington, DC: Association for the Care of Children's Health.

Sherman, J. J. (1996). Medicare's mental health benefits: coverage, use, and expenditures. *Journal of Aging & Health, 8*(1), 54–71.

Shiboski, C. H., Palacio, H., Neuhaus, J. M., & Greenblatt, R. M. (1999). Dental care access and use among HIV-infected women. *American Journal of Public Health, 89*(6), 834–839.

Shinn, M., Weitzman, B. C., Stojanovic, D., Knickman, J. R., Jiménez, L., Duchon, L., James, S., & Krantz, D. H. (1998). Predictors of homelessness among families in New York City: From shelter request to housing stability. *American Journal of Public Health, 88*(11), 1651–1657.

Shiono, P. H., & Behrman, R. E. (1995). Low birth weight: analysis and recommendations. *Future of Children, 5*(1), 4–18.

Shore, M. F. (1996). An overview of managed behavioral health care. *New Directions for Mental Health Services, 72,* 3–12.

Short, P. F., & Freedman, V. A. (1998). Single women and the dynamics of Medicaid. *Health Services Research, 33*(5 Pt. 1), 1309–1336.

Short, P. F., & Leon, J. (1990). *Use of home and community services by persons ages 65 and older with functional difficulties* (DHHS Publication No. PHS 90–3466). Washington, DC: U.S. Government Printing Office.

Shortell, S. M., Gillies, R. R., & Anderson, D. A. (1994). The new world of managed care: Creating organized delivery systems. *Health Affairs. 13*(5), 46–64.

Shortell, S. M., Gillies, R. R., Anderson, D. A., Erickson, K. M., & Mitchell, J. B. (1996). *Remaking health care in America: Building organized delivery systems.* San Francisco: Jossey-Bass.

Showstack, J., Lurie, N., Leatherman, S., Fisher, E., & Inui, T. (1996). Health of the public: The private-sector challenge. *Journal of the American Medical Association, 276*(13), 1071–1074.

Shulsinger, E. (1990). Needs of sheltered homeless children. *Journal of Pediatric Health Care, 4*(3), 136–140.

Shy, K. K., Luthy, D. A., Bennett, F. C., & Whitfield, M. (1990). Effects of electronic fetal-heart-rate monitoring, as compared with periodic auscultation, on the neurologic development of premature infants. *New England Journal of Medicine, 322,* 588–593.

Siddharthan, K. (1990). HMO enrollment by Medicare beneficiaries in heterogeneous communities. *Medical Care, 28,* 918–927.

Siddharthan, K., & Ahern, M. (1996). Inpatient utilization by undocumented immigrants without insurance. *Journal of Health Care for the Poor and Underserved, 7*(4), 355–363.

Silverman, J. (1989). The contribution of social services to preventing youth suicide. In M. L. Rosenberg & K. Baer (Eds.), *Report of the Secretary's Task Force on Youth Suicide: Vol. 4: Strategies for the prevention of youth suicide* (DHHS Publication No. ADM 89–1624) (pp. 168–170). Alcohol, Drug Abuse, and Mental Health Administration. Washington, DC: U.S. Government Printing Office.

Simon, J. L. (1991). The case for greatly increased immigration. *Public Interest, 102,* 89–118.

Simpson, D. D., Joe, G. W., Fletcher, B. W., Hubbard, R. L., & Anglin, M. D. (1999). A national evaluation of treatment outcomes for cocaine dependence. *Archives of General Psychiatry, 56*(6), 507–514.

Singer, B. H., & Manton, K. G. (1998). The effects of health changes on projections of health service needs for the elderly population of the United States. *Proceedings of the National Academy of Sciences of the United States of America, 95*(26), 15618–15622.

Singer, M. (1994). AIDS and the health crisis of the U.S. urban poor: The perspective of critical medical anthropology. *Social Science & Medicine, 39*(7), 931–948.

Skogan, W. G. (1990). The polls—a review: The national crime survey redesign. *Public Opinion Quarterly, 54,* 256–272.

Slap, G. B., Vorters, D. F., Chaudhuri, S., & Centor, R. M. (1989). Risk factors for attempted suicide during adolescence. *Pediatrics, 84,* 762–772.

Smith, J. P., & Edmonston, B. (Eds.). (1997). *The new Americans: Economic, demographic, and fiscal effects of immigration.* Washington, DC: National Academy Press.

Smith, K. B. (1997). Explaining variation in state-level homicide rates: Does crime policy pay? *Journal of Politics, 59*(2), 350–367.

Söderlund, N., Lavis, J., Broomberg, J., & Mills, A. (1993). The costs of HIV prevention strategies in developing countries. *Bulletin of the World Health Organization, 71*(5), 595–604.

Solomon, M. Z., & DeJong, W. (1989). Preventing AIDS and other STDs through condom promotion: A patient education intervention. *American Journal of Public Health, 79,* 453–458.

Soumerai, S. B., McLaughlin, T. J., Ross-Degnan, D., Casteris, C. S., & Bollini, P. (1994). Effects of a limit on Medicaid drug-reimbursement benefits on the use of psychotropic agents and acute mental health services by patients with schizophrenia. *New England Journal of Medicine, 331*(10), 650–655.

Southern Regional Project on Infant Mortality. (1989). *A bold step: The South acts to reduce infant mortality.* Washington, DC: Author.

Spector, W. D. (1990). Functional disability scales. In B. Spilker (Ed.), *Quality of life assessment in clinical trials* (pp. 115–129). New York: Raven Press.

Spilker, B., Molinek, F. R., Jr., Johnston, K. A., Simpson, R. L., Jr., & Tilson, H. H. (1990). Quality of life bibliography and indexes. *Medical Care, 28*(Suppl.), DS1-DS77.

Spohn, P. H., Bergthold, L., & Estes, C. L. (1988). From cottages to condos: The expansion of the home health care industry under Medicare. *Home Health Care Services Quarterly, 8*(4), 25–55.

Stack, S. (1987). The sociological study of suicide: Methodological issues. *Suicide and Life-Threatening Behavior, 17,* 133–150.

Stack, S. (1996–1997). The effect of labor force participation on female suicide rates: An analysis of individual data from sixteen states. *Omega, 34*(2), 163–169.

Starfield, B. (1989). Preventive interventions in the health and health-related sectors with potential relevance for youth suicide. In M. L. Rosenberg & K. Baer (Eds.), *Report of the Secretary's Task Force on Youth Suicide: Vol. 4: Strategies for the prevention of youth suicide* (DHHS Publication No. ADM 89–1624) (pp. 145–167). Alcohol, Drug Abuse, and Mental Health Administration. Washington, DC: U.S. Government Printing Office.

Starfield, B. (1996). Public health and primary care: A framework for proposed linkages. *American Journal of Public Health, 86*(10), 1365–1369.

Stark, E. (1990). Rethinking homicide: Violence, race, and the politics of gender. *International Journal of Health Services, 20*, 3–26.

Stein, M. D., Fleishman, J., Mor, V., & Dresser, M. (1993). Factors associated with patient satisfaction among symptomatic HIV-infected persons. *Medical Care, 31*(2), 182–188.

Stein, R.E.K. (Ed.). (1989). *Caring for children with chronic illness: Issues and strategies.* New York: Springer.

Steinmetz, S. K. (1988). *Duty bound: Elder abuse and family care.* Thousand Oaks, CA: Sage.

Stephen, E. H., Foote, K., Hendershot, G. E., & Schoenborn, C. A. (1994). *Health of the foreign-born population: United States, 1989–90.* (DHHS Publication No. PHS 94–1250). Washington, DC: U.S. Government Printing Office.

Stephens, D., Dennis, E., Toomer, M., & Holloway, J. (1991). The diversity of case management needs for the care of homeless persons. *Public Health Reports, 106*, 15–19.

Stephens, R. C., Feucht, T. E., & Roman, S. W. (1991). Effects of an intervention program on AIDS-related drug and needle behavior among intravenous drug users. *American Journal of Public Health, 81*, 568–571.

Sterling, T. D., & Weinkam, J. J. (1989). Comparison of smoking-related risk factors among black and white males. *American Journal of Industrial Medicine, 15*, 319–333.

Stewart, A. L., Greenfield, S., Hays, R. D., Wells, K., Rogers, W. H., Berry, S. D., McGlynn, E. A., & Ware, J. E., Jr. (1989). Functional status and well-being of patients with chronic conditions. *Journal of the American Medical Association, 262*, 907–913.

Stimson, G. V., Eaton, G., Rhodes, T., & Power, R. (1994). Potential development of community oriented HIV outreach among drug injectors in the UK. *Addiction, 89*(12), 1601–1611.

Stone, R. I. (1989). The feminization of poverty among the elderly. *Women's Studies Quarterly, 17*, 20–45.

Stone, R. I., & Murtaugh, C. M. (1990). The elderly population with chronic functional disability: Implications for home care eligibility. *Gerontologist, 30*, 491–496.

Stone, R. I., & Short, P. F. (1990). The competing demands of employment and informal caregiving to disabled elders. *Medical Care, 28*, 513–526.

Stoto, M. A., Almario, D. A., & McCormick, M. C. (Eds.). (1999). *Reducing the odds: Preventing perinatal transmission of HIV in the United States.* Washington, DC: National Academy Press.

Stratton, K., Howe, C., & Battaglia, F. C. (Eds.). (1996). *Fetal alcohol syndrome: Diagnosis, epidemiology, prevention, and treatment.* Washington, DC: National Academy Press.

Straus, M. A., Gelles, R. J., & Steinmetz, S. K. (1981). *Behind closed doors: Violence in the American family.* Newbury Park, CA: Sage Publications.

Straus, M. B. (Ed.). (1988). *Abuse and victimization across the life span.* Baltimore, MD: Johns Hopkins University Press.

Strauss, A., & Corbin, J. M. (1988). *Shaping a new health care system: The explosion of chronic illness as a catalyst for change.* San Francisco: Jossey-Bass.

Streiner, D. L., & Adam, K. S. (1987). Evaluation of the effectiveness of suicide prevention programs: A methodological perspective. *Suicide and Life-Threatening Behavior, 17*, 93–106.

Substance Abuse and Mental Health Services Administration. (1994). *Preliminary estimates from the Drug Abuse Warning Network: 1993 preliminary estimates of drug-related emergency department episodes* (Advance Report, No. 8.). Washington, DC: U.S. Government Printing Office.

Substance Abuse and Mental Health Services Administration. (1996). *Mental health estimates from the 1994 National Household Survey on Drug Abuse.* (DHHS Publication No. SMA 96–3103). Washington, DC: U.S. Government Printing Office.

Substance Abuse and Mental Health Services Administration. (1997). *Substance use among women in the United States* (DHHS Publication No. SMA 97–3162). Washington, DC: U.S. Government Printing Office.

Substance Abuse and Mental Health Services Administration. (1998a). *Mid-year 1997 preliminary emergency department data from the Drug Abuse Warning Network* (DHHS Publication No. SMA 98–3252). Washington, DC: U.S. Government Printing Office.

Substance Abuse and Mental Health Services Administration. (1998b). *National household survey on drug abuse: Main findings 1996* (DHHS Publication No. SMA 98–3200). Washington, DC: U.S. Government Printing Office.

Substance Abuse and Mental Health Services Administration. (1998c). *Preliminary results from the 1997 National Household Survey on Drug Abuse* (DHHS Publication No. SMA 98–3251). Washington, DC: U.S. Government Printing Office.

Substance Abuse and Mental Health Services Administration. (1998d). *Prevalence of substance use among racial and ethnic subgroups in the United States, 1991–1993* (DHHS Publication No. SMA 98–3202). Washington, DC: U.S. Government Printing Office.

Substance Abuse and Mental Health Services Administration. (1998e). *Services research outcomes study* (DHHS Publication No. SMA 98–3177). Washington, DC: U.S. Government Printing Office.

Substance Abuse and Mental Health Services Administration. (1999a). *Cost savings from the treatment of substance abuse problems: Lessons for prevention from the cost-offset literature* (DHHS Publication No. 98–3236). Washington, DC: U.S. Government Printing Office.

Substance Abuse and Mental Health Services Administration. (1999b). *Drug Abuse Warning Network: Annual medical examiner data 1997* (DHHS Publication No. SMA 00–3377). Washington, DC: U.S. Government Printing Office.

Substance Abuse and Mental Health Services Administration. (1999c). *National household survey on drug abuse: Main findings 1997* (DHHS Publication No. SMA 99–3295). Washington, DC: U.S. Government Printing Office.

Substance Abuse and Mental Health Services Administration. (1999d). *National household survey on drug abuse: Population estimates 1998* (DHHS Publication No. SMA 99–3327). Washington, DC: U.S. Government Printing Office.

Substance Abuse and Mental Health Services Administration. (1999e). *Summary of findings from the 1998 National Household Survey on Drug Abuse* (DHHS Publication No. SMA 99–3328). Washington, DC: U.S. Government Printing Office.

Substance Abuse and Mental Health Services Administration. (1999f). *Year-end 1998 emergency department data from the Drug Abuse Warning Network* (DHHS SMA 00–3376). Washington, DC: U.S. Government Printing Office.

Surles, R. C., & Shore, M. F. (1996). The public sector—private sector interface: current issues, future trends. *New Directions for Mental Health Services, 72,* 71–79.

Swartz, M., Carroll, B., & Blazer, D. (1989). In response to "Psychiatric diagnosis as reified measurement": An invited comment on Mirowsky and Ross. *Journal of Health and Social Behavior, 30,* 33–34.

Szilagyi, P. G., & Schor, E. L. (1998). The health of children. *Health Services Research, 33*(4 Pt. 2), 1001–1039.

Szwarcwald, C. L., Bastos, F. I., Viacava, F., & de Andrade, C. L. (1999). Income inequality and homicide rates in Rio de Janeiro, Brazil. *American Journal of Public Health, 89*(6), 845–850.

Taeuber, C. M., & Siegel, P. M. (1990, Nov.). *Counting the nation's homeless population in the 1990 census.* Paper presented at the Conference on Enumerating Homeless Persons: Methods and Data Needs, Washington, DC.

Takahashi, L. M. (1997). The socio-spatial stigmatization of homelessness and HIV/AIDS: Toward an explanation of the NIMBY syndrome. *Social Science and Medicine, 45*(6), 903–914.

Tanda, G., Pontieri, F. E., & Di Chiara, G. (1997). Cannabinoid and heroin activation of mesolimbic dopamine transmission by a common mu1 opioid receptor mechanism. *Science, 276*(5321), 2048–2050.

Tatara, T., & Kuzmeskus, L. B. (1997). *Summaries of the statistical data on elder abuse in domestic settings for FY 95 and FY 96.* Washington, DC: National Center on Elder Abuse.

Taube, C. A., Goldman, H. H., & Salkever, D. (1990). Medicaid coverage for mental illness: Balancing access and costs. *Health Affairs, 9*(1), 5–18.

Taylor, B. M. (1989). *New directions for the National Crime Survey* (Tech. Rep.). Office of Justice Programs, Bureau of Justice Statistics. Washington, DC: U.S. Department of Justice.

Taylor, S. E., Repetti, R. L., & Seeman, T. (1997). Health psychology: What is an unhealthy environment and how does it get under the skin? *Annual Review of Psychology, 48*, 411–447.

Tell, E. J., Wallack, S. S., & Cohen, M. A. (1987). New directions in life care: An industry in transition. *Milbank Quarterly, 65*, 551–574.

Thamer, M., Richard, C., Casebeer, A. W., & Ray, N. F. (1997). Health insurance coverage among foreign-born US residents: The impact of race, ethnicity, and length of residence. *American Journal of Public Health, 87*(1), 96–102.

Thamer, M., & Rinehart, C. (1998). Public and private health insurance of US foreign-born residents: Implications of the 1996 welfare reform law. *Ethnicity and Health, 3*(1–2), 19–29.

Thompson, M. S., & Meyer, H. J. (1989). The costs of AIDS: Alternative methodological approaches. In L. Sechrest, H. Freeman, & A. Mulley (Eds.), *Conference Proceedings: Health Services Research Methodology: A Focus on AIDS* (DHHS Publication No. PHS 89–3439) (pp. 95–106). Washington, DC: U.S. Government Printing Office.

Thompson, R. S. (1998). Domestic violence identification: Outcomes/effectiveness [Abstract]. *AHCPR Research Activities, 222*, 25.

Thompson-Hoffman, S., & Storck, I. F. (Eds.). (1991). *Disability in the United States: A portrait from national data.* New York: Springer.

Thyen, U., Thiessen, R., & Heinsohn-Krug, M. (1995). Secondary prevention—serving families at risk. *Child Abuse and Neglect, 19*(11), 1337–1347.

Tilden, V. P., Schmidt, T. A., Limandri, B. J., Chiodo, G. T., Garland, M. J., & Loveless, P. A. (1994). Factors that influence clinicians' assessment and management of family violence. *American Journal of Public Health, 84*(4), 628–633.

Tims, F. M., & Leukefeld, C. G. (Eds.). (1988). *Relapse and recovery in drug abuse* (DHHS Publication No. ADM 88–1473). Washington, DC: U.S. Government Printing Office.

Tobler, N. S. (1986). Meta-analysis of 143 adolescent drug prevention programs: Quantitative outcome results of program participants compared to a control or comparison group. *Journal of Drug Issues, 16*, 537–567.

Tolan, P. (1988). Socioeconomic, family, and social stress correlates of adolescent antisocial and delinquent behavior. *Journal of Abnormal Child Psychology, 16*, 317–331.

Tolley, K., & Gyldmark, M. (1993). The treatment and care costs of people with HIV infection or AIDS: Development of a standardised cost framework for Europe. *Health Policy, 24*(1), 55–70.

Tommasini, N. R. (1994). Private insurance coverage for the treatment of mental illness versus general medical care: A policy of inequity. *Archives of Psychiatric Nursing, 8*(1), 9–13.

Toole, M. J., & Waldman, R. J. (1990). Prevention of excess mortality in refugee and displaced populations in developing countries. *Journal of the American Medical Association, 263*, 3296–3302.

Torrens, P. R. (Ed.). (1985). *Hospice programs and public policy*. Chicago: American Hospital Publishing.

Torrey, E. F., Bigelow, D. A., & Sladen-Dew, N. (1993). Quality and cost of services for seriously mentally ill individuals in British Columbia and the United States. *Hospital and Community Psychiatry, 44*(10), 943–950.

Toseland, R. W., & Rossiter, C. M. (1989). Group interventions to support family caregivers: A review and analysis. *Gerontologist, 29*, 438–448.

Trautman, P. D. (1989). Specific treatment modalities for adolescent suicide attempters. In M. R. Feinleib (Ed.), *Report of the Secretary's Task Force on Youth Suicide: Vol. 3: Prevention and interventions in youth suicide* (DHHS Publication No. ADM 89–1623) (pp. 253–263). Alcohol, Drug Abuse, and Mental Health Administration. Washington, DC: U.S. Government Printing Office.

Trepper, T. S., Nelson, T. S., McCollum, E. E., & McAvoy, P. (1997). Improving substance abuse service delivery to Hispanic women through increased cultural competencies: A qualitative study. *Journal of Substance Abuse Treatment, 14*(3), 225–234.

True, W. R., Xian, H., Scherrer, J. F., Madden, P. A., Bucholz, K. K., Heath, A. C., Eisen, S. A., Lyons, M. J., Goldberg, J., & Tsuang, M. (1999). Common genetic vulnerability for nicotine and alcohol dependence in men. *Archives of General Psychiatry, 56*(7), 655–661.

Tucker, W. (1987). Where do the homeless come from? *National Review, 39*(18), 32.

Turner, C. F., Miller, H. G., & Moses, L. E. (Eds.). (1989). *AIDS: Sexual behavior and intravenous drug use*. Washington, DC: National Academy Press.

Turner, R. J., Grindstaff, C. F., & Phillips, N. (1990). Social support and outcome in teenage pregnancy. *Journal of Health and Social Behavior, 31*, 43–57.

Turshen, M. (1996). Unhealthy paradox: A nation of immigrants debates harsh immigration controls. *Current Issues in Public Health, 2*, 61–67.

Twaddle, A. C., & Hessler, R. M. (1977). *A sociology of health*. St. Louis, MO: Mosby–Year Book.

Tweed, D. L., & George, L. K. (1989). A more balanced perspective on "Psychiatric diagnosis as reified measurement": An invited comment on Mirowsky and Ross. *Journal of Health and Social Behavior, 30*, 35–37.

Tweed, J. L., Schoenbach, V. J., George, L. K., & Blazer, D. G. (1989). The effects of childhood parental death and divorce on six-month history of anxiety disorders. *British Journal of Psychiatry, 154*, 823–828.

U.S. Bureau of the Census. (1991). *Statistical abstract of the United States, 1991* (111th ed.). Washington, DC: U.S. Government Printing Office.

U.S. Bureau of the Census. (1999a). *Health insurance coverage, 1998*. Current Population Reports, No. P60–208. Washington, DC: U.S. Government Printing Office.

U.S. Bureau of the Census. (1999b). *Legal immigration, fiscal year 1998* [On-line]. Available: http://www.ins.usdoj.gov/graphics/aboutins/statistics/index.htm [Accessed Mar. 7, 2000. Last updated May 1999].

U.S. Bureau of the Census. (1999c). *Money income in the United States, 1998*. Current Population Reports, No. P60–206. Washington, DC: U.S. Government Printing Office.

U.S. Bureau of the Census. (1999d). *Poverty in the United States, 1998*. Current Population Reports, No. P60–207. Washington, DC: U.S. Government Printing Office.

U.S. Bureau of the Census. (1999e). *Statistical abstract of the United States, 1999* (119th ed.). [On-line]. Available: http://www.census.gov/prod/www/statistical-abstract-us.html [Accessed Feb. 22, 2000. Last updated July 27, 1999].

U.S. Commission on Security and Cooperation in Europe. (1990). *Staff report on homelessness in the United States*. Washington, DC: U.S. Commission on Security and Cooperation in Europe.

U.S. Conference of Mayors. (1999). *A status report on hunger and homelessness in America's cities, 1999: A twenty-six-city survey, December 1999*. Washington, DC: Author.

U.S. Department of Health and Human Services. (1998). *Healthy people 2010 objectives: Draft for public comment* (Gov Doc No HE 1.2: P 39/ Draft 0445). Washington, DC: U.S. Government Printing Office.

U.S. Department of Health and Human Services. (1999). *Mental health: A report of the Surgeon General: Executive summary.* Washington, DC: U.S. Government Printing Office.

U.S. Department of Housing and Urban Development. (1984). *A report to the Secretary on the homeless and emergency shelters.* Office of Policy Development and Research. Washington, DC: U.S. Government Printing Office.

U.S. Department of Housing and Urban Development. (1989). *A report on the 1988 national survey of shelters for the homeless.* Office of Policy Development and Research. Washington, DC: U.S. Department of Housing and Urban Development.

U.S. Department of Housing and Urban Development. (1991). *The 1990 annual report of the Interagency Council on the Homeless.* Interagency Council on the Homeless. Washington, DC: U.S. Department of Housing and Urban Development.

U.S. Department of Justice. (1998). *Sourcebook of criminal justice statistics, 1998* [On-line]. Available: http://www.albany.edu/sourcebook/1995/tost_1.html [Accessed Jan. 17, 2000].

Upsal, M. S. (1990). Volunteer peer support therapy for abusive and neglectful families. *Public Health Reports, 105,* 80–84.

Urrutia-Rojas, X., & Aday, L. A. (1991). A framework for community assessment: Designing and conducting a survey in an Hispanic immigrant and refugee community. *Public Health Nursing, 8*(1), 20–26.

van der Feltz-Cornelis, C. M., Lyons, J. S., Huyse, F. J., Campos, R., Fink, P., & Slaets, J. P. (1997). Health services research on mental health in primary care. *International Journal of Psychiatry in Medicine, 27*(1), 1–21.

Van Devanter, N. (1999). Prevention of sexually transmitted diseases: The need for social and behavioral science expertise in public health departments. *American Journal of Public Health, 89*(6), 815–818.

Velentgas, P., Bynum, C., & Zierler, S. (1990). The buddy volunteer commitment in AIDS care. *American Journal of Public Health, 80,* 1378–1380.

Vertrees, J. C., Manton, K. G., & Adler, G. S. (1989). Cost effectiveness of home and community-based care. *Health Care Financing Review, 10*(4), 65–78.

Viano, D. C. (1990). A blueprint for injury control in the United States. *Public Health Reports, 105,* 329–333.

Vinokur, A. D., Price, R. H., & Caplan, R. D. (1996). Hard times and hurtful partners: How financial strain affects depression and relationship satisfaction of unemployed persons and their spouses. *Journal of Personality and Social Psychology, 71*(1), 166–179.

Wagner, E. H. (1997). Managed care and chronic illness: health services research needs. *Health Services Research, 32*(5), 702–714.

Wagner, J. D., Menke, E. M., & Ciccone, J. K. (1994). The health of rural homeless women with young children. *Journal of Rural Health, 10*(1), 49–57.

Waitzkin, H., Britt, T., & Williams, C. (1994). Narratives of aging and social problems in medical encounters with older persons. *Journal of Health & Social Behavior, 35*(4), 322–348.

Walker, E. A., Unutzer, J., Rutter, C., Gelfand, A., Saunders, K., VonKorff, M., Koss, M. P., & Katon, W. (1999). Costs of health care use by women HMO members with a history of childhood abuse and neglect. *Archives of General Psychiatry, 56*(7), 609–613.

Wallace, D., & Wallace, R. (1998). Scales of geography, time, and population: The study of violence as a public health problem. *American Journal of Public Health, 88*(12), 1853–1858.

Wallace, S. P. (1990). The no-care zone: Availability, accessibility, and acceptability in community-based long-term care. *Gerontologist, 30,* 254–261.

Wallerstein, N. (1992). Powerlessness, empowerment, and health: Implications for health promotion programs. *American Journal of Health Promotion, 6*(3), 197–205.

Wallerstein, N., & Bernstein, E. (1994). Introduction to community empowerment, participatory education, and health. *Health Education Quarterly, 21*(2), 141–148.

Waltman, D. (1995). Key ingredients to effective addictions treatment. *Journal of Substance Abuse Treatment, 12*(6), 429–439.

Ware, J. E., Jr. (1986). The assessment of health status. In L. H. Aiken & D. Mechanic (Eds.), *Applications of Social Science to Clinical Medicine and Health Policy* (pp. 204–228). New Brunswick, NJ: Rutgers University Press.

Ware, J. E., Jr. (1989). Measuring health and functional status in mental health services research. In C. A. Taube, D. Mechanic, & A. A. Hohmann (Eds.), *The future of mental health services research* (DHHS Publication No. ADM 89–1600) (pp. 289–301). National Institute of Mental Health. Washington, DC: U.S. Government Printing Office.

Ware, J. E. Jr., Bayliss, M. S., Rogers, W. H., Kosinski, M., & Tarlov, A. R. (1996). Differences in four-year health outcomes for elderly and poor, chronically ill patients treated in HMO and fee-for-service systems. Results from the Medical Outcomes Study. *Journal of the American Medical Association, 276*(13), 1039–1047.

Warren, N., Bellin, E., Zoloth, S., & Safyer, S. (1994). Human immunodeficiency virus infection care is unavailable to inmates on release from jail. *Archives of Family Medicine, 3*(10), 894–898.

Watters, J. K., & Biernacki, P. (1989). Targeted sampling: Options for the study of hidden populations. *Social Problems, 36,* 416–430.

Watters, J. K., Estilo, M. J., Clark, G. L., & Lorvick, J. (1994). Syringe and needle exchange as HIV/AIDS prevention for injection drug users. *Journal of the American Medical Association, 271*(2), 115–120.

Weine, S. M., Becker, D. F., McGlashan, T. H., Laub, D., Lazrove, S., Vojvoda, D., & Hyman, L. (1995). Psychiatric consequences of "ethnic cleansing": Clinical assessments and trauma testimonies of newly resettled Bosnian refugees. *American Journal of Psychiatry, 152*(4), 536–542.

Weinick, R. M., & Monheit, A. C. (1999). Children's health insurance coverage and family structure, 1977–1996. *Medical Care Research & Review, 56*(1), 55–73.

Weinreb, L., & Bassuk, E. L. (1990). Health care of homeless families: A growing challenge for family medicine. *Journal of Family Practice, 31,* 74–80.

Weinreb, L., Goldberg, R., Bassuk, E., & Perloff, J. (1998). Determinants of health and service use patterns in homeless and low-income housed children. *Pediatrics, 102*(3 Pt. 1), 554–562.

Weisner, C., & Schmidt, L. (1993). Alcohol and drug problems among diverse health and social service populations. *American Journal of Public Health, 83*(6), 824–829.

Weisner, C., & Schmidt, L. A. (1995). Expanding the frame of health services research in the drug abuse field. *Health Services Research, 30*(5), 707–726.

Weissert, W. G., & Cready, C. M. (1989a). A prospective budgeting model for home- and community-based long-term care. *Inquiry, 26,* 114–129.

Weissert, W. G., & Cready, C. M. (1989b). Toward a model for improved targeting of aged at risk of institutionalization. *Health Services Research, 24,* 485–510.

Weissert, W. G., Cready, C. M., & Pawelak, J. E. (1988). The past and future of home- and community-based long-term care. *Milbank Quarterly, 66,* 309–388.

Weissert, W. G., & Harris, K. M. (1998). Health and social service use by the frail elderly. In S. M. Allen & V. Mor (Eds.), *Living in the community with disability: Service needs, use, and systems* (pp. 42–72). New York: Springer.

Weissman, G., McClain, M., Hines, R., Harder, P., Gross, M., Marconi, K. M., & Bowen, G. S. (1994). Creating an agenda for research and evaluation: HIV service delivery, the Ryan White CARE Act, and beyond. *Journal of Public Health Policy, 15*(3), 329–344.

Weissman, G., Melchior, L., Huba, G., Altice, F., Booth, R., Cottler, L., Genser, S., Jones, A., McCarthy, S., Needle, R. et al. (1995). Women living with substance abuse and HIV disease: Medical care access issues. *Journal of the American Medical Women's Association,* *50*(3–4), 115–120.

Weitzman, B. C. (1989). Pregnancy and childbirth: Risk factors for homelessness? *Family Planning Perspectives, 21*(4), 175–178.

Wells, K., & Tracy, E. (1996). Reorienting intensive family preservation services in relation to public child welfare practice. *Child Welfare, 75*(6), 667–692.

Wells, K. B., & Brook, R. H. (1989). The quality of mental health services: Past, present, and future. In C. A. Taube, D. Mechanic, & A. A. Hohmann (Eds.), *The future of mental health services research* (DHHS Publication No. ADM 89–1600) (pp. 203–224). National Institute of Mental Health. Washington, DC: U.S. Printing Office.

Wells, K. B., Keeler, E., & Manning, W. G., Jr. (1990). Patterns of outpatient mental health care over time: Some implications for estimates of demand and for benefit design. *Health Services Research, 24,* 773–789.

Wells, K. B., Manning, W. G., Jr., & Valdez, R. B. (1989). *The effects of a prepaid group practice on mental health outcomes of a general population: Results from a randomized trial* (R-3834-NIMH-HFCA). Santa Monica, CA: RAND.

Wenzel, S. L., Bakhtiar, L., Caskey, N. H., Hardie, E., Redford, C., Sadler, N., & Gelberg, L. (1995). Homeless veterans' utilization of medical, psychiatric, and substance abuse services. *Medical Care, 33*(11), 1132–1144.

Wenzel, S. L., Koegel, P., & Gelberg, L. (1996). Access to substance abuse treatment for homeless women of reproductive age. *Journal of Psychoactive Drugs, 28*(1), 17–30.

West, J. (Ed.). (1991). The Americans with Disabilities Act: From policy to practice. *Milbank Quarterly, 69*(Suppl. 1/2).

Westermeyer, J. (1987). Prevention of mental disorder among Hmong refugees in the United States: Lessons from the period 1976–1986. *Social Science and Medicine, 25,* 941–947.

Westermeyer, J. (1990). Methodological issues in the epidemiological study of alcohol-drug problems: Sources of confusion and misunderstanding. *American Journal of Drug and Alcohol Abuse, 16,* 47–55.

Westermeyer, J., Callies, A., & Neider, J. (1990). Welfare status and psychosocial adjustment among 100 Hmong refugees. *Journal of Nervous and Mental Disease, 178,* 300–306.

Whitaker, C. J. (1989). *The redesigned national crime survey: Selected new data.* Office of Justice Programs, Bureau of Justice Statistics, Special Report. Washington, DC: U.S. Department of Justice.

Whiteis, D. G. (1998). Third world medicine in first world cities: Capital accumulation, uneven development and public health. *Social Science and Medicine, 47*(6), 795–808.

Wholey, D. R., Burns, L. R., & Lavizzo-Mourey, R. (1998). Managed care and the delivery of primary care to the elderly and the chronically ill. *Health Services Research, 33*(2 Pt. Ii), 322–353.

Wickizer, T. M., & Lessler, D. (1998). Do treatment restrictions imposed by utilization management increase the likelihood of readmission for psychiatric patients? *Medical Care, 36*(6), 844–850.

Wiener, J. M., & Hanley, R. J. (1990). The bumpy road to long-term care reform. *Caring, 9*(3), 12–16.

Wiener, J. M., & Rubin, R. M. (1989). The potential impact of private long-term care financing options on Medicaid: The next thirty years. *Journal of Health Politics, Policy and Law, 14,* 327–340.

Wilkinson, R. G. (1996). *Unhealthy societies: The afflictions of inequality.* New York: Routledge.

Wilkinson, R. G., Kawachi, I., & Kennedy, B. P. (1998). Mortality, the social environment, crime and violence. *Sociology of Health and Illness, 20*(5), 578–597.

Williams, B. C., Phillips, E. K., Torner, J. C., & Irvine, A. A. (1990). Predicting utilization of home health resources: Important data from routinely collected information. *Medical Care, 28,* 379–391.

Williams, D. R., & Collins, C. (1995). U.S. socioeconomic and racial differences in health: Patterns and explanations. *Annual Review of Sociology, 21,* 349–386.

Williams, K. R., Scarlett, M. I., Jiménez, R., Schwartz, B., & Stokes-Nielson, P. (1991). Improving community support for HIV and AIDS prevention through national partnerships. *Public Health Reports, 106*(6), 672–677.

Willis, A. G., Willis, G. B., Manderscheid, R. W., Male, A., & Henderson, M. (1998). Mental illness and disability in the U.S. adult household population. In R. W. Manderscheid & M. J. Henderson (Eds.), *Mental health, United States, 1998* (pp. 113–123) (DHHS Publication No. SMA 99–3285). Center for Mental Health Services. Substance Abuse and Mental Health Services Administration. Washington, DC: U.S. Government Printing Office.

Wilson, C. V. (1993). Substance abuse and managed care. *New Directions for Mental Health Services,* (59), 99–105.

Wilson, I. B., Sullivan, L. M., & Weissman, J. S. (1998). Costs and outcomes of AIDS care: Comparing a health maintenance organization with fee-for-service systems in the Boston Health Study. *JAIDS: Journal of Acquired Immune Deficiency Syndromes, 17*(5), 424–432.

Wilson, W. J. (1980). *The declining significance of race: Blacks and changing American institutions* (2nd ed.). Chicago: University of Chicago Press.

Wilson, W. J. (Ed.). (1989). The ghetto underclass: Social science perspectives. *Annals of the American Academy of Political and Social Science, 501.*

Wilson, W. J. (1990). *The truly disadvantaged: The inner city, the underclass, and public policy.* Chicago: University of Chicago Press.

Wilson, W. J. (1996). *When work disappears: The world of the new urban poor.* New York: Knopf.

Wing, J. K., Beevor, A. S., Curtis, R. H., Park, S. B., Hadden, S., & Burns, A. (1998). Health of the Nation Outcome Scales (HoNOS). Research and development. *British Journal of Psychiatry, 172,* 11–18.

Winkenwerder, W., Kessler, A. R., & Stolec, R. M. (1989). Federal spending for illness caused by the human immunodeficiency virus. *New England Journal of Medicine, 320,* 1598–1624.

Witkin, M. J., Atay, J. E., Manderscheid, R. W., DeLozier, J., Male, A., & Gillespe, R. (1998). Highlights of organized mental health services in 1994 and major national and state trends. In R. W. Manderscheid & M. J. Henderson (Eds.), *Mental health, United States, 1998* (pp. 143–175) (DHHS Publication No. SMA 99–3285). Center for Mental Health Services. Substance Abuse and Mental Health Services Administration. Washington, DC: U.S. Government Printing Office.

Wolfinger, N. H. (1998). The effects of parental divorce on adult tobacco and alcohol consumption. *Journal of Health and Social Behavior, 39*(3), 254–269.

Wolfner, G. D., & Gelles, R. J. (1993). A profile of violence toward children: A national study. *Child Abuse and Neglect, 17*(2), 197–212.

Wood, D. L., Valdez, R. B., Hayashi, T., & Shen, A. (1990). Health of homeless children and housed, poor children. *Pediatrics, 86,* 858–866.

Woods, R. E. (Ed.). (1998). Special Projects of National Significance Program: Ten models of adolescent HIV care. *Journal of Adolescent Health, 23*(2 Suppl.).

Worden, J. K., Flynn, B. S., Merrill, D. G., Waller, J. A., & Haugh, L. D. (1989). Preventing alcohol-impaired driving through community self-regulation training. *American Journal of Public Health, 79,* 287–290.

World Health Organization. (1948). Constitution of the World Health Organization. In *Handbook of basic documents.* Geneva: Author.

Wright, J. D., & Weber, E. (1987). *Homelessness and health.* Washington, DC: McGraw-Hill's Healthcare Information Center.

Wright, R. J., Wright, R. O., & Isaac, N. E. (1997). Response to battered mothers in the pediatric emergency department: A call for an interdisciplinary approach to family violence. *Pediatrics, 99*(2), 186–192.

Wurtele, S. K. (1987). School-based sexual abuse prevention programs: A review. *Child Abuse and Neglect, 11*, 483–495.

Wyatt, R. J. (1986). Scienceless to homeless. *Science, 234*(4782), 1309.

Wyshak, G., & Modest, G. A. (1996). Violence, mental health, and substance abuse in patients who are seen in primary care settings. *Archives of Family Medicine, 5*(8), 441–447.

Yelin, E. H., Greenblatt, R. M., Hollander, H., & McMaster, J. R. (1991). The impact of HIV-related illness on employment. *American Journal of Public Health, 81*, 79–84.

Yen, I. H., & Kaplan, G. A. (1998). Poverty area residence and changes in physical activity level: evidence from the Alameda County Study. *American Journal of Public Health, 88*(11), 1709–1712.

York, R., Grant, C., Gibeau, A., Beecham, J., & Kessler, J. (1996). A review of problems of universal access to prenatal care. *Nursing Clinics of North America, 31*(2), 279–292.

Yudkowsky, B. K., & Fleming, G. V. (1990). Preventive health care for Medicaid children. *Health Care Financing Review, Annual Supplement*, 89–96.

Yuen, F. (1994). Evaluations in mental health services: Some methodological considerations. *Journal of Nursing Management, 2*(6), 287–291.

Zaid, A., Fullerton, J. T., & Moore, T. (1996). Factors affecting access to prenatal care for U.S. / Mexico border-dwelling Hispanic women. *Journal of Nurse-Midwifery, 41*(4), 277–284.

Zierler, S., & Krieger, N. (1997). Reframing women's risk: social inequalities and HIV infection. *Annual Review of Public Health, 18*, 401–436.

Zill, N., & Schoenborn, C. A. (1990). *Developmental learning, and emotional problems: Health of our nations's children, United States, 1988* (DHHS Publication No. PHS 91–1250). Washington, DC: U.S. Government Printing Office.

Zima, B. T., Bussing, R., Forness, S. R., & Benjamin, B. (1997). Sheltered homeless children: Their eligibility and unmet need for special education evaluations. *American Journal of Public Health, 87*(2), 236–240.

Zlotnick, C., Kronstadt, D., & Klee, L. (1998). Foster care children and family homelessness. *American Journal of Public Health, 88*(9), 1368–1370.

Zolopa, A. R., Hahn, J. A., Gorter, R., Miranda, J., Wlodarczyk, D., Peterson, J., Pilote, L., & Moss, A. R. (1994). HIV and tuberculosis infection in San Francisco's homeless adults: Prevalence and risk factors in a representative sample. *Journal of the American Medical Association, 272*(6), 455–461.

NAME INDEX

SUBJECT INDEX

A

Abusing families: described, 45, 47–49, 83, 86; health care access by, 194–195; health care costs of, 214–215; health care quality for, 234–235; health care research on, 256–258; health care services for, 146–150; indicators of, 46t, 84t–85t; personal, social, and human resources of, 109–111; principal programs and services for, 147t; public and private payers for, 174

Access to Community Care and Effective Services, 154

ADA (American with Disabilities Act) [1990], 184

ADAMHA (Alcohol, Drug Abuse, and Mental Health Administration), 253

ADL (activities of daily living): due to chronic conditions, 61, 65; limitation in, 24–25. *See also* Chronically ill/disabled

Administration for Children, Youth and Families, 47, 83, 103

Adolescent Family Life Program, 174

Adolescents: AIDS education to, 187–188; births by, 21, 60; social status and alcohol/substance abuse by, 105–106

AFDC (Aid to Families with Dependent Children), 161, 163, 175, 176, 203

African Americans: age as vulnerability issue for, 55; economic/social disadvantages of, 96; high-risk mothers/infants, 57–60; homicide rates of male, 82; race/ethnicity as vulnerability issue for, 56

Age issues, 55

Agency for Healthcare Research and Quality, 224

AHSP (Robert Wood Johnson Foundation AIDS Health Services Program), 129

AIDS (acquired immunodeficiency syndrome), 4. *See also* HIV/AIDS population

AIDS Clinical Trials Group (1994), 131

AIDS Drug Assistance Programs, 168

AIDS education, 187–188

Alcohol, Drug Abuse, and Mental Health block grant, 135

Alcohol, Drug Abuse and Mental Health, Community Development, and Social Services, 170

Alcoholics Anonymous, 141, 142, 231

Alcohol/substance abusers: described, 36–37, 42, 73, 75, 81; health care access by, 190–192; health care quality for, 230–232; health care research on, 251–254; indicators of, 38t–42t, 76t–80t; neurological mechanisms of, 105–107; principal programs and services for, 138t; public and private payers of, 171–173; in U.S. household population, 75

Alzheimer's disease, 36, 70

American Managed Behavioral Healthcare Association, 229

American Medical Association, 276

American Medical Association Council on Scientific Affairs, 235

American Psychiatric Association Task Force, 135

American Public Health Association, 103, 276

Analytic research: on abusing families, 257; on alcohol or sub-

I